MEDICAL MONITORING IN
THE HOME AND WORK ENVIRONMENT

Medical Monitoring
in the
Home and Work Environment

EDITORS

**Laughton E. Miles, M.D.,
Ph.D., F.R.A.C.P.**

*Clinical Monitoring Center
Palo Alto, California*

**Roger J. Broughton, M.D.,
Ph.D., F.R.C.P.(C)**

*Ottawa General Hospital
University of Ottawa
Ottawa, Canada*

Raven Press ⚜ New York

Raven Press, 1185 Avenue of the Americas, New York, New York 10036

Library of Congress Cataloging-in-Publication Data

Medical monitoring in the home and work environment / editors.
    Laughton E. Miles, Roger J. Broughton.
        p.   cm.
    Includes bibliographical references.
    ISBN 0-88167-595-4
    1. Patient monitoring.   2. Ambulatory medical care.   I. Miles,
Laughton E.   II. Broughton, Roger J.
        [DNLM: 1. Monitoring.   Physiologic.   WB 142 M489]
    RC71.3.M44   1989
    616.07'54—dc20
    DNLM/DLC
    for Library of Congress   89-24228
                                                                         CIP

Papers or parts thereof have been used as camera-ready copy as submitted by the authors whenever possible; when retyped, they have been edited by the editorial staff only to the extent considered necessary for the assistance of an international readership. The views expressed and the general style adopted remain, however, the responsibility of the named authors. Great care has been taken to maintain the accuracy of the information contained in the volume. However, neither Raven Press nor the editors can be held responsible for errors or for any consequences arising from the use of information contained herein.

The use in this book of particular designations of countries or territories does not imply any judgment by the publisher or editors as to the legal status of such countries or territories, of their authorities or institutions, or of the delimitation of their boundaries.

Some of the names of products referred to in this book may be registered trademarks or proprietary names, although specific reference to this fact may not be made; however, the use of a name with designation is not to be construed as a representation by the publisher or editors that it is in the public domain. In addition, the mention of specific companies or of their products or proprietary names does not imply an endorsement or recommendation on the part of the publisher or editors.

Authors were themselves responsible for obtaining the necessary permission to reproduce copyright materials from other sources. With respect to the publisher's copyright, material appearing in this book prepared by individuals as part of their official duties as government employees is only covered by this copyright to the extent permitted by the appropriate national regulations.

9   8   7   6   5   4   3   2   1

Preface

Long-term physiological monitoring and other forms of clinical evaluation of patients in their own environment seem destined to revolutionize health care. Recent developments in microelectronics, computer software, biomedical sensors, and new materials have fostered rapid growth in this field, and the escalating cost of health care, increasing consumer advocacy, and heightened attention to the consequences of clinical decision-making and therapeutic intervention have become powerful motivating forces behind the implementation of long-term monitoring. This approach allows clinical data to be obtained during many physiological states (e.g., sleep, exercise, eating, and emotional stress), over more than a 24-hour period (thereby taking into account circadian variations), and in various environments.

By continuous surveillance of physiological data, monitoring equipment can decide to interrogate the patient, activate an alarm, or intervene by dispensing medication or modifying the patient's behavior. Not only are the data obtained often more valid and clinically relevant than single measurements or inpatient studies, but also the data collection, recovery, and analysis tend to be more cost-effective and labor-saving and the treatment more timely. Frequently, such information may be sufficient to ensure the optimum clinical outcome without more expensive tests in a special facility.

This book introduces the fundamental considerations and concepts involved in long-term monitoring and describes a variety of existing clinical applications. It assesses the impact of diagnostic tests on clinical decision-making and patient outcome and reviews the role of the clinical history and clinical data base, the current state of biomedical sensor technology, and the use of portable microcomputers, biomedical telemetry, and active remote monitoring. The chronobiologic approach, so-called "closed-loop" systems, and emergency or alarm systems are also illustrated. The clinical applications include monitoring daytime as well as 24-hour sleep/wake functions, exercise physiology, and circadian dyschronosis. Finally, its usefulness in evaluating cardiovascular disorders, impotence, sleep disorders in general and sleep apnea in particular, and gastrointestinal disorders is also reviewed.

This volume will be useful to all those interested in long-term physiological monitoring and clinical evaluation in the home, work, educational, and recreational environments. It is especially relevant to those involved in chronobiology; sleep disorders; emergency medicine; space, aviation, or military medicine; behavioral, occupational, or environmental medicine; exercise physiology; sports and rehabilitation medicine; biomedical engineering; and home health care and clinical decision-making. Those in more general clinical specialties such as neurology, cardiopulmonary disease, pediatrics, geriatrics, gastroenterology, pharmacology, psychiatry, and psychology will also find the volume helpful. We believe that the techniques and concepts advocated in this book will some day have a major impact on the validity, efficacy, and cost of health care.

The Editors

Acknowledgments

This book was undertaken as a result of discussions held following a scientific meeting entitled "Monitoring and Evaluation of Sleep/Wake Disorders in the Home and Work Environment" organized by the Clinical Monitoring Center of Palo Alto, California, and held in San Francisco in March of 1987.

Its publication would not have been possible without the meticulous and enthusiastic editorial assistance of Alexa Kwiatkowski of the Clinical Monitoring Center, and financial support from the following companies: Ambulatory Monitoring, Inc., Sleep Care, Inc., Somnitec, Inc., Spectrum Medical Products, Inc., and Vitalog Monitoring, Inc.

Contents

The Chronobiologic Approach

"Closed-Loop" Systems

Monitoring Daytime Function

24-Hour Sleep–Wake/Activity Monitoring

Applications in Exercise Physiology

Applications in Circadian Dyschronosis

Applications in Cardiology

Applications in Sleep Disorders (General)

Applications in Sleep Apnea

Evaluation of Impotence

Applications in Gastrointestinal Disorders

Emergency Systems

Contributors

Torbjorn Akerstedt
IPM and Karolinska Institute
Box 60205
S-10401 Stockholm, Sweden

Sonia Ancoli-Israel
Department of Psychiatry
University of California, San Diego
Veterans Administration Medical Center
3350 La Jolla Village Drive
San Diego, California 92161

Earl Bakken
Medtronic, Inc.
7000 Central Avenue, NE
Minneapolis, Minnesota 55432

Roger J. Broughton
Human Neurosciences Research Unit
Ottawa General Hospital
University of Ottawa
Ottawa, Canada K1H 8L6

Kent F. Burnett
Department of Counseling Psychology
University of Wisconsin, Madison
Madison, Wisconsin 53706

Mary A. Carskadon
Department of Psychiatry
Bradley Hospital
1011 Veterans Memorial Parkway
East Providence, Rhode Island 02915

Rosalind D. Cartwright
Rush-Presbyterian-St. Luke's Medical
  Center
1653 West Congress Parkway
Chicago, Illinois 60615

Kun-Mu Chen
Department of Electrical Engineering
Michigan State University
East Lansing, Michigan 48824

Deanna G. Cheung
Hypertension Center
Veterans Administration Medical Center
University of California, Irvine
Long Beach, California 90822

Jesper Clausen
Sleep Laboratory
Department of Clinical Neurophysiology
Copenhagen County Hospital
2600 Glostrup
Copenhagen, Denmark

Linda J. Connell
NASA Ames Research Center
Aerospace Human Factors Research
  Division
Moffett Field, California 94035

Germaine Cornelissen
Chronobiology Laboratories
University of Minnesota
Minneapolis, Minnesota 55455

Charles A. Czeisler
Department of Medicine
Harvard Medical School
Brigham and Women's Hospital
221 Longwood Avenue
Boston, Massachusetts 02115

Patrick Delmore
Medtronic, Inc.
7000 Central Avenue, NE
Minneapolis, Minnesota 55432

Sabri Derman
Sleep Disorders Center
Department of Psychiatry
University of Texas Health Science Center
San Antonio, Texas 78212

Alan B. Douglass
Veterans Administration Medical Center
2215 Fuller Road
Ann Arbor, Michigan 48105

Wayne Dunham
Human Neurosciences Research Unit
Ottawa General Hospital
University of Ottawa
Ottawa, Canada K1H 8L6

Saul B. Freedman
Hallstrom Institute of Cardiology
University of Sydney and Royal Prince
Alfred Hospital
Missenden Road, Camperdownts
New South Wales, 2050 Australia

Margaret Gatz
Psychology Department
University of Southern California
Los Angeles, California 90089-1061

R. Curtis Graeber
NASA Ames Research Center
Aerospace Human Factors Research
Division
Moffett Field, California 94035

Lois Watanabe Gregg
Department of Psychiatry
University of California
San Diego, California 92161

Christian Guilleminault
Stanford University
Stanford, California 94305

Erna Halberg
Chronobiology Laboratories
University of Minnesota
Minneapolis, Minnesota 55455

Franz Halberg
Chronobiology Laboratories
University of Minnesota
Minneapolis, Minnesota 55455

Julia Halberg
St. Paul-Ramsey Medical Center
St. Paul, Minnesota 55101

Robert Houser
Department of Psychiatry
Bradley Hospital
1011 Veterans Memorial Parkway
East Providence, Rhode Island 02915

Wu Jinyi
Chengdu College of Traditional Chinese
Medicine
Chengdu, Sichuan, People's Republic of
China

Kahlil Kayed
Clinical Neurophysiology Section
Akershus Central Hospital
1474 Nordbyhagen, Norway

Dorothy H. Kelly
Pediatric Pulmonary Laboratory
Massachusetts General Hospital
Boston, Massachusetts 02114

Wen H. Ko
Electronics Design Center
Case Western Reserve University
Cleveland, Ohio 44106

Daniel F. Kripke
Department of Psychiatry
University of California
San Diego, California 92161

Michael Langemark
Department of Neurology and Department
of Clinical Neurophysiology
Copenhagen County University Hospital
2900 Hellerup, Denmark

Lea Leinonen
Department of Physiology
Helsinki University
SF-00170 Helsinki, Finland

Benjamin Littenberg
Department of Medicine
Stanford University
Veterans Administration Medical Center
Palo Alto, California 94304

Mary Beth Masterson
Stanford University
Stanford, California 94305

Jonathan H. Mermin
Neuroendocrinology Laboratory
Division of Endocrinology
Brigham and Women's Hospital
221 Longwood Avenue
Boston, Massachusetts 02115

Laughton E. Miles
Clinical Monitoring Center
Palo Alto, California 94304
and
Vitalog Monitoring, Inc.
Redwood City, California 94063

Michael R. Neuman
Departments of Obstetrics and Gynecology
and Biomedical Engineering
Cleveland Metropolitan General Hospital
Case Western Reserve University
3395 Scranton Road
Cleveland, Ohio 44109

Joel M. Neutel
Hypertension Center
Veterans Administration Medical Center
University of California, Irvine
Long Beach, California 90822

William C. Orr
Baptist Medical Center of Oklahoma
*   Foundation*
3300 Northwest Expressway
Oklahoma City, Oklahoma 73112-4481

Cynthia Pearson
Psychology Department
University of Southern California
Los Angeles, California 90089-1061

Thomas Penzel
Marburg University
D-3550 Marburg, F.R.G.

J. Herman Peter
Marburg University
D-3550 Marburg, F.R.G.

Martin Rivers
Human Neurosciences Research Unit
Ottawa General Hospital
University of Ottawa
Ottawa, Canada K1H 8L6

Salvador Sanchez de la Pena
Chronobiology Laboratory
University of Minnesota
Minneapolis, Minnesota 55455

Ante Santic
Department of Electrical Engineering
University of Zagreb
Unska 17
Zagreb 41000, Yugoslavia

Lawrence E. Scheving
University of Arkansas for Medical
*   Sciences*
Department of Anatomy No. 510
4301 W. Markham
Little Rock, Arkansas 72205

Marymae Seward
Psychology Department
University of Southern California
Los Angeles, California 90089-1061

Deborah E. Sewitch
Sleep Disorders Center
The Griffin Hospital
Derby, Connecticut 06418
and
Department of Psychiatry
Yale University School of Medicine
New Haven, Connecticut 06519

Jack R. Smith
Electrical Engineering Department
University of Florida
Gainesville, Florida 32611

Harold C. Sox, Jr.
Department of Medicine
Dartmouth-Hitchcock Medical Center
Hanover, New Hampshire 03756

Claudio Stampi
Human Neurosciences Research Unit
Ottawa General Hospital
University of Ottawa
Ottawa, Canada K1H 8L6

Riccardo Stoohs
Marburg University
D-3550 Marburg, F.R.G.

C. Barr Taylor
Laboratory for the Study of Behavioral
*   Medicine*
Stanford University School of Medicine
Stanford, California 94305

Lawrence F. Van Egeren
Department of Psychiatry
Michigan State University
A227 East Fee Hall
East Lansing, Michigan 48824

Michael A. Weber
Hypertension Center
Veterans Administration Medical Center
University of California, Irvine
Long Beach, California 90822

Gordon Wildschiodtz
Sleep Laboratory
Department of Clinical Neurophysiology
Copenhagen County Hospital
2600 Glostrup
Copenhagen, Denmark

Medical Monitoring in the Home and Work Environment,
edited by Laughton E. Miles and Roger J. Broughton.
Raven Press, New York © 1990.

INTRODUCTION

Laughton E. Miles and *Roger J. Broughton

Clinical Monitoring Center, Palo Alto California 94304; and *Human
Neurosciences Research Unit, Ottawa General Hospital, University of
Ottawa, Ottawa, Canada K1H8L6

Advances in technology often occur years before they find practical application. Even so, factors such as the high cost of health care, consumer advocacy, and advances in clinical decision-making, should provide a considerable incentive to exploit the recent developments in microelectronics, computer software, biomedical sensors, and new materials.

Some reasons for the slow utilization of existing technology are evident. The medical profession has tended to regard the consumerism movement in health care with some suspicion and anxiety, and rarely is new medical technology directed explicitly towards a reduction in the cost of health care delivery. Furthermore, professional societies involved in health care, and individuals responsible for establishing health care policy, tend to have a conservative attitude towards new devices and procedures. This is partly due to a legitimate attempt to protect the general public; but by their very nature, many organizations have an investment in the status quo.

From a practical medical viewpoint, there should be a strong incentive to define the minimum information needed to achieve the optimal clinical outcome, and to find ways of obtaining that information in the appropriate environment by a convenient and cost-effective method.

Most clinical evaluations are relatively brief and occur during the usual work day, yet dysfunctions often vary dramatically throughout the 24 hours. The symptoms and signs of illness in the doctor's office or hospital ward can be misleading or irrelevant; and illness typically has its impact because of the way it effects people in their usual environment and activities. Marital conflicts, work stress, tragedies and disappointments, as well as physical exercise, fulfillment, and ecstasy, are all features of life with which health and disease must inevitably interact. Furthermore, it is known that most physiological and biochemical systems have an innate rhythmicity to be taken into account when making measurements.

It seems obvious therefore, that an individual's disease (or health) status should ideally be determined by monitoring appropriate physiological parameters and behaviors throughout 24 hours (perhaps as long as a week) while that person functions in his or her normal environment, carrying out usual sleep, work, educational, recreational, nutritional, sexual, and other activities. Conversely, a restrictive facility and short term tests should only be used when a controlled environment or special procedure is necessary or cost-effective.

It is important to emphasize that the rationale for monitoring humans in their usual "free-ranging" environment is not limited to diagnostic or surveillance procedures. At times an "alarm" or emergency function is important. Other devices employ so-called "closed-loops" in which the physiological monitor detects some event or trend, alerts and interrogates the patient, and (as a result of both the recorded data and the interrogation) offers the patient advice, treatment, or behavioral modification. In these applications the monitor must also contain an output device or "actuator".

The chapters in this book have been arranged in order to present and discuss some of these concepts and to demonstrate clinical applications. Note that many presentations cover more than one aspect.

The fundamental justification for evaluating patients in their normal environment is usually established by consideration of clinical decision making and patient outcome; yet few physicians are aware of the issues involved in determining these endpoints. It is therefore appropriate that the first chapter in the book, by Benjamin Littenberg and Harold Sox, addresses the assessment of diagnostic technologies.

Any clinical evaluation requires an effective medical history obtained by interrogation, questionnaires or abstraction from previous medical records; and given current technologies, the information should be contained in an effective and accessible database. This aspect is considered with reference to sleep disorders, by Alan Douglas, Mary Carskadon and Robert Houser.

The technical aspects of medical monitoring in the home and work environment are in rapid evolution and are of great importance. Wen Ko reviews the recent advances in sensor technology. Laughton Miles describes the use of portable programmable microcomputers with special reference to the Vitalog physiological monitoring systems; and he also offers a new quality-control/technical-validation/clinical-decision-making scheme.

Michael Neuman and Ante Santic review the advantages and problems of biomedical telemetry systems, while Kun-Mu Chen describes a unique method for active remote monitoring of heart rate and respiration using the reflection of microwaves. Remarkably, this system can detect living organisms through solid brick walls.

The very important chronobiological considerations are reviewed by Franz Halberg and his colleagues. Lawrence Scheving describes the concept of autorhythmometry, whereby simple equipment can be used even by children to characterize individual circadian rhythms and identify early signs of disease. By education and self awareness, individuals can learn to take increasing responsibility for their own health care.

Conceptually advanced "Closed-Loop" systems are described in the chapters by Kent Burnett and Barr Taylor (using heart rate and body movement monitoring with patient interrogation) and by Rosalind Cartwright (using a monitor which can modify the behavior of patients suffering from obstructive sleep apnea only in the supine position).

Torbjorn Akerstedt describes the problems of monitoring sleepiness in occupations in which alertness is critically important. Roger Broughton and his colleagues review their extensive experience in 24-hour sleep-wake monitoring of normals and patients with various medical conditions. During a study of computer-based monitoring of physical activity in subjects undergoing 24 hour blood pressure monitoring, Lawrence Van Egeren demonstrates the value of a manual diary which can be automatically scanned by a computer.

A chapter by Jonathan Mermin and Charles Czeisler describes the use of a solid-state monitor to carry out circadian studies of body temperature and physical exercise in cyclists engaged in a race across the USA.

Applications in chronobiology research are described by Linda Connell and Curtis Graeber (in aviation medicine) and Daniel Kripke and Lois Gregg (concerning the circadian effects of environmental light on depression.)

Several chapters describe purely clinical applications. The first two cover long-term non-invasive monitoring of hypertension (Michael Weber et al.) and myocardial ischemia (Saul Freedman). Many of the remaining chapters relate to the relatively new specialty of sleep disorders medicine.

Tapani Salmi and Lea Leinonen describe the use of a movement-sensitive sleeping surface for the evaluation of cardio-respiratory abnormalities and other sleep disorders. Jack Smith describes techniques for transferring "classic" EEG-polysomnography to the home environment. Deborah Sewitch reports a comparison of the Oxford Medilog 9000 tape recorder and the Telediagnostic (transtelephonic) system for monitoring sleep in the patient's home. Khalil Kayed demonstrates an approach for the evaluation of sleep disorders by recording patients in their own home using either the Vitalog HMS-3000 (Lunch-Box) monitor, the Oxford Medilog 9000, or the new Oxford Multi-Parameter Analysis (MPA) monitor.

Reflecting the current interest in sleep apnea, Christian Guilleminault with colleagues from Marburg, West Germany, describe their system for stepwise evaluation of patients with special reference to a device for monitoring heart rate and snoring. Sonia Ancoli-Israel reports the evaluation of patients suspected of sleep apnea using a 4 channel Medilog tape recorder; and Gordon Wildschiodtz, Jesper Clausen and Michael Langemark from Denmark, describe the all-solid-state "Somnolog" system for monitoring sleep EEG, snoring, and other physiological data. In more specialized applications, Sabri Derman reviews the use of home monitors for evaluation of penile erectile impairment; and William Orr discusses the role of ambulatory monitors in the evaluation of gastrointestinal disease.

Finally, the use of equipment designed to detect medical emergencies is discussed by Dorothy Kelly in respect to infant monitoring; and Cynthia Pearson, Maymae Seward and Margaret Gatz, describe the "Lifeline" system and other personal emergency response systems.

Major advances in clinical medicine are not restricted to manipulating genes and antibodies or the promise of room-temperature superconductors. Some years ago, the science-fiction author Issac Asimov described a "Fantastic Voyage" through the human blood stream in which a miniaturized vehicle containing a group of intrepid adventurers removed atherosclerotic plaques and repaired a cerebral aneurysm. We now know that such an odyssey is effectively feasible through techniques of "virtual-reality" already utilized by companies such as VPL Research of Redwood City, California, and the development of mechanical devices such as the microscopic turbine recently constructed at the University of California at Berkeley.

Much is already possible. This volume aims to convince the reader that effective methods currently exist for long term physiological monitoring and clinical evaluation in the home, work, recreational and educational environments. It advances the proposition that such methods will eventually redefine health care by providing most of the information necessary to optimize the clinical outcome, and (in many situations) by also providing a cost-effective approach for treatment and behavioral modification.

Medical Monitoring in the Home and Work Environment,
edited by Laughton E. Miles and Roger J. Broughton.
Raven Press, New York © 1990.

ASSESSING DIAGNOSTIC TECHNOLOGIES

Benjamin Littenberg and *Harold C. Sox, Jr.

Department of Medicine, Stanford University
Veterans Administration Medical Center
Palo Alto, California 94304
*Department of Medicine
Dartmouth-Hitchcock Medical Center
Hanover, New Hampshire 03756

INTRODUCTION

The goals of this paper are to present some of the theoretical and logical concepts behind recent efforts to evaluate medical diagnostic technologies and to discuss the major methods available. This paper is not a review of decision analysis or an introduction to the basic concepts of diagnostic accuracy measurement. These topics are well reviewed elsewhere (3,11,12). The paper will, (a) outline the goals of technology assessment, (b) define "technology" and outline some of the major ways we evaluate technologies, and (c) discuss the concept of a "gold standard."

THE LOGIC OF TECHNOLOGY ASSESSMENT

Medical activity has two main goals. One is to improve understanding; the other is patient care. These two goals are related in subtle and complex ways, but for now can be thought of separately. We seem to be closer to achieving both these goals than in the past. How do we know if we are making progress?

Progress in understanding is evaluated by a complex process that is the domain of scientists. In broad outline, we might imagine that the scientist proposes a theory, does experiments to test the theory, and then uses the experimental results to reject, revise or expand the theory. Science is good if it leads to verification, revision or expansion of the scientific model.

Patient care has different goals and therefore a different mode of evaluation. The goal of patient care is to relieve suffering and prolong life in a manner appropriate to the setting and acceptable to the patient and society. A patient has a problem in the form of bothersome symptoms and/or a risk of premature death. The patient may not care so much for explanations of etiology and drug mechanism as for relief. A good technology will relieve the patient's problem.

To the patient, relief is the main thing, but not the only thing. The cure is sometimes worse than the disease. A good technology will not only relieve the problem, it will do so with minimal cost and risk, and will be socially and morally acceptable to the patient. Costs are wide-reaching and can include money, time, inconvenience, pain, anxiety, social isolation and other subtle factors.

Using penicillin for pneumonia, for example, seems a pretty clear case. The drug is cheap, easy to take, reasonably safe and markedly efficacious in relieving symptoms due to pneumococci. On balance, the benefits clearly out-weigh the risks and costs. Penicillin is one example of a medical technology. Medical Technology means the "techniques, drugs, equipment, and procedures used by health-care professionals in delivering medical care to individuals, and the systems within which such care is delivered" (4). This definition explicitly includes drugs, but also applies to operations, tests, the health care delivery system, the personnel involved, and even the dress and attitude of the doctor.

Much of the advance in medical technology assessment over the last century has been in therapeutics, especially drugs. The preferred method for evaluating a therapeutic technology is the randomized clinical trial (RCT). The United States Food and Drug Administration insists on at least two RCTs before a new drug can be sold in the United States. A host of other methods, of generally lesser power, are also available. Most physicians feel best about using a therapeutic technology when they know that strong evidence in the form of RCTs supports its use.

Diagnostic technologies are much more complex to evaluate than therapies. Consider the chest x-ray in a patient suspected of having a pneumonia. Clearly, the radiograph has costs and even some risks. Equally clearly, it has large benefits in some cases. How are these costs, risks and benefits distributed?

It is clear that not all individuals will benefit from a diagnostic technology and that we usually cannot predict which of the many candidate patients for the technology will actually receive some advantage. For instance, among patients with suspected pneumonia, some will not have the disease and would be better off without the risk and expense of the test. Others may have pneumonia but will get better without treatment and thus don't gain very much from the diagnostic exercise. Others truly have pneumonia and need treatment, but will have a normal X-ray and may have therapy delayed by the test, rather than enhanced. However, there are certainly some pneumonia patients who need the therapy urgently; and the X-ray offers a way of promptly identifying and treating them. These people get the lion's share of the benefits, but the costs and risks are spread around a larger group.

It is important to note that diagnostic tests do not stand on their own like therapeutic technologies sometimes do. Diagnostic technologies have little impact unless there is an effective intervention for the patients diagnosed. An accurate test for an untreatable condition is not very appealing (excepting that the test may itself be therapeutic as a source of reassurance or a placebo). If the therapies are inadequate, the diagnostic tests are not likely to help the patient very much. To evaluate a diagnostic test fully, one must evaluate the test's total impact on the patient, including the role of associated therapies.

Even the simple pneumonia problem presented here becomes quite complex and demonstrates that we need a lot of information to decide if the test is any good. For instance, can the test generate reliable reports? How often will the test be positive or negative? How often will it correctly identify the patient's true state of illness? How often will the therapy help? How often will it hurt? What is the rate of spontaneous cure? How do patient and disease characteristics affect these estimates? There are many variables that must be known before a thorough evaluation is possible.

FOUR LEVELS OF DIAGNOSTIC TECHNOLOGY ASSESSMENT

To organize all the information needed to assess a diagnostic technology, we have divided them into four categories. Diagnostic technology assessment should address (a) **biologic plausibility**, (b) **technical feasibility**, (c) **diagnostic accuracy**, and, most importantly, (d) **clinical impact**.

First are questions about biologic plausibility. Do we have some understanding of the mechanics of the test? Can we imagine that it should work? Is it in step with biologic theory? New diagnostic tests that cannot be explained in terms of what is already known about the disease in question are unlikely to be useful in clinical practice. The requirement for biologic plausibility can help to protect us against over-ambitious claims for new tests.

The dexamethasone suppression test for depression provides a good example of a technology that was widely used without close attention to biological plausibility (6). The theoretical basis of the test was very poorly worked out. Although it is true that some depressed people have abnormalities of the pituitary-adrenal axis, these are probably secondary to alterations in diet and sleep patterns that occur in many conditions other than depression. Adrenal suppression is related to emotional depression in a fairly round-about manner. Because there are many causes of pituitary-adrenal alterations, and because not all depressed patients will have the expected alterations in sleep and diet patterns, one would expect that not all patients with depression will fail to suppress and not all non-suppressors are depressed. There appear to be good biologic reasons to suspect that the dexamethasone suppression test will fail to distinguish depressed from non-depressed patients in many situations.

We needn't insist that every last detail of a diagnostic technology have a plausible biologic explanation before we adopt the technology. We might not be using electrocardiograms or urinalyses if we demanded complete biologic understanding. However, biologic plausibility serves as an important restraint on our enthusiasm for new technologies.

Biologic theory covers a lot of clever ideas that have no practical applicability. Therefore, we must also examine the technical feasibility of the test. Is the test practical in clinical settings? Is equipment available? Are the results internally consistent, repeatable, and reliable? Are the costs reasonable? If the test results fluctuate wildly from day to day, or can be obtained only in one specially equipped laboratory, the test has very limited technical feasibility.

Let us use the dexamethasone test again as an example. None of the early enthusiastic reports of this technology noted the great variability in bioavailability of dexamethasone. There is so much variability in dexamethasone absorption among different people that as many as one-third of normal patients do not absorb enough drug to suppress their adrenal-pituitary axis. This technical problem makes it extremely difficult to interpret the test results in a clinical setting. In addition, there are major problems in the measurement of the study end-point (serum cortisol). Technical problems don't necessarily render a test useless, but they do need to be addressed before the technology is disseminated.

If issues about technical feasibility are resolved, we turn our attention to questions about <u>diagnostic accuracy:</u> How often does the test correctly indicate the underlying pathophysiology? These data are hard to come by. They are often reported in the form of true-positive rates, specificity, predictive values and the like. Methods to generate these data are difficult to execute, prone to bias, and require large populations of clinical subjects. Well-done diagnostic accuracy studies are disturbingly infrequent.

As an example of diagnostic accuracy in action, consider the partial thromboplastin time, a test for abnormal coagulation (13). Many physicians order clotting studies on all patients scheduled for invasive procedures. However, the sensitivity for post-operative bleeding is only 8%. Sensitivity is the frequency of abnormal test results in patients with the disease. A sensitivity of 8% means that only 1 in 13 bleeding episodes are predicted. To further confuse things, the specificity is only 87%. Since specificity is the frequency of normal test results in patients without the disease, a specificity of 87% means that 1 in 8 non-bleeders have an abnormal test. These numbers form the underlying bases of analyses that are being used by third-party payers and hospital review committees in an attempt to define clinical circumstances where the test is appropriate. Likewise, carcinoembryonic antigen, the CEA test, has fallen out of favor for diagnosing most cancers since we have learned that it has very low sensitivity and specificity and therefore is not often clinically useful (2).

One of the common causes of over-estimation of diagnostic accuracy is the problem of spectrum bias (7). By choosing a limited spectrum of patients in whom to try the new test, you can get misleading results. For instance, if a test for coronary disease is evaluated only in subjects with severe classic angina, it will usually appear to perform well. The very sick subjects usually have several different disease manifestations for the test to detect, and the abnormalities are often so severe that they are easy to detect. But those are the easy cases: we don't need a test for subjects who are easy to diagnose. In clinical practice, we need the most help with patients who have confusing clinical presentations and are difficult to diagnose. The younger person with atypical chest pain is difficult for the clinician to diagnose, because the diagnostic clues are few in number and conflict with one another. If these patients are excluded from the analysis, the results may be very misleading when the test is applied to a general population.

However, even if a diagnostic test is accurate, there is another level of assessment that should be undertaken. This has to do with <u>clinical impact:</u> Does this technology improve patient outcome? Do people live longer? Are they happier? At the least, is medical management influenced by the technology? Does the information generated by the test have a beneficial impact on patient care? These questions have rarely been answered for diagnostic technologies. In part, these questions are difficult because useful measures of clinical outcome (other than mortality) have not been available. How much is it worth to set someone's mind at ease or to make a diagnosis that will direct a therapy that improves comfort but not life-expectancy?

There are only a few examples of analyses that take clinical impact into account. An analysis of upper GI X-ray tests (5) found that patient management decisions were influenced by the test in 7% of cases. In no case did normal X-rays result in stopping empiric therapy; and only 14% of abnormal x-rays resulted in an addition to therapy. The doctors appeared to manage the patients without much reference to the test results.

The four levels of diagnostic technology assessment serve as a framework for evaluating diagnostic tests. Although it is possible to have a useful test that does not satisfy all aspects of all four levels, failure to fulfill the four levels should serve as a warning that there may be serious problems with the diagnostic technology.

METHODS OF DIAGNOSTIC TECHNOLOGY ASSESSMENT

What are the methods that are available to clinicians and researchers to decide whether a medical test satisfies the four levels of diagnostic technology assessment? We will discuss four of the main methods of technology assessment and outline some advantages and disadvantages of each. Diagnostic tests are usually part of a strategy or package of activities used to help a patient. The strategy may start with diagnosis, but often will not be helpful unless therapy and long-term care are successful. Some assessment methods apply to complete strategies of diagnosis, therapy, and follow-up. Other methods can be used to assess a part of the strategy, such as the diagnostic accuracy of the test. Methods that evaluate complete management strategies are generally more powerful, but the methods that address only parts of the strategy are often easier to apply and provide useful information.

The Randomized Clinical Trial

The first method is the randomized clinical trial of a complete strategy. To perform a trial, you design a strategy that includes a package of diagnostic and therapeutic maneuvers and randomly assign some subjects to get that package and others to get a different package. Then you carefully follow what happens to each group and record all the benefits and all the costs.

There are few examples of this level of comprehensive assessment applied to diagnostic technologies. One attempt to do this is a 1981 study of the impact of a package of ECG plus serum cardiac enzymes in a population of chest pain patients selected to be at very low risk for coronary disease (10). Using a randomized, prospective, controlled design, the study compared the strategy of testing plus physician- or nurse-practitioner-care to care without testing. Because there was little coronary disease in the group, impact of therapy was not an issue, and the impact of the test on mortality was nil. However, in this select group, the test had significant effects on short-term disability as well as satisfaction with the quality of care.

The advantages of this complete approach are that it provides information on clinical impact, which is the highest level of assessment. It is easily translated into clinical use: clinicians should adopt the strategy that performed best. Randomized, prospective designs are widely believed to be the strongest method of evaluation, have the best chance at reducing bias, and are appealing to the clinician/investigator for their elegance and power.

Randomized trials have disadvantages. They can be technically difficult, very costly and time-consuming. They often require sophisticated outcome measures that may not be readily available. Because the results are usually generated in only one patient population, they may not be generalizable to other populations, slightly different strategies, or other clinical settings. Finally, these studies are not decomposable: it is difficult to determine which parts of the strategy work and which don't.

Partial Evaluation by Prospective Trial

The second method of assessment is partial evaluation by prospective trial. A partial evaluation is a limited approach because it assumes that you need to know only one or two important parameters to evaluate the technology. For instance, you might be satisfied with an AIDS screening test if you knew the sensitivity of the test. Therefore, you can concentrate your resources on answering just one limited question. Partial evaluations are often used to measure some facet of technical feasibility or diagnostic accuracy such as specificity or inter-observer variability. For some of the more widely evaluated technologies, you can find dozens of these limited reports. A recent review of exercise thallium testing for coronary artery disease found 56 reports of sensitivity and specificity (1). However, other aspects of this technology, such as clinical impact, have not been studied as often.

The advantages of partial trials are that they are cheaper, faster and simpler than a complete evaluation of clinical impact. They can provide important data for model building. And, because they can often be done with rigorous attention to methodology, they can provide reliable and precise data.

Unfortunately, partial trials can rarely provide a total evaluation of a diagnostic technology (most problems have more than one unknown). Even though less complex than complete evaluations, they can become large and complicated in their own right, with substantial expense and time needed to complete the trial. They are subject to the same problems of bias and limited generalizability as other methods. Most disturbing, a partial evaluation may mislead the decision-maker if it is represented as the "whole" answer.

Model Building

The third major method is model building. A model is a representation of a real-world situation in a setting that allows for easy study, manipulation, and comparison. The representation may be made of wood, plastic, guinea pigs, thoughts, words, images, numbers or equations. Models generally exist on paper, in a computer or in a laboratory.

To use models for diagnostic technology assessment, one constructs an imaginary (usually mathematical) representation of all the inputs required by the technology (money, time, etc.) and all the expected impacts (lives saved, side-effects incurred, mistakes caused or avoided, etc.). It is then necessary to estimate the importance of each input and impact. The estimates come from published trials (often of the partial type described above), surveys and in-house records, consensus of experts, informed opinion or just raw guesses. The model is used to predict the costs, risks and benefits if the technology is adopted. Under the names decision analysis, cost-effectiveness analysis and cost-benefit analysis, these mathematical models have gained favor among third-party payers, government analysts, and others influential in health policy. Tests that would require very large study populations to evaluate empirically, such as screening tests for uncommon diseases, are often evaluated in this way.

Modeling is relatively fast and inexpensive. Rather than collect thousands of clinical cases and observe them for years, a "thought-experiment" on a micro-computer might take a few milliseconds. Even with programming and background research, these models are typically available in days to months rather than months to decades. Models are effective devices for communication and education. The mathematical nature of the model leaves little room for ambiguity and often demonstrates the nature of a clinical problem more powerfully than any verbal or written form. One decision tree can be worth a thousand words. Models also serve to point up the most important parts of a problem. Often, the mere act of designing the model reveals some hidden aspect of the problem. Finally, and perhaps most powerfully, mathematical models allow decomposition (sensitivity analysis). You can easily alter some critical variable and repeat the "experiment" to observe the effect of that variable on the result. Sometimes you discover that a very controversial factor has little impact on the results even when its value varies over a wide range of values. When the results are insensitive to a variable, it frees up your physical and intellectual resources for other aspects of the problem.

There are several disadvantages of modeling. The model is never complete and never perfect. Although it shares these defects with clinical trials, models are often attacked because of their assumptions or because a variable was omitted from the model. Fortunately, models can be modified easily. A more serious problem is that models are only as good as the modeler's data. A model cannot provide reasonable predictions without some high-quality empirical data.

Expert Opinion

The last method of diagnostic technology assessment we will discuss is expert opinion. There is a specialized form of this method called the "consensus conference." Experts' opinions and consensus conferences are the most commonly applied methods when trying to answer questions of clinical impact, such as "What are the indications for this test?" The National Institutes of Health have sponsored a series of about 60 highly publicized consensus conferences that have been very influential in establishing standards of practice and reimbursement policies.

Using experts, you can get an answer to most questions quickly and inexpensively. Convening a panel of experts is much less costly and time-consuming than a clinical trial or even mathematical modeling. And where a model might explicitly require large amounts of precise data, experts are often called upon to provide a judgement without complete data in hand. Expert panels have been extremely persuasive.

The disadvantages of expert opinion and consensus panels are very troublesome. Experts often make decisions in opaque and sometimes biased ways. Too often, the reports from expert panels provide too little justification for the conclusions. After the panel has dispersed, we cannot cross-examine the experts and there are often no data left behind to support their conclusions. Experts are often long-standing practitioners of the method in question and may harbor biases that affect their recommendations. When the experts are forced to reach a consensus in a short time and without the opportunity to provide a written analysis of their reasoning, expert opinion can be subject to a variety of disturbing biases.

There are ways to improve consensus methods. The 1986 National Heart, Lung, and Blood Institute National Conference on Antithrombotic Therapy explicitly described the type and quality of the data the experts considered and graded each recommendation according to the strength of the supporting evidence (8). This assessment was reached after months of research in the medical literature and debate among the participants.

The American College of Physicians (9) has sponsored a particularly successful forum for expert opinion called The Clinical Efficacy Assessment Project (CEAP). CEAP recommendations start out with a commissioned, comprehensive review of a clinical problem by a physician with expertise in clinical epidemiology or decision analysis. These papers often contain detailed reviews of clinical trials and other data sources. The papers are widely circulated for review and comment by sub-specialty experts, clinicians, and other analysts. When a consensus has been achieved, the papers are again reviewed for publication in *The Annals of Internal Medicine.* This process sacrifices the speed of the two-day consensus conference, but usually provides an explicit, clearly-reasoned clinical strategy that is fully referenced and explained. In the CEAP process, consensus is used as a means to ensure that the clinical issue is fully explored.

GOLD STANDARDS

The four methods of technology assessment, including their many variations, are often used to evaluate a new test (index method) by comparing it's results to those of a reference test. The reference test, often called the "gold-standard," serves to tell us the true state of the patient, i.e. whether the patient really has the disease. It is hoped that the new method of diagnosis (the index test) will yield the same results as the gold standard test. The two methods rarely agree completely. Errors in diagnostic accuracy are expressed as imperfect sensitivity or specificity. Choosing the gold standard is the most important issue in assessing a new technology. If the reference test doesn't really represent the true state of the patient, we can be badly misled about the value of the index test. For example, "instant" tests for chlamydia infection are usually compared to culture methods. But cultures aren't perfect. Many investigators suspect that cultures are often negative in patients who really have the disease. If the new test detects these infections, they will be labeled "false-positives" and the index test, which is actually more accurate, will appear to have low specificity.

What makes a good gold-standard? The answer to this question lies in the goals of clinical care. The "true state" of the patient may not always be exactly what we want to know. Often, we want our tests to predict which patients need therapy and which don't. A gold-standard test is one that provides information that directly affects prognosis or therapy. "Hyperuricemia," for example, is not a useful diagnosis unless the patient complains of some dysfunction, symptom or anxiety that is associated with the elevated urate level. A new diagnostic test that accurately predicts the uric acid level is of limited usefulness (even though it has perfect sensitivity and specificity) if it does not predict symptomatic gout well. What we want are tests that predict clinical disease, symptoms, prognosis or response to therapy.

Choose your gold standards accordingly. The reference test should accurately predict the clinical outcome of interest. Often, to decide if your reference test is any good, you would do well to run a validation trial where the gold test is compared to long-term clinical outcome. This approach is expensive, difficult, time-consuming and well worthwhile.

CONCLUSIONS

Diagnostic technologies are in the service of clinical medicine and should be designed to ultimately impact clinical care. We have identified four levels of evaluation that a test should go through before we accept it as a useful technology. First, biologic validity is the scientific rationale behind the test. Second, technical feasibility is the ability of the test to be applied in clinical situations and to reliably report its results. Third, diagnostic accuracy is the ability of the test to accurately report the underlying pathophysiology. Finally, if biological plausibility, technical feasibility and diagnostic accuracy are satisfactory, new tests should still be evaluated to assess their clinical impact: Does this technology further the goals of clinical medicine in reducing mortality and morbidity? We may still decide to keep the test even if it doesn't meet all these criteria, but we will do so with a better knowledge of its strengths and weaknesses.

ANNOTATED BIBLIOGRAPHY

1. Detrano, R., Janosi, A., Lyons, K.P., Marcondes, G., Abbassi, N. and Froelicher, V.F. (1988): Factors Affecting Sensitivity and Specificity of a Diagnostic Test: The Exercise Thallium Scintigram. *Am. J. Med.*, 84:699-710. [A review of the many papers on one diagnostic modality. Because most of the literature has focused on diagnostic accuracy, without reference to the other levels of assessment, even a test that has received a lot of attention is probably under-evaluated.]

2. Fletcher, R.H. (1986): Carcinoembryonic Antigen. *Ann. Intern. Med.*, 104:66-73. [A review of this serum marker test with guidelines for use. This article is included in Common Diagnostic Tests (11) and served as the basis for the Blue Cross and Blue Shield Association Guidelines.]

3. Griner, P.F., Mayewski, R.J., Mushlin, A.I. and Greenland, P. (1981): Selection and Interpretation of Diagnostic Tests and Procedures: Principles and Application. *Ann. Intern. Med.*, 94:553-600. [A well-written tutorial on the principles of assessing diagnostic accuracy.]

4. Institute of Medicine (1985): *Assessing Medical Technologies.* National Academy Press, Washington, D.C. [A combination handbook and textbook covering the wide range of technology assessment in medicine. This is the basic reading for beginning technology assessors.]

5. Marton, K.I., Sox, H.C., Wasson, J. and Duisenberg, C.E. (1980): The Clinical Value of the Upper Gastrointestinal Tract Roentgenogram Series. *Arch. Intern. Med.*, 140:191-195. [One of the few studies to address the management impact of a diagnostic technology.]

6. Nierenberg, A.A. and Feinstein, A.R. (1988): How to Evaluate a Diagnostic Marker Test: Lessons from the Rise and Fall of Dexamethasone Suppression Test. *JAMA*, 259:1699-1702. [A review of the history of this marker test with insight into where the assessment went wrong.]

7. Ransohoff, D.F. and Feinstein, A.R. (1978): Problems of Spectrum and Bias in Evaluating the Efficacy of Diagnostic Tests. *N. Engl. J. Med.*, 299:926-930. [An exposition of the impact of some common biases on the reported accuracy of test.]

8. Sackett, D.L. (1986): Rules of Evidence and Clinical Recommendations on the Use of Antithrombotic Agents. *Arch. Intern. Med.*, 146:464-465. [A brief description of the methodology of one type of consensus conference. The accompanying papers provide the experts' findings on various applications of antithrombotic drugs.]

9. Schwartz, J.S., Ball, J.R. and Moser, R.H. (1982): Safety, Efficacy and Effectiveness of Clinical Practices: A New Initiative. *Ann. Intern. Med.*, 96:246-247. [A brief introduction to the American College of Physicians' Clinical Efficacy Assessment Project.]

10. Sox, H.C., Margulies, I. and Sox, C.H. (1981): Psychologically Mediated Effects of Diagnostic Tests. *Ann. Intern. Med.*, 95:680-685. [This paper demonstrates that a diagnostic test, in the right setting, could have important therapeutic effects without adding any other therapeutic maneuvers.]

11. Sox, H.C. editor (1987): *Common Diagnostic Tests: Use and Interpretation.* American College of Physicians, Philadelphia. [A collection of 15 papers from *The Annals of Internal Medicine* that each address a common test, review the literature and provide guidelines for use. The Blue Cross and Blue Shield Association adopted these statements and they have become very influential in

reimbursement policy. The introduction provides a review of probability theory in the use of diagnostic tests.]

12. Sox, H.C., Blatt, M.A., Higgins, M.C. and Marton, K.I. (1988): *Medical Decision Making*. Butterworths, Boston, [A new textbook for medical students and physicians that covers decision making, test ordering, cost-benefit analysis, outcome measurement and related issues. A good starting place.]

13. Suchman, A.L. and Griner, P.F. (1986): Diagnostic Uses of the Activated Partial Thromboplastin Time and Prothrombin Time. *Ann. Intern. Med.*, 104:810-816. [This article is included in Common Diagnostic Tests (11) and served as the basis for the Blue Cross and Blue Shield Association Guidelines.]

Medical Monitoring in the Home and Work Environment,
edited by Laughton E. Miles and Roger J. Broughton.
Raven Press, New York © 1990.

HISTORICAL DATA BASE, QUESTIONNAIRES, SLEEP AND LIFE CYCLE DIARIES

Alan B. Douglass, *Mary A. Carskadon and Robert *Houser

Veterans Administration Medical Center
2215 Fuller Road, Ann Arbor, Michigan 48105
*Department of Psychiatry, Bradley Hospital
1011 Veterans Memorial Parkway
East Providence, Rhode Island 02915

INTRODUCTION

The intended audience for this chapter is the clinician without formal training in sleep disorders medicine who finds himself in the position of having to assess patients for their sleep complaints. Researchers without a clinical background may also find the information useful, but they are cautioned that patients with a primary complaint of excessive sleepiness or persistent insomnia would likely be better served if they saw a specialist in sleep disorders medicine rather than undergoing only the procedures described below.

The medical concept of triage is important when patients with sleep disorders are assessed in outpatient or ambulatory monitoring settings. Sleep disorders are still sufficiently unfamiliar to medical professionals that many persons with quite severe sleep disorders remain unidentified. Therefore, any screening procedure for sleep disorders might be the first opportunity for a person to make known his complaints of disordered sleep. Once known, this information should be used to begin an assessment of the severity of the illness, to document it by physiological monitoring, and to make referrals to the proper agencies.

PATIENT HISTORY

There can be no substitute for a personal contact with every patient. At the very least, persons being assessed for sleep disorders should be asked:

1. "Do you snore severely, so that others complain?"
2. "Do you fall asleep in situations where most people would not?"
3. "Do you feel muscle weakness if you laugh, get angry, or emotional in any way?"
4. "Are you awakened at night by leg cramping or calf pain?"

Although far from pathognomonic or definitive, the first question is often positively answered by persons with obstructive sleep apnea, the second by anyone with a sleep disorder causing excessive somnolence, the third by narcoleptics, and the fourth by persons suffering nocturnal myoclonus (periodic movements in sleep). For further reading about signs and symptoms, a brief introduction to sleep disorders is available (9), and also the detailed nomenclature (1) of the sleep disorders.

Unfortunately, a wide range of medical and psychiatric disorders can present as a sleep symptom, and the reader is cautioned that a full medical workup of many of these patients will be required. Clinicians currently working in sleep disorders medicine often comment on the multidisciplinary nature of their practice, since it crosses the specialties of pulmonary medicine, psychiatry, and neurology. It is likely that clinicians trained in any one of these specialties will overdiagnose the disorders they are familiar with when confronted with the patients complaining of a sleep disorder, because of the similar constellation of symptoms produced by sleep disorders of very different etiologies. Also to be considered is the preference of patients and physicians alike for an organic diagnosis rather than a psychiatric one, if at all possible!

In general, physicians will wish to consider cardiovascular, neurological, and endocrinological disorders in their differential diagnosis of patients complaining of sleep abnormalities. These can usually be ruled out by appropriate laboratory tests. The kind of symptoms which patients present to psychologists or psychiatrists are less easy to evaluate by existing laboratory tests. Often negative night and day sleep monitoring is required before the complaint can safely be regarded as purely psychogenic.

From the above discussion, it should be obvious that the "medical model" is the appropriate initial approach to a patient with sleep complaints, whether or not other methods are used later.

In the available space, it will be impossible to give a detailed list of symptoms to ask about, or a flow-chart of how these symptoms are combined into working diagnoses for investigation. A clinical experience with sleep disorders patients is required for this sort of synthesis. It is possible to alert the clinician to some of the more notable clinical observations:

1. Every patient should have current drug use carefully documented. Sedative/hypnotic drugs are often prescribed for sleep complaints, yet if used for 6 months or in increasing doses, these drugs suppress delta-wave (deep) sleep, and also REM, so that they may become a cause of insomnia, not a cure for it.

2. Abusers of amphetamines may try to feign narcolepsy in order to get legal prescriptions. Anorexia nervosa patients sometimes attempt the same, hoping that the amphetamine will suppress appetite.

3. Clinical levels of apparent depression can be produced by sleep apnea or nocturnal myoclonus.

4. Deterioration of cognitive functions sufficient to be detectable on psychological testing can result from sleep apnea. In very severe apnea cases, the clinical picture can resemble dementia, yet the symptoms resolve with resolution of the apnea.

5. Poor school performance in children can in some cases be caused by sleep apnea and the resulting daytime sleepiness. The same is true of

narcolepsy. In children under 10, daytime sleepiness is likely to present as behavioral agitation or even hyperactivity in the classroom, rather than actual sleep in class.

6. Visual hallucinations are common in narcolepsy, often accompanied by tactile or auditory components. While typically seen at sleep onset or offset (hypnagogic, hypnopompic hallucinations), many severe narcoleptics are on the verge of sleep continuously, and so can hallucinate during the day. They can be misinterpreted as being psychotic, especially at the age when the hallucinations first begin, which is typically around puberty.

7. Severe daytime sleepiness often involves the patient falling asleep when driving, resulting in a swerve into the ditch on the highway. Others fall asleep when stopped at red lights. Still others continue a trip past the intended destination ("automatic behavior"). With no further information, such a symptom could result from narcolepsy, sleep apnea, or severe nocturnal myoclonus.

8. Many persons with nocturnal myoclonus can give a history of a close relative with similar nocturnal leg cramping. A similar strong family history is found in narcolepsy.

9. Snoring becomes significant if the bed partner has had to move to another room due to the noise, or if people in other parts of the house are disturbed by it despite closed doors. Such snoring is very suggestive of the near-asphyxia of obstructive sleep apnea. Hypertension, a short thick neck, and obesity are also common features of the disease.

10. Many patients with the major disorders of excessive somnolence will fall asleep, if left alone in the waiting room.

11. Many patients with narcolepsy can identify a year, usually the seventh to tenth grade, when their school marks fell precipitously and remained low despite the patient's feeling that "I knew the material". In retrospect, this usually marks the onset of uncontrollable daytime sleepiness.

12. The symptom of cataplexy is the single most useful one to differentiate narcolepsy from other causes of severe hypersomnolence. The uninitiated should be careful, however, because the symptom is often found in a partial form of weakness or droopiness only, without a dramatic complete fall to the floor. Also, depending on one's definition of narcolepsy, it is possible to have a "narcoleptic" Multiple Sleep Latency Test (MSLT) and not have clinical cataplexy.

QUESTIONNAIRES

Many facilities using ambulatory monitoring will find that assessment of the patient by questionnaire fits in well with the clinic's philosophy. Numerous questionnaires are available, and can be divided into roughly four categories: psychological, physical, sleep disorders, and sleep/wake diaries. Before drafting an entirely new questionnaire, an investigator must seriously consider whether he is "re-inventing the wheel". Also, those new to this area should consider that most psychological questionnaires are copyrighted, sold by the copy, and sold only under the understanding that a licensed professional psychologist will administer and interpret them. Some questionnaires are also available as computer programs which allow the patient to answer at a personal computer console. This type of questionnaire has the advantage of offering immediate scoring of the responses by the computer, a significant manpower saving in large clinics.

Psychological Questionnaires

Often a quick assessment of depression is required. Common choices would include the Carroll (5), Beck (3), or Hamilton (13) rating scales. Of these, the only the Hamilton requires a trained rater to give the test. A more complete psychological assessment of the patient's thoughts, moods, and personality can be achieved using self-report paper and pencil tests such as the SCL-90 (the shortest one), the MMPI, or Cattell's 16- PF. These instruments are so complex that the results really must be interpreted by a clinical psychologist. The assessment of intelligence or brain function is even more complicated, requiring a clinical psychologist both to administer and to interpret the tests. The WAIS and the Halstead-Reitan neuropsychological test battery fall into this category.

Physical Health Questionnaires

As much as the medical doctor must be careful in assessing psychological status using only a paper and pencil test, psychologists and others must remain alert to the fact that surveys of physical health are no substitute for a history and physical exam by a physician. There is the added problem that the missed physical illness provokes litigation more often than an erroneous assessment of personality. This said, the Cornell Medical Index (4) is as good as any instrument. For research purposes, it also serves to standardize the format of the patient's response.

Sleep Disorder Questionnaires

To date, the only major published questionnaire which addresses all of clinical sleep disorders is the SQAW (12), but it is a very long instrument which patients have some difficulty in completing. One of us (ABD) has been working with the SQAW authors in an attempt to shorten this questionnaire and to derive clinical scale scores from it, which were not part of the original SQAW. An initial description of this modification is available (10), but the revised questionnaire is not yet completed. The best-known questionnaire about a sleep symptom is the Stanford Sleepiness Scale (14), which assesses the amount of sleepiness at a given moment. Other instruments exist for special situations, such as a post-sleep inventory (19), or one for drug trials (18).

Sleep Diaries

A sleep diary or sleep log is a day-by-day report of sleeping and waking patterns, usually given as self-report, but occasionally completed by an observer in the case of children or demented patients. It is an inexpensive and efficient way to monitor daily sleep behavior, as well as many other diurnal and nocturnal activities and events (see Table 1). Such diaries offer a wide range of applications to clinicians in the ambulatory monitoring

VARIABLES OF INTEREST

SLEEP

Bed time
Sleep time
Rise time
Total sleep time
Naps-
    duration
    time
Means of awakening-
    alarm
    spontaneous
    other

WAKE

Exercise
Work schedule
Class schedule
Intake-
    food
    caffeine
    alcohol
    medication
    nicotine
    illicit drugs

SYMPTOMS

Awakenings-
    number
    length
    time
Abnormal behaviors
Parasomnias-
    somnambulism
    somniloquy
    enuresis
    night terrors
    nightmares

Excessive daytime sleepiness
Cataplexy
Automatic behavior
Sleep paralysis
Hypnogogic hallucinations

SUBJECTIVE RATINGS

Mood
Stress
Sleep quality
Alertness upon arising
Sleepiness

TABLE 1. Examples of the specific information the clinician
or researcher might ask for on a sleep diary.

setting, and to researchers. Accordingly, they will be considered in some detail.

SLEEP DIARIES

Clinical Applications

From a clinical perspective, the sleep log is a valuable adjunct for not only diagnostic evaluation, but also to assess treatment compliance and follow-up. As a diagnostic tool, the sleep diary is frequently an extremely useful supplement to interview and sleep habits questionnaire information, providing time- oriented information that may reveal relationships not obvious to the patient or inaccessible through other data gathering methods. The sleep diary can also provide a gauge of the severity of a complaint - - in terms of frequency of occurrence and degree to which the symptoms may disrupt the patient's daily life.

While a thorough interview usually picks up relevant activities or events that occur every day, the sleep diary is often most important when significant events or activities occur at less than daily intervals. Thus, a pattern providing clues to the etiology of a particular complaint may emerge for the first time on a diary. A patient may report serious difficulty falling asleep about three or four nights a week, for example, but fail to note the relationship of this sleep difficulty to "low-activity" days sitting in the office and drinking large amounts of coffee. Another common example is the parental report of a child who wets the bed or has night terrors two or three nights a week. The sleep diary may reveal that the wet or disturbed nights are those on which the child has skipped a nap, has had less sleep than usual the night before, or has had a very active day -- each of which may have etiologic significance (11).

Information given at interview or on a questionnaire may often be skewed by the patients' own preconceptions or by their perception of the physician's interests or biases. Sleep diary information may be more accurate than such information for a number of reasons. Patients with complaints of disturbed sleep may, for example, recall and thus focus on those nights that are the worst, using them as "prototypes" for describing their symptoms. As a result, it may appear that these nights are typical, when in fact their frequency has been exaggerated. By contrast, patients who are excessively sleepy may underreport symptoms because they have difficulty remembering sleep attacks and other symptoms retrospectively. Parents, too, may exaggerate or underreport their child's symptoms depending upon how it impacts on their own sleep/wake patterns and how well they are able to cope. Documenting the symptoms on a diary may give the patient or parent, as well as the physician, added perspective on the sleep problem.

Initial evaluation of patients with sleep-wake schedule disturbances generally requires that a sleep diary be completed for several weeks. Such schedule disruptions may not become apparent at the initial interview because they are not consistently obvious upon cross-sectional interrogation. This is true for patients of all ages.

Another area in which the sleep-wake diary is extremely useful is the monitoring of patient behavior before a scheduled laboratory assessment. A careful record of the patient's sleeping and medication pattern for at least a week before sleep lab testing is suggested. It is well known that a number of drugs, not only those which may be prescribed specifically for sleep problems, affect the nocturnal distribution of sleep stages. For example, tricyclic antidepressants generally suppress REM sleep, and acute withdrawal from these compounds results in a "rebound" of REM sleep (15). Prior sleep-wake patterns also affect the distribution of sleep stages. For example, chronically disturbed or restricted sleep can lead to the abnormal occurrence of REM sleep at sleep onset (6) posing the risk of a false-positive diagnosis of narcolepsy. Thus, the pattern of nocturnal sleep cannot be fully appreciated, if the sleep and drug histories are not clearly delineated. Daytime tests of alertness, such as the Multiple Sleep Latency Test (MSLT) are also affected by previous sleep and by drugs. It has been shown that the MSLT is not only influenced by the immediately preceding night's sleep, but can also be affected by the sleep pattern for as many a seven nights (6).

If monitoring of sleep, activity level, or other physiological variables is performed on an ambulatory basis, then not only is a pretesting diary important, but also an accurate behavioral log for the testing days. Such logs are needed not only to detail the patient's sleep-wake pattern and other activities, but also to enumerate events that may refer specifically to the physiological recording device. It is essential to know when the patient took it off to bathe. If the ambulatory monitoring is targeted to specific events such as seizures or cataplexy, then logging the occurrence of these symptoms is important to correlate the recording with the patient's perceptions.

Once a specific treatment has begun, the sleep diary assists the clinician to monitor patient compliance to instructions. For example, a patient with a circadian rhythm disturbance such as Delayed Sleep Phase Syndrome must postpone sleep daily until sleep occurs at a desired time, at which time an invariant schedule must be maintained (8). An accurate sleep log will reveal deviations from the prescribed schedule. In a number of settings in which behavior modification is used, it has been found that treatment instructions are followed more closely when patients are required to maintain a concrete record of activities (16).

Sleep diaries can be useful on a long-term basis to examine treatment progress, to monitor re-emergence of symptoms, and to promote self management. In the field of sleep disorders medicine, in which diagnosis results from symptoms not always accessible to laboratory testing, and where treatment is often done through self-management, a tool that gives a detailed subjective account of daily patterns is invaluable to the physician. The sleep diary keeps both the clinician and the patient informed of treatment progress.

Research Applications

Researchers use sleep logs in a number of ways that overlap with the clinical applications (e.g., pre- laboratory information), as well as several wider applications. Thus sleep diaries have been used to screen study

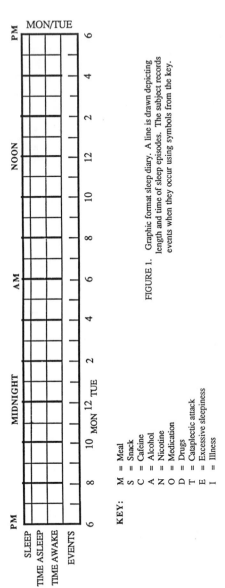

FIGURE 1. Graphic format sleep diary. A line is drawn depicting length and time of sleep episodes. The subject records events when they occur using symbols from the key.

KEY:

M	=	Meal
S	=	Snack
C	=	Cafeine
A	=	Alcohol
N	=	Nicotine
O	=	Medication
D	=	Drugs
T	=	Cataplectic attack
E	=	Excessive sleepiness
I	=	Illness

volunteers, to establish baseline sleep patterns for volunteers, and to monitor compliance with a study schedule. Another major research application is to examine sleep-wake patterns in large samples. In such studies, the diary often plays a gross data collection role. Without it, the only way to record data on the variables listed in Table 1 is with physiological monitoring or direct observation, which is not feasible for studying large samples. Nevertheless, diaries provide a more dynamic and more accurate estimation of sleep behavior across groups of individuals than might be available from one-time sleep habits questionnaires.

Sleep diaries are also used for longitudinal studies of a large sample to examine in a naturalistic setting the impact of a life transition, such as retirement, on sleep habits. Baseline and follow-up sleep levels of sailors on rotating watch systems (2,7) or pilots on transmeridian flights have been examined with sleep diaries (17). Shift workers in hospitals and factories provide ample material for research on sleep pattern disruption. A nursing example might be to monitor the number of arousals from sleep during sleep episodes before, during, and after a week of night shift rotation.

FORMATS

Its wide array of applications has caused the sleep diary to take on a range of formats. They can be grouped into three general categories: "Graphic"; in which sleep episodes are recorded on a time line; "Chart"; the times of activities listed in grid form; and "Questionnaire"; short responses to a series of questions.

Equally important as selecting the format is determining which variables, in addition to estimates of sleep episodes, need to be logged; and over what time period the diary should be maintained. At a minimum, patients are usually requested to log medication use, meal time, alcohol ingestion, and exercise periods for one week. Physicians generally choose the graphic format (Fig. 1.) because it provides an "analog" view of the sleep-wake data, a visual representation of patterns that can be easily compared across days. The patient's complaint will usually provide cues to the other activities that need to be logged. For instance, if excessive sleepiness and cataplexy are at issue, the patient should have specific instructions to note sleep attacks and cataplectic episodes. One might also consider adding the Stanford Sleepiness Scale (14) to be completed at intervals across the day.

The researcher dealing with large subject populations is often not interested in an analog view of a single individual's pattern. Instead, the aim is the accurate and speedy collection of large amounts of data. While the clinician is interested in relative sleep times, the researcher wants exact numbers -- data that are most easily taken from the chart and questionnaire formats (Fig. 2.).

	Monday
Respond after waking up	
What time did you fall asleep?	
What time did you wake up today?	
How long did you sleep last night?	
How many times did you wake up for more than ten minutes?	
What woke you up today? Alarm Spontaneous Other	A S O
What time did you have to get up?	
Respond during day	
Intake: 1. Food Nicotine Caffeine Medicine Alcohol Drugs	F N C M A D
2. Food Nicotine Caffeine Medicine Alcohol Drugs	F N C M A D
3. Food Nicotine Caffeine Medicine Alcohol Drugs	F N C M A D
4. Food Nicotine Caffeine Medicine Alcohol Drugs	F N C M A D
5. Food Nicotine Caffeine Medicine Alcohol Drugs	F N C M A D
6. Food Nicotine Caffeine Medicine Alcohol Drugs	F N C M A D
7. Food Nicotine Caffeine Medicine Alcohol Drugs	F N C M A D
8. Food Nicotine Caffeine Medicine Alcohol Drugs	F N C M A D
Activity: 1. Exercise Sleepiness	E S
2. Exercise Sleepiness	E S
3. Exercise Sleepiness	E S
Respond before bed	
If you have a job, what hours did you work today? Start - End -	
Did you nap today? Start - End -	
Were you sick today?	
If you circled Medicine or Drugs today please specify.	

FIGURE 2.   Chart format sleep diary. The complete diary has one example day and seven response days.

SUMMARY

The sleep diary provides valuable information on multiple levels. Whether one is attempting to assess the level of functioning of a patient with narcolepsy, or to understand the causes of night terrors, a sleep diary can enhance the battery of information and provide a detailed, subjective account of daily functioning.

REFERENCES

1. Association of Sleep Disorders Centers (1978): Diagnostic Classification of Sleep and Arousal Disorders, First Edition, Prepared by the Sleep Disorders Classification Committee, H.P. Roffwarg, Chairman. *Sleep*, 2:1-137.

2. Beare, A.N., Bondi, K.R., Biersner, R.J. and Naitoh, P. (1981): Work and Rest On Nuclear Submarines. *Ergonomics*, 24(8):593-610.

3. Beck, A.T. (1967) *Depression: Clinical, Experimental and Theoretical Aspects.* Hoebner Medical Division, Harper and Row, New York.

4. Brodam, K., Erdmann, A.J. and Wolf, H.G. (1956). *The Cornell Medical Index Health Questionnaire Manual.* Cornell University Medical College, New York.

5. Carroll, B.J., Feinberg, M., Smouse, P.E., Rawson, S.G. and Greden, J.F. (1981): The Carroll Rating Scale for Depression. *Br. J. Psychiat.*, 138:194-200.

6. Carskadon, M.A. and Dement, W.C. (1981): Cumulative Effects of Sleep Restriction on Daytime Sleepiness. *Psychophysiology*, 18:107-113.

7. Colquhoun, W.P., Rutenfranz, J., Goethe, H., Neidhart, B., Condon, R., Plett, R. and Knauth, P. (1988): Work At Sea: A Study of Sleep and of Circadian Rhythms In Physiological and Psychological Functions In Watchkeepers On Merchant Vessels. *Int. Arch. Occup. Environ. Health.*, 60:321-329.

8. Czeisler, C.A., Richardson, G.S., Coleman R.M., Zimmerman J.C., Moore-Ede, M.C., Dement, W.C. and Weitzman, E.D. (1981): Chronotherapy: Resetting the Circadian Clocks of a Patient with Delayed Sleep Phase Syndrome. *Sleep*, 4:1-21.

9. Douglass, A.B. (1986): Sleep disorders. *Medicine North America*, 36:5293-5298.

10. Douglass, A.B., Bornstein, R.A., Nino-Murcia, G, Keenan, S., Miles, L., Zarcone, V.P., Guilleminault, C. and Dement, W.C. (1986): Creation of the ASDC Sleep Disorders Questionnaire. *Sleep Res.*, 15:117.

11. Ferber, R. (1985): *Solve Your Child's Sleep Problems.* Simon and Schuster, New York.

12. Guilleminault, C. editor (1982): *Sleeping and Waking Disorders: Indications and Techniques.* Addison Wesley, Menlo Park.

13. Hamilton, M. (1967): Development of a Rating Scale for Primary Depressive Illness. *Br. J. Soc. Clin. Psychol.*, 6:278-296.

14. Hoddes, E., Zarcone, V., Smythe, H., Phillips, R. and Dement, W.C. (1973): Quantification of Sleepiness: A New Approach. *Psychophysiology*, 10:431-436.

15. Kay, D.C., Blackburn, A.B., Buckingham, J.A. and Karacan, I. In: *Human Pharmacology of Sleep*, edited by R.L. Williams and I. Karacan. John Wiley and Sons, New York.

16. Lacks, P. (1987): *Behavioral Treatment for Persistent Insomnia.* Pergamon Press, New York

17. Nicholson, A.N. (1972): Duty Hours and Sleep Patterns In Aircrew Operating World-Wide Routes. *Aerospace Med.*, 43(2):138-141.

18. Parrott, A.C. and Hindmarch, I. (1980): The Leeds Sleep Evaluation Questionnaire in Psychopharmacological Investigations - A Review. *Psychopharmacol*, 71:173-179.

19. Webb, W.B., Bonnet, M. and Blume, G. (1976): A Post-Sleep Inventory. *Percept. Motor Skills*, 43:987-993.

Medical Monitoring in the Home and Work Environment,
edited by Laughton E. Miles and Roger J. Broughton.
Raven Press, New York © 1990.

SOLID STATE TRANSDUCERS

Wen H. Ko

Electronics Design Center
Case Western Reserve University
Cleveland, Ohio 44106

INTRODUCTION

In the development of advanced medical instrumentation and therapeutic systems, one of the limiting factors is the transducer (sensors and actuators) that interfaces the patient with the instrument system. During the last decade much attention has been focused on the development of input sensors and output actuators to provide transducers for instrumentation used in various areas including measurement technology, industrial automation, aero space and biomedical measurements. Both physical and chemical transducers have been developed. This article will review solid state transducers, discuss their performance, and outline transducer technology, intelligent transducers and future trends in transducer research. A limited reference list, mostly in physical transducers, was selected subjectively by the author either because the paper describes a principle discussed herein or because it represents the advanced technology on a particular subject.

There are many types of transducers currently used in biomedical measurements. Present transducers cannot satisfy the increasing demand for high performance including: sensitivity, stability, size and weight and ease of operation. Furthermore, with the advances in both artificial intelligence and electronic technology during the last decade, new and better control systems for biomedical instruments are being designed using reliable, low cost, sophisticated VLSI circuits. These VLSI components and microprocessors make possible reliable, high performance systems to carry out complex control and signal manipulation functions. However, all these systems demand new or better transducers.

With solid state electronic and micromachining technology, transducers can be designed and mass produced which can offer potentially: (a) uniformity of device performance, (b) higher reliability than individually assembled devices, (c) low cost when mass produced, (d) integration with electronic circuits that interface with other signal processing or computing circuits, and (e) better performance.

The application of silicon integrated circuits and micromachining technology to the development of high performance, long-term stable, computer compatible microsensors for control applications has been the focus of efforts and has shown great potential and promise. Table I lists some of the solid state transducers reported in the literature that can be integrated with electronic circuits on the chip and that may have significance in biomedical systems. Several transducers are discussed below as selected examples.

PHYSICAL TRANSDUCERS

Temperature

Patient and environmental temperatures are measured with thermal resistive devices--thermistor; thermoelectrical devices--thermocouple; p-n junction diodes; temperature sensitive resonant circuits, infrared radiation and chemical devices -- liquid crystals and others. Most of these principles can be applied to solid state sensors fabricated on semiconductor substrates.

P-n junction temperature sensors are now commercially available. For normal junction diodes with a constant current flowing through, the p-n junction voltage decreases about 2 to 3 mV/^{o}C as the temperature rises. Junction sensors with an integrated circuit interface can give direct voltage readings corresponding to temperature in ^{o}F or ^{o}C at the output [39]. The sensitivity of special junction devices is generally -1.2 V/^{o}C or -10%/^{o}C which is comparable to thermistors in sensitivity [54]. Many of these devices are commercially available from National, Motorola, PM1 Intensil (AD-590) and Analog Devices. Microstructured thermopile infrared detectors have been fabricated on silicon substrates for noncontact temperature measurement or IFR detection with a responsiveness of 6V/W and a time constant of 15 ms [34].

A p-n junction array was made to measure the temperature profile in the body during cancer therapy [1]. The change of the energy band gap with temperature in semiconductor materials can be measured by the Optical Absorption Spectrum Edge. When incorporated with fiberoptics it provides a means for measuring body temperature with nonconductive devices. Liquid crystals or other materials that change their absorption characteristics with temperature can also be used with optical fibers to provide a nonconductive method for determining localized temperature.

Position and Motion

Position and displacement are measured with potentiometric devices, strain gauges, linear voltage differential transformers, capacitive displacement devices and ultrasonic devices. Velocity is measured with ultrasonic or optical Doppler effects, electro- magnetic devices and integration of acceleration or differentiation of displacement. Acceleration is measured by a mass and its acceleration force. A two-dimensional position detector in the form of a six to eight millimeter rectangular chip of silicon crystal that can determine the two-dimensional coordinates of a light spot projected on the surface of the device with good linearity was reported [40,42]. Figure 2 illustrates that the displacement or position of a refracting surface can be accurately measured by optical reflection. An analog signal can be obtained at the output with an accuracy below a few microns [18].

TABLE 1. Solid State Transducers

PARAMETERS MEASURED	PRINCIPLES USED	REFERENCES
Electrical Potential and Impedance	Active Electrodes with Amplifier Micro-Electrode	30 67
Temperature and Infrared Radiation	Junction Diode with IC Bulk Barrier Diode Thermopiles on Si	39 54 34
Sound and Ultrasound	ZnO on MOSFET Amplifier PVF$_2$ with FET Amplifier ZnO Integrated Into Gate of MOSFET	52 62 69
Light	LED and Diode Lasers CCD and Photodetectors	
Magnetic Field	Multicollector Transistor Carrier Domain Movement Magnetoresistance	70 43 45
Fluid Flow	"Hot Wire Anemometer" with IC Double Bridge Detector Pyroelectric Detector	23 65 49
Two-Demensional Position	Light Sport Position Sensitive Photodetectors on Si or on GaAs	36,40,42
Pressure	Deformation of Si Diaphragm by Capacitance or Piezoresistance Changes with IC Resonant Diaphragm with ZnO on Si in the Feedback Loop	26,27 6,59 57
Acceleration	Inertia Force on Micromachined Cantilevel Beams, on Si with IC, or on GaAs	51 22,60
Force	P-N Junction Stress Effects	53
Actuators	Piezoelectric Wafer Operated Ink Jets Electrostatic Shutter Display Electrostatic Force on Skin	41 14 4
Moisture, Humidity	Charge Flow Transistor Oxide Films	55 46,50
Gas Concentration	MOSFET with Pd or Pt Gate	37,44,46
Chemical Species in Air	Si Wafer Gas Chromatograph Oxide Films, Potentiometric	45,46,63 12,16,47
Ionic Concentration in Electrolytes	Ion Sensitive Diode Ion Sensitive FET	5,66 9,38,56
Chemical Ions and Molecules, Solution	Chemically Sensitive FET Optical Absorbing of Fluorescent Indicators	24,45,46 21,61

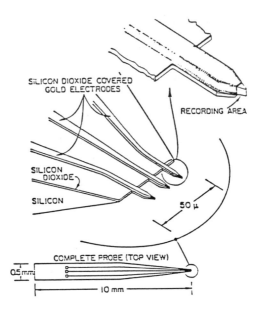

FIG. 1. A multi-probe microelectrode for biopotential recording (67).

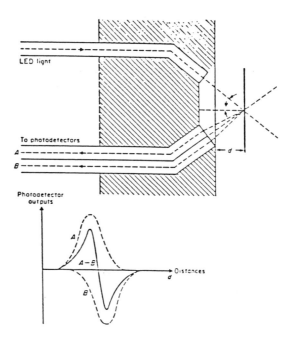

FIG. 2. Principle of optical displacement detector (18).

The device was used to measure the motion of a stape in a cat's ear. A silicon chip mass and spring accelerometer, 2 x 3 x 0.6 mm in size, weighing less than 0.02 gms was reported with a frequency response of 1000 Hz [51,60]. Several designs using piezoelectric films were reported to sense the inertia force [47]. These devices can be used in biological and physiological prostheses and sensory aids.

Figure 3 shows the principle and structure of an externally attachable capacitive sensor used to measure the knee angle (the knee is a complex joint and it is difficult to measure the angle with conventional sensors). The sensor can provide needed feedback signals for computer controlled walking [33].

Pressure

Methods for pressure transduction include measuring mechanical elastic properties of tubes and diaphragms, and using piezoresistive, capacitive and optical methods to convert mechanical deformation of metal, glass and silicon diaphragms into electrical signals representing pressure. Most of the present solid state sensors use piezoresistivity of silicon material to fabricate miniature force and pressure transducers. Figure 4 depicts a silicon diaphragm piezoresistive device for both gauge and absolute pressure. It measures 1 x 3 x 0.5 mm in size. Long-term baseline stability of 0.1% to 0.3% per month at 300 Torr Full Scale in body environment was observed [35]. The problem of packaging this device for biomedical applications still needs to be improved. Several miniature silicon capacitive pressure transducers with some signal processing circuits integrated on the chip were reported [6,26,59,68]. A design with a bipolar oscillator, capacitance bridge and follower circuits integrated on the capacitor chip is shown in Figure 5 [27,29]. The optical reflection technique described in the paragraph "position and motion" has also been used to convert diaphragm deflection caused by pressure change into an electrical signal.

Flow

Fluid flow has been measured with electromagnetic devices, ultrasonic and optical Doppler devices, fiberoptics, pressure gradient and thermal dilution methods [10]. There are many review articles and textbooks discussing the established ultrasonic, electromagnetic and dilution techniques for flow measurement. Therefore, they are not discussed herein. Figure 6 illustrates a thermal transport device fabricated on a silicon chip that measures the temperature differences at the up and down streams of a heat source, referring back to the flow velocity [23]. Integrated circuits can be fabricated on the flow sensor chip to perform simple processing functions [65].

Actuators

Solid state micro-actuator research is relatively new. Existing designs include cantilevel beams, ink jets [41], electrostatic motors [14], and display. These principles and techniques can be used to design drug pumps and flow

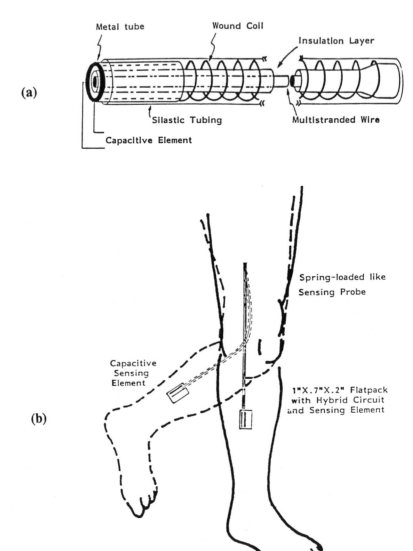

FIG. 3. (a) Body position sensor. (b) Knee angle sensor.

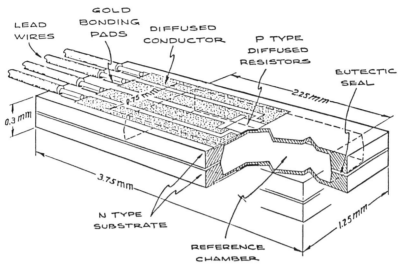

FIG. 4. Silicon diaphragm piezoresistive pressure sensor for absolute pressure measurement (27).

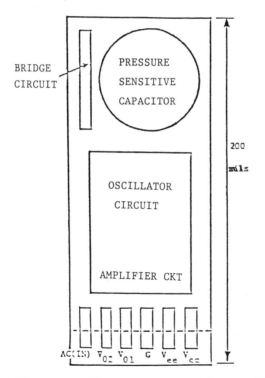

FIG. 5. A silicon capacitive pressure transducer with bipolar signal processing circuit on the chip.

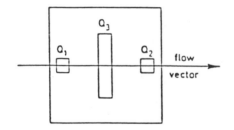

Basic chip layout.

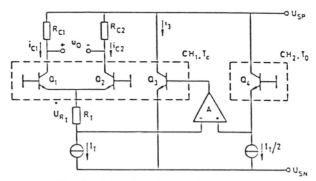

Circuit of the direction-sensitive flow transducer.

FIG. 6. Silicon integrated flow sensor (23).

control devices. Work on miniature drug pumps has been reported in the literature, as has a constant flow valve to control small amounts of fluid [58].

CHEMICAL TRANSDUCERS

Solid state chemical sensors have been developed in the following areas.

Humidity Sensor

Humidity can be measured by the change of (a) impedance of plastic material absorbing water vapor, (b) the surface impedance (resistance and capacitance) of insulators, such as Al_2O_3, with closely spaced electrodes and (c) the dew point when the sensor temperature is lowered. One solid state humidity sensor used a silicon chip on top of the Peltier cooling element. The chip contained two inter-digitated electrode structures forming a capacitor. As the temperature is lowered, water vapor starts to condense on the structure, drastically changing its capacitance due to the large dielectric constant of water [50]. Other designs utilized porous oxide layers sandwiched between a base metal and a top electrode [46]. The charge flow transistor oscillator also offers an interesting alternative as a humidity sensor [55].

Gas Sensors

H_2 gas can be monitored with Pd or Pt gate MOSFET [37, 44]. At $150^{\circ}C$, 10 ppm of H_2 can be detected. Other reducing and oxidizing gases can be monitored by the impedance of SnO_2, ZnO, TiO_2 and other oxide surfaces [12,16,63,]. The combustive gas monitor used in gas heated homes and various laboratories to sense various gases with improved sensitivity and selectivity. A gas chromatographic air analyzer was fabricated on a silicon wafer using solid state electronic techniques [63]. Similar techniques can be used to design gas sensor arrays that measure the smell and freshness of fish and vegetables.

Ion Sensors

Ion Sensitive Field Effect Transistors, ISFET, is an M-O-S FET with the gate electrode removed to the reference electrode and with the insulator exposed to the electrolyte. It can be used to measure ionic concentration in body electrolytes. Concentrations such as pH, K^+, Na^+, Ca^{++}, Ma^{++}, Cl^-, F^-, etc. can be measured with various modified insulators or by adding a membrane to the gate insulator [5,9,24,38,56,66]. Thin and thick film sensors for PO_2, PCO_2 and other gas and ionic species in solution are also being developed using silicon substrates and photolithography. Multiple sensors and reference electrodes can be integrated on the chip with the exposed area on the order of 10 um^2, thus alleviating many problems due to flow and protein deposition. Fiberoptics have been used for oxygen saturation measurement in blood. Improvement in signal analysis and sensor design should lead to the development of on-line catheter-type monitoring devices.

Enzyme and Molecular Sensors

By enclosing, trapping or absorbing enzymes, antibodies, and microorganisms on the surface of chemical sensors, the product of the enzymatic and other biochemical reactions can be sensed as a means of detecting the presence of biochemical materials on the substrate [21,24,61]. The on-line determination of proteins and moleculars will greatly improve environmental health and some phases of laboratory processes. Stability and packaging are the major current problems encountered with these types of sensors.

Combining solid state electronic technology and micromachining methods to produce new and improved chemical sensors opens a vast new area limited only by the creative approaches taken and the manner in which innovative concepts are implemented.

NEW TECHNOLOGIES - MICROMACHINING

In order to design new transducers, new technology will be needed. The field of micromachining where silicon or other materials in micrometer dimensions can be fabricated has been growing for the last decade [17,53].

The major micromachining functions are:

1.   Etching and Etch Stop.   Wet etching, using chemical and electrochemical techniques, has been developed for silicon, metal and other materials [2,66]. Dry etching techniques using plasma, ion beam and spark erosion have been developed. Silicon diaphragms thinner than 1 micron with an area greater than 1 $(mm)^2$, micro-cavities, beams, and bridges in micron scales, have been fabricated in laboratories.

2. Bonding. Silicon can be electrostatically bonded to pyrex glass (#7740) to form a hermetically sealed unit with a junction flatness below a micrometer [13]. Other bonding techniques use SiO_2, sputtered glass, both #7740 and low melting temperature glasses, as a sealing layer to bond silicon to silicon substrates or silicon to metal [7,17,32]. Metal compounds have also been used as brazing material to seal silicon to metal, ceramics, etc.

3. Selective Deposition. Many techniques can selectively deposit layers of conductive, semiconductive and insulating materials of various properties on the substrate.   These include: evaporation, sputtering, ion beam sputtering, plasma and chemical vapor deposition (CVD) [3,20,25]. Single crystal silicon, polysilicon, SiO_2, Si_3N_4, Al_2O_3 and organic films have been deposited on silicon and other substrates to form three-dimensional micro-structures [19].   Single chip multiple sensors can also be fabricated with these techniques.

4. Feedthrough, Holes and Packaging. In transducer design there is need for insulated electrical connections between bonded layers which require holes and micro-chambers fabricated on the substrate and particularly require a method to package those transducers for implant or indwelling applications where the devices have to be in communication with the biological system. At the same time, leads and signal processing circuits have to be protected from the corrosive and highly conductive fluids in the body.

INTELLIGENT TRANSDUCERS

The concept of intelligent or integrated transducers is to fabricate part of the signal processing circuitry on the same chip with the transducer. Such an approach is being made practical and many integrated sensors are being designed.

The functions of integrated transducers, besides transduction, are:

1. Impedance transformation and amplification
2. Compensation and error correction
3. Coding and modulation to provide digital output
4. Signal averaging and redundancy
5. Reliability checking fault detection and alarm
6. Remote sensing and telemetry
7. Power reduction scheme and time sharing
8. System parameter integration

The development of implantable pressure transducers at Case Western Reserve University can be used to illustrate the evolution of integrated sensors [27,26]. Pressure is a common biomedical parameter that is important to cardiovascular, respiratory and locomotive systems. The same sensor with small modifications, can be used to measure force, stress, strain, displacement, acceleration, flow, etc. However, high sensitivity (mm H_2O), long term implantable pressure sensors with time stability of 1% per year and suitable size and weight for small animals are still to be developed. In the past decade significant progress has been made. As a result, many high performance industrial pressure transducers are now available. With careful design, implantable biomedical sensors are within reach.

Figure 4 illustrates a piezoresistive pressure transducer, with a built in reference chamber designed to measure absolute pressure [31]. This device has reached 3%/year stability after 3 months aging, at 300 mm Hg full scale range and is being used to measure body fluid pressure with additional packaging.

To overcome some sensitivity and stress interference limitations, capacitive pressure transducers using microelectronic techniques were studied [27]. The performance is better than similar piezoresistive devices. However, they need an oscillator as power supply and the output impedance is high - (200kHz).

Figure 5 shows a capacitive pressure transducer integrated with the 1/2 MHz oscillator and an emitter follower amplifier as an integrated sensor. Other work at Case Western Reserve has yielded capacitive sensors with dc input and output at + 1.5 volt swing with a sensitivity of 1 volts/10^{-14} farad, or an equivalent sensitivity of 20 mv/mmH_2O at a short term noise level of ± 2mv.

This evolution in pressure sensor development is believed to be the general direction for other solid state microsensors [29]. The sensors being designed now will be able to go directly to the last stage after sufficient experience is accumulated.

FUTURE TRENDS

Besides utilizing new principles and materials, research work should be directed toward the packaging of biomedical transducers to meet the previously stated requirements. Methods need to be found for incorporating first stage signal processing circuitry into sensors so that the requirements for packaging can be reduced and the signal transmission improved thereby producing a new family of integrated transducers.

Several transducers can be integrated on a single chip or in a single package, so that they can be correlated with computing devices to give better reliability and confidence or a more useful indication of the subject's health status.

The new generation of transducers should be computer compatible, highly reliable, and easily interfaced to other systems. The concept of integrating electronic signal processing circuits on the transducer chip to generate intelligent transducers is being pursued. The combination of integrated transducers (sensors and actuators) with microcomputers and VLSI chips is expected to change our concept and approach to measurement technology and biomedical instrument design. Functional approaches to assess the status of the environment and form a basis for decision, instead of measuring individual parameters, is the trend of future research and development.

SUMMARY

This paper reviewed the development of solid state sensors and actuators during the last decade. Both solid state physical and chemical sensors suitable for use in the medical diagnosis and therapy, as well as prosthesis control, were discussed. The principles, device structure and performance of physical transducers for temperature, pressure, displacement, acceleration, flow, display, fluid injection and controlled fluid flow valves were summarized. Chemical sensors for humidity, combustive gases, ionic concentration in electrolytes and biological molecules concentration were also outlined for their potential applications in health care and medical research.

The technology of micro-machining, one of the bases for solid state transducers, was discussed with examples given to illustrate its capabilities and remaining problems.

The possibility of integrating signal processing circuits on or near the transducer chip to fabricate "intelligent sensors" was presented along with the functions that can be incorporated on the transducers.

Future trends in solid state transducer research and the possibility of beneficial collaboration between users and designers, as well as between material scientists, technologists, device designers and packaging engineers, was discussed.

ACKNOWLEDGEMENTS

The assistance of my colleagues at the Electronics Design Center and its staff is genuinely appreciated.

This work was partially supported by NIH grants RR80057, RR02024 and NS-19174.

REFERENCES

1. Barth, P. and Angell, J. (1982): Thin Linear Thermometer Arrays for Use in Localized Cancer Hyperthermia. *IEEE Trans. Electron Devices*, 29:144.

2. Bassous, E. (1978): Fabrication of Nevel 3-D Microstructure by Aniso Tropic Etching of (100) and (110) Silicon. *IEEE Trans. Electron Devices*, 25:1178.

3. Bean, J. (1981): Silicon Molecular Beam Epitaxy as a VLSI Processing Technique. *Technical Digest*, p. 6.

4. Bel, N. (1980): Integrated Capacitive Imaging Display for the Blind. Proc. 4th European Conf. Electronics, Germany, edited by W. Kaiser and W. Proebster, p. 549. North Holland Pub. Co., Netherlands.

5. Bergveld, P. (1972): Development, Operation and Application of the Ion Sensitive Field Effect Transistor as a Tool for Electrophysiology. *IEEE Trans. Biomed. Eng.*, 19:342.

6. Borky, J. and Wise, K. (1979): Integrated Signal Conditioning for Silicon Pressure Sensors. *IEEE Trans. Electron Devices*, 26(12):1906.

7. Brooks, A. and Donovan, R. (1972): Low Temperature Electrostatic Silicon to Silicon Seals Using Sputtered Borosilicate Glass. *J. Electrochem. Soc.*, 119:545.

8. Chen, P. et al. (1982): Integrated Silicon Microbeam PI-FET Accelerometer. *IEEE Trans. Electron Devices*, 29(1):27.

9. Cheung, P., Ko, W., Fung, C. and Wong, A. (1978): Theory, Fabrication, Testing and Clinical Response of Ion Selective Field Effect Transistor Devices. In: *Theory, Design and Biomedical Applications of Solid State Chemical Sensors*, edited by P. Cheung, et al., pp. 91-118. CRC Press, Florida.

10. Cobbold, R. (1974): Transducers for Biomedical Measurements. John Wiley, New York.

11. Coburn, J. (1981): Plasma assisted etching. *Plasma Chemistry and Plasma Processing,* 2(1):1.

12. Croset, M., Schnell, P., Velasco, G. and Sielka, J. (1977): Study of Calcia-Stabilized Zirconia Thin Film Sensors. *J. Vac. Sci. Technol.*, 14:777.

13. Eugelkrout, D., et. al. (1982): Current Research in Adhesiveless Bonding of Cover Glass to Solar Cells. *Sixteenth IEEE Photovoltaic Spec. Conf.,* p. 108.

14. Fan, L. S., Tai, Y. C. and Muller, R. S. (1988): Integrated Movable Micromechanical Structures for Sensors and Actuators. *IEEE Trans. E. D.*, 35:6, pp. 724-731.

15. Flamm, D. and Donnelly, V. (1981): The Design of Plasma Etchants. *Plasma Chemistry and Plasma Processing*, 1(4):317.

16. Fouletier, J. (1982): Gas Analysis With Potentiometric Sensors. *Sensors and Actuators*, 3:295.

17. Fung, C.D., Cheung, P.W., Ko, W.H. and Fleming, D.G., editors (1985): *Micromachining and Micropackaging of Transducers*. Elsevier Scientific Publishing Co., Amsterdam.

18. Green, L. and Ko, W. (1980): Optical Displacement Measurement Device. EDC Design Memo 297-A, Case Western Reserve University.

19. Guckel, H. and Burns, D. (1984): Planar Processed Polysilicon Sealed Cavities for Pressure Transducer Arrays. *Technical Digest,* p. 223.

20. Herring, R. (1979): Advances in Reduced Pressure Silicon Epitaxy. *Solid State Technol.,* 22:75.

21. Higgins, I. et al. editor. *J. Biosensors,* Elsevier, Netherlands.

22. Hok, B., Ovren, C. and Gustafsson, E. (1983): Batch Fabrication of Micromechanical Elements in GaAs-A1 $xGA_{1-x}As$. *Sensors and Actuators* , 4:341.

23. Huijsing, J., Schuddemat, J. and Verhoef, W. (1982): Monolithic Integrated Direction-Sensitive Flow Sensor. *IEEE Trans. Electron Devices,* 29(1):133.

24. Janata, J. and Huber, R. (1980): Chemically Selective Field Effect Transistors in Ion-Selective Electrode. In: *Analytical Chemistry,* edited by H. Freiser, Vol. 2 pp. 31-79. Plenum Press, New York.

25. Kern, W. and Bau, V. (1978): *Chemical Vapor Deposition of Inorganic Thin Films in Thin Film Processes,* edited by J. Vossen and W. Kern. Academic Press, New York.

26. Ko, W., et al. (1983): Capacitive Pressure Transducers With Integrated Circuits. *Sensors and Actuators* 4:403, 1983.

27. Ko, W., Bao, M. and Hong, Y. A High-Sensitivity Integrated-Circuit Capacitive Pressure Transducer. *IEEE Trans. Electron Devices,* 29 (1):48.

28. Ko, W., Bergmann, B. and Plonsey, R. (1977): Data Acquisition System for Body Surface Potential Mapping. *J. of Bioengineering,* 2:38-46.

29. Ko, W. and Fung, C. (1982): VLSI and Intelligent Transducers. *Sensors and Actuators,* 2:239.

30. Ko, W. and Hynecek, J. (1974): In: *Dry Electrodes and Electrode Amplifiers. In Biomedical Electrode Technology,* edited by H. Miller and D. Harrison, p. 169. Acad. Press, New York.

31. Ko, W., Hynecek, J. and Boettcher, S. (1979): Development of a Mini Ature Pressure Transducer for Biomedical Applications. *IEEE Trans. Electron Devices,* 26:1986.

32. Ko, W., Suminto, J. and Yeh, G. (1985): Bonding Techniques for Microsensors. *In Micromachining and Micropackaging of Transducers.* Elsevier Scientific Publishing Co., Amsterdam.

33. Ko, W., Wang, S. and Marsolais, E. (1984): Altitude Sensor for Angle Measurement in Neural Prosthesis. *Proc. 37th ACEMB,* p.106. Los Angeles, California.

34. Lahiji, G. and Wise, K. (1982): A Batch-Fabricated Silicon Thermo Pile Infrared Detector. *IEEE Trans. Electron Devices*, 29(1):14.

35. Leung, A., Ko, W., Spear, T. and Bettice, J. (1985): Intracranial Pressure Telemetry System Using Semicustom Integrated Circuits. Part I. Overall Development. *IEEE Trans. BME.*

36. Lubke, K., Rieder, G. and Thim, H. (1983): A High-Speed High-Resolution Two-Dimensional Position-Sensitive GaAs Schottky Photodetector. *Sensors and Actuators*, 4:317.

37. Lundstrom, K., Shivaman, M. and Svensson, C. (1975): A Hydrogen Sensitive Pd-Gate MOS Transistor. *J. App. Phys.*, 46:3876.

38. Matsuo, T. and Wise, K. (1974): An Integrated Field Effect Electrode for Biopotential Recording. *IEEE Trans. Biomed. Eng.*, 21:485.

39. Meijer, G. (1980): An IC Temperature Transducer With an Intrinsic Reference. *IEEE Trans. Sol. St. Cir.*, SC-15:370.

40. Noorlag, D. and Middelhoek, S. (1979) Two Dimensional Position Sensitive Photodetector With High Linearity Made With Standard IC Technology. *IEEE J. Sol. St. Elec. Dev.*, 3:75.

41. Petersen, K.E. (1979): Silicon as a Mechanical Material. *Proc. IEEE* , 70:420.

42. Petersson, G. and Lindholm, L. (1978): Position Sensitive Light Detectors With High Linearity. *IEEE J. Sol. St. Circ.*, SC-13:392.

43. Popovic, R. and Balter, H. (1983): Dual-Collector Magnetotransistor Optimized With Respect to Injection Modulation. *Sensors and Actuators*, 4:155.

44. Poteat, T. and Lalevic, B. (1982): Transition Metal-Gate MOS Gaseous Detectors. *IEEE Trans. Electron Devices*, 29:123.

45. Proc. 1st and 2nd Sensor Symposium. IEE Society, Japan; (1981-82), edited by S. Kataoka.

46. Proc. Internat. Meet. Chemical Sensors, Kodansha, Japan; (1983), edited by T. Seiyama.

47. Proc. 2nd Internat. Conf. Solid State Sensors and Actuators, Delft, The Netherlands; (1983/84): *Sensors and Actuators*, Vol. 4.

48. Prohaska, O., et. al. (1979): A 16-Fold Semi-Microelectrode for Intracortical Recording of Field Potentials. *Electroenceph. Clinical Neurophysiology*, 47:629.

49. Rahnamai, H. and Zemel, J. (1981): Pyroelectric anemometer:

Preparation and Flow Velocity Measurements. *Sensors and Actuators* , 2:3.

50. Regtien, P. (1981): Solid State Humidity Sensors. *Sensors and Actuators*, 2:85-95.

51. Royance, L. and Angell, J. (1979): A Batch-Fabricated Silicon Accelerometer. *IEEE Trans. Electron Devices*, 26(12):1911.

52. Royer, M., et al. (1983): ZnO on Si Integrated Acoustic Sensor. *Sensors and Actuators* 4:357.

53. Sansen, W., Vandeloo, P. and Puers, B. (1982): A Force Transducer Based on Stress Effects in Bipolar Transistors. *Sensors and Actuators*, 3:343.

54. Schaffer, H. and Koeder, O. (1983): A Sensitive All Silicon Temperature Transducer. *Sensors and Actuators*, 4:661.

55. Senturia, S., Garverick, S. and Togashi, K. (1981): Monolithic Integrated Circuit Implementations of the Charge Flow Transistor Oscillator Moisture Sensor. *Sensors and Actuators*, 2:59-72.

56. Siu, W. and Cobbold, R. (1979): Basic Properties of the Electrolyte-SiO_2-Si System: Physical and Theoretical Aspects. *IEEE Trans. Electron Devices*, 26:1805-1815

57. Smits, J., et al. (1983): Resonant Diaphragm Pressure Measurement System With ZnO on Si Excitation. *Sensors and Actuators*, 4:565.

58. Spencer, W. (1981): A Review of Programmed Insulin Delivery Systems. *IEEE Trans.*, 28:3.

59. Sugiyama, S., Takigawa, M. and Igarashi, I. (1983): Integrated Piezo-Resistive Pressure Sensor With Both Voltage and Frequency Output. *Sensors and Actuators*, 4:113.

60. Suminto, J. T., Yeh, G. J., Spear, T. M. and Ko, W. H. (1987): Silicon Diaphragm Capacitive Sensor for Pressure, Flow, Acceleration and Altitude Measurement *Digest of Int. Solid-State Sensors & Actuators Conf., Tokyo, Japan. (p.336)*.

61. Suzuki, S., editor (1984): *Biosensors*. Tokyo, Japan.

62. Swartz, R. and Plummer, J. (1979): Integrated Silicon-PVF_2 Acoustic Transducer Arrays. *IEEE Trans. Electron Devices*, 26(12):1921.

63. Terry, S., Jerman, J. and Angell, J. (1979): A Gas Chromatographic Air Analyzer Fabricated on a Silicon Wafer. *IEEE Trans. Electron Devices*, 26:1880.

64. Theunissen, M. et. al. (1970): Application of Preferential Electro

Chemical Etching of Silicon to Semiconductor Device Technology. *J. Electrochem. Society,* 117(7):959.

65. Van Putten, A. (1983): An Integrated Silicon Double Bridge Anemometer. *Sensors and Actuators,* 4:387.

66. Wen, C., Chen, T. and Zemel, J. (1979): Gate Controlled Diodes for Ionic Concentration Measurement. *IEEE Trans. Electron Devices,* 26:1945.

67. Wise, K., Angell, J. and Starr, A. (1970): An Integrated-Circuit Approach to Extracellular Microelectrodes. *IEEE Trans. Biomed. Eng.,* BME-17:238.

68. Yamada, K., Nishihara, M. and Kanzawa, R. (1983): A Piezoresistive Integrated Pressure Sensor. *Sensors and Actuators,* 4:63.

69. Yeh, Y., Muller, R. and Kwan, S. (1977): Detection of Acoustic Waves With a PI DMOS Transducer. *J. App. Phys.,* 16-1 suppl.:517. Japan.

70. Zieren, V. and Duyndam, D. (1982): Magnetic-Field-Sensitive Multi Collector N-P-N Transistors. *IEEE Trans. Electron Devices,* 29(1):83.

Medical Monitoring in the Home and Work Environment,
edited by Laughton E. Miles and Roger J. Broughton.
Raven Press, New York © 1990.

A PORTABLE MICROCOMPUTER FOR LONG-TERM PHYSIOLOGICAL MONITORING IN THE HOME AND WORK ENVIRONMENT

Laughton E. Miles

Clinical Monitoring Center, Palo Alto, Calfornia 94304
and Vitalog Monitoring, Inc., Redwood City, California 94063

INTRODUCTION

During the past 15 years, advances in microelectronics, sensor technology and computer software, have allowed the development of small, light-weight, all-solid-state physiological monitors, suitable for recording data for long periods of time from biomedical sensors attached to free-ranging humans or other animals. These intelligent devices consume very little electrical power, and tend to be more reliable than devices such as tape recorders which have moving parts. On the other hand, for some applications, solid-state monitors are limited by their consumption of battery power or amount of data storage.

This paper reviews the many applications of a programmable, portable microcomputer with multiple physiological inputs, versions of which have been manufactured by Vitalog Corporation (now Vitalog Monitoring Inc.) since 1978.

LONG-TERM PHYSIOLOGICAL MONITORING OF FREE-RANGING HUMANS AND OTHER ANIMALS

A small (6.0 x 3.4 x 1.3 inch) portable version of the Vitalog physiological monitoring system(PMS-8™) has been used to monitor free-ranging animals or humans in a variety of environments, for up to one week on a single battery charge (see Figure 1). Applications have been extraordinarily diverse, involving such specialized studies as stress and anxiety research, cardiac rehabilitation, executive fitness, military combat, exercise physiology, environment medicine, jet lag, shift work, chemotherapy, chronic pain, drug side-effects, nutrition, insomnia, psychiatric disorders, antarctic exploration, high altitude research, and both U.S. and Soviet Space Flight Missions. Several applications are reported in this volume (see Chapters by Burnett and Barr Taylor; Mermin and Czeisler; Connell and Graeber; Kripke and Gregg; and Kayed).

The hardware and software were originally designed for use with the Apple II computer (5), but the currently available software (VitaKRON™) is used with IBM-PC/AT computers. It is based on the concept of

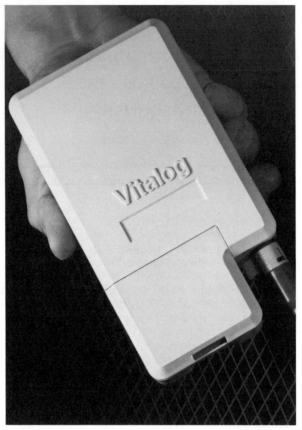

FIG. 1. The PMS-8 portable multichannel physiological monitor.

individual sensor software modules which may be customized by the user as to sampling rate, numerical precision, real-time processing, data-encoding etc. Using this software, up to nine different modules can be selected, combined, and down-loaded into the monitor at the time the recording is initiated. In this way any given sensor can use independent recording variables or, if necessary, modify its recording algorithm according to some other sensor input. A popular configuration uses three (individually specified) temperature channels, one body movement channel, a heart rate channel, and a patient event marker.

The data can be graphically displayed on a video screen, and by pressing particular keys it is possible to include "windows" specifying the data and absolute time at the position of a cursor. The location of the display and the degree of data compression can be varied (by channel or by screen); and other channels (sensors) can be substituted. Six channels of data can be printed in "chart-recorder mode" (See Figure 2); and the data is also available for numerical listing and export to other software programs for alternative analyses.

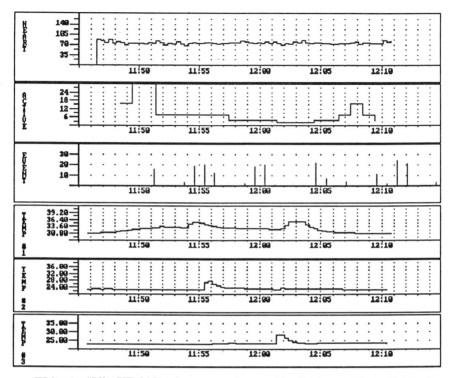

FIG. 2. "VitaKRON" chart-recorder-mode display with individually specified channels, time and data windows and other features.

CARDIO-RESPIRATORY MONITORING IN THE HOME ENVIRONMENT

The Vitalog HMS3000™ home cardio-respiratory monitoring system (see Figure 3) is designed to measure chest and abdominal respiratory effort (using calibrated Vitalog inductive plethysmography (VIP) sensors), paradoxical breathing, air flow, heart rate, oximetry, body movement, leg movement, eye movement, and sleeping position. The basic monitor, together with its sensor interface unit, a battery-operated oximeter, an LCD electrical multimeter, and a single multi-sensor cable, is contained in a small (30 cm x 22 cm x 12 cm) aluminum "Lunch-Box" (6,8). When not in use, the sensors and cables are contained in a pouch in the lid of the "Lunch-Box".

When the recording is terminated, the data is recovered by connecting the monitor to an IBM-PC/AT compatible computer; but the "Lunch-Box" also provides real-time analog and digital outputs which can be directly interfaced with a polygraph or other recorder. Furthermore, the faceplate also provides an input for an external oximeter, and input connectors for any alternative or additional sensors developed by the user.

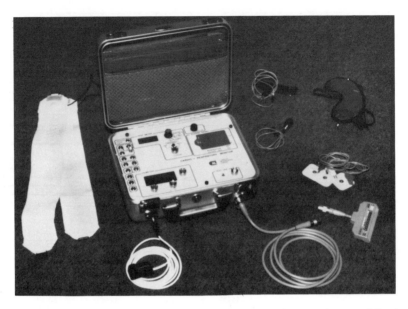

FIG. 3. Vitalog HMS-3000 ("Lunch-Box") Cardio-Respiratory Monitor, with sensors.

The integral impedence/voltmeter makes it easy to check the 4.5 Amp/Hr NiCad battery, and ensure that the ECG electrodes have a suitable electrical connection to the skin. During calibration and start-up, an optical isolation device protects the patient from the 115-240 VAC electricity in the IBM computer.

The currently available system utilizes new data collection and data analysis software (VITACORE V4.3 and VITARESP V4.3) developed by Vitalog Monitoring Inc. However, the Clinical Monitoring Center also uses other software and a hand-held spirometer (Boehringer Labs. Inc) to provide, (a) more quantitative calibration of the respiration sensor, (b) screening pulmonary function tests (Vital Capacity and FEV-1), and (c) inspection of the ECG wave form.

Because non-invasive respiration recordings are commonly distorted and uncalibrated by movement artefact, physical displacement of the sensors and changes in body position, computerized analyses (including apnea detection) of an overnight respiration record are often unreliable or misleading. The VITARESP computer program addresses this problem by utilizing the concept of a local inspiratory reference amplitude (IRA), against which changes in the respiration signal can be compared. The preliminary IRA values allotted by the computer are manually reviewed on a video screen in a first editing pass which also allows specification of wake, sleep, REM, artefact, and brief arousals. The computer then scores the record for apneas and hypopneas, paradoxical breathing, oximetry, heart rate, body position, body movement, leg movement or eye movement. The scored record is displayed on a video screen for final editing. Events are identified by a bar code, and numerically characterized in a continuously

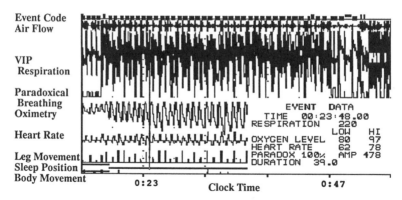

FIG. 4. Display of data recorded from patient with obstructive sleep apnea, using VitaRESP software.

updated screen window according to the position of a moveable cursor (see Figure 4).

The program can randomly access and display the longest event in each category, or any location in the record, in detail which can vary from 5 minutes to 180 minutes per screen. The analysis software then summarizes the data numerically (including any variation by body position); and automatically generates oximetry histograms, compressed plots, examples from the record, and a list of all breathing abnormality with associated physiological changes.

The Clinical Monitoring Center uses a special version of this report generation software to automatically access the results, archive the data, and prepare a final report to the referring physician, using a medical information system based on the PARADOX Relational Data Base Program (Version 3.0) from Borland International, Scotts Valley, California.

The Sensors

The patented "VIP" chest and abdominal respiration sensors use an inductive plethysmography technique, and can be calibrated to measure absolute tidal volume (7). Compared to the Respitrace™ version (Ambulatory Monitoring, Inc. Ardsley, New York) the VIP sensors are more robust, have fewer connectors, are easier to apply (one size can fit most adults), and are less likely to be inappropriately deformed during use. Because the transformer coil is an integral part of each respiration band, the sensors are less affected by movement artefact.

The airflow interface can be adapted to accept either thermistor, thermocouple, or acoustic (throat microphone) inputs, changing its function by software menu selection and a three-way switch.

The "Lunch-Box" includes an oximeter as an internal device especially configured for outpatient recordings, but the monitor can also accept the analog output from an external oximeter.

In the past, most recordings were carried out using a body movement

TABLE 1.

EVALUATION OF SLEEP APNEA USING THE VITALOG HOME MONITOR

TOTAL RECORDINGS   =   2,293

FIRST RECORDINGS   =   1,963   (1,857 with SEVERITY RATINGS)

                       18.2 % FEMALE

                       81.7 % MALE

		N	1	2	3	4	5
FEMALE	#	106	119	30	49	26	9
	%	31.3	35.1	8.8	14.5	3.4	2.6
MALE	#	189	529	216	277	140	167
	%	12.5	34.8	14.2	18.2	9.2	11.0

sensor based on an omnidirectional array of 360-degree mercury tilt switches; but this sensor has now been replaced by a more reliable and quantitative dual-axis piezo-resistive accelerometer made from micromachined silicon. A second accelerometer can be used in place of the eye-movement sensor in order to measure leg movements.

Body sleeping position is usually measured by a specially designed multiconductor mercury tilt switch; but the same piezo-resistive accelerometer used for measuring movement can also provide accurate and reliable body position data.

The three-lead ECG sensor allows calculation of a local steady-state heart rate which has been validated during exercise testing and Holter monitoring studies (1).

Eye movements are measured by an Infra-Red LED system. Unless the sensor is carefully positioned, the signal can be relatively insensitive, or include respiration and pulse rate artefact. Piezo-electric sensors used by other investigators may be more effective. The ability to detect REM sleep during monitoring of patients with sleep apnea is often believed to be worthwhile, although the resulting information is quite unlikely to modify any therapeutic decisions or cause the recording to be repeated.

Applications of the "Lunch Box" Design

At the Clinical Monitoring Center, various versions of the Vitalog Monitor have been used to evaluate more than 2000 patients suspected of having obstructive sleep apnea. Table 1 shows the distribution of 1-5 level severity estimates made on the basis of these recordings.

Detailed information relating to the effect of sleeping position on breathing abnormalities and hypoxemia, has been obtained in 936 patients (10) (see Table 2). Overall, the supine position showed the most breathing abnormalities, the most falls in oxygen saturation, the lowest average "low-

TABLE 2.

SLEEPING POSITION IN PATIENTS REFERRED FOR EVALUATION OF SLEEP APNEA

NUMBER   =   936   83 % MALES
(ALL > 240 min TST)   17 % FEMALES

	SUPINE	RIGHT-SIDE	PRONE	LEFT-SIDE	TOTAL
MINUTES	147	122	45	84	398
%	36.9	30.6	11.3	21.1	

oximetry" value, and the longest time below 85 % saturation; and this was true in all severity grades except the normal group. The study showed that it is usually possible to evaluate the physiological changes during sleep in the supine position when patients are recorded without supervision in their own (usual) environment. For example, 88 % of the patients spent at least 20 minutes in the supine position. Other sleeping positions are less certain, but this may not be important since breathing and oximetry abnormalities are usually similar in all non-supine positions, and some non-supine position is almost always recorded. It is likely that night-to-night variability of apnea/hypopnea is reduced, and the evaluation of therapeutic efficacy more reliable, when the data is normalized for sleeping position. Furthermore, in many individuals, modifying the sleeping position can be an effective and non-invasive treatment for sleep apnea (see Cartwright, this volume).

The "Lunch-Box" has primarily been used to evaluate people with loud and disruptive snoring and patients with obstructive sleep apnea. It has proved to be very suitable for a new protocol which has allowed safe, reliable, and cost-effective calibration of Nasal-CPAP treatment in more than 80 patients, without requiring supervised polysomnography (9). It has also been used as a convenient and effective recording oximeter. Patients prefer the "Lunch-Box" over previous versions of the Vitalog monitor; and recordings are rarely repeated because of defective hardware or sensors.

We do repeat the test (with-out any additional fee), if the respirations become grossly uncalibrated, if a sensor becomes dislodged, malpositioned or (in the case of the oximeter finger-probe) impaired by low blood perfusion; or if we have reason to believe that the recording does not represent the patient's usual sleep. Occasionally there are problems because of patient errors, poor cooperation, or indiscreet activity (eg. staying awake all night at a party).

Validation Studies

Published validation studies using early versions of the Vitalog cardio-respiratory monitor demonstrated that estimates of the overall number of events per hour of sleep, were as reliable as those made using supervised inpatient EEG-polysomnography (3,11,12). Validating the classification of individual events (apneas v. hypopneas, central v. obstructive) was less successful, but these distinctions are also difficult within supervised polysomnography (2), partly due to the fact that no major clinical organization has proposed or established unequivocal event definitions. Validation studies utilizing software earlier than VITARESP version 4.0, have indicated that the Vitalog monitor under-estimated the number of central apneas (3). In more recent versions of the software, this problem has been addressed by excluding any paradoxical breathing occurring during event termination.

The Vitalog monitor relies upon calibrated chest and abdominal inductive plethysmography sensors for measuring tidal volume and identifying airway obstruction by paradoxical breathing. However, the system now includes a direct measure of airflow, because an event could be wrongly classified as an obstructive hypopnea rather than obstructive apnea, if the chest and abdominal compartments become unbalanced.

On the other hand, an apparent improvement in the distinction between central apneas and obstructive apneas may not have much clinical impact. Some patients are observed to have undoubted obstructive apnea during part of the night, yet show many central events or a major "central-component" elsewhere. More elaborate and invasive polysomnographic recordings usually do no more than confirm the relative lack of respiratory effort, yet the events in question usually respond to treatment with nasal-CPAP. Therefore, most experts believe that such "central" apnea, even if confirmed by monitoring esophageal pressure or diaphragmatic EMG, is secondary to (or associated with) the abnormality causing airway obstruction, and should not be taken as evidence that treatment of the obstruction is unnecessary.

At the present time, the most serious opportunity for mis-classification and mis-scoring occurs when the overall amplitude of the respiration signal is artificially small. When this occurs the calculation of paradoxical breathing is impaired, and events may be falsely located and/or misclassified as non-obstructive. Artificially high amplitudes are less of a problem, but can obscure true events and produce false evidence of paradoxical breathing. We are attempting to overcome these problems by utilizing a new respiration interface which automatically adjusts the gain and balance during sleep.

The Role of the Vitalog Monitor and Other Home Monitoring Systems in the Diagnosis and Management of Sleep Apnea

The clinical role of the Vitalog monitor and other systems for unsupervised home cardio-respiratory monitoring during sleep has been controversial, in part because of concerns about the validity of the data, in part because of a disagreement as to whether classic EEG-sleep stage information is needed in order to treat sleep apnea. (Note that the Vitalog monitor does not provide a continuous record of the EEG, EOG, EMG, or ECG wave-forms.

There has also been concern about the possible abuse of cheaper devices and more cost-effective diagnostic services by individuals outside the control or influence of the academic sleep disorders community and overnight sleep-recording facilities. The situation is complicated by the recent emphasis on cost-containment and efficacy, and the current uncertainty regarding indications for treatment of sleep apnea.

Unfortunately, no study of the impact of such home monitoring devices on clinical decision-making and patient-outcome is available, and "gold-standards" have proven to be notoriously unreliable. In one study, heuristic severity estimates obtained from scoring and reviewing Vitalog recordings were no different from estimates obtained from evaluation of simultaneous polysomnographic recordings (12).

A case can be made that sleep apnea patients may require supervised EEG-polysomnography if; (a) the patient seems more sleepy than the apnea justifies; (b) the patient needs continuous supervision in order to obtain a technically satisfactory recording; (c) it is necessary to confirm a suitable or accurate total sleep time in an atypical recording; (d) one needs to characterize a movement disorder simulating or influencing apnea; (e) an apparent central component needs more detailed evaluation by measuring intrathoracic pressure; (f) it is necessary to confirm a mainly or exclusively REM sleep related problem; (g) an attempt is to be made to relate a known and serious nocturnal cardiac arrhythmia to a specific breathing abnormality; (h) some intervention is planned (eg. nasal CPAP treatment) and the patient has serious cardiac or pulmonary disease.

These situations can all be anticipated from the clinical history or the results of home monitoring; and most are relatively rare or of doubtful clinical relevance.

The Clinical Monitoring Center's experience as a referral-based, fee-for-service home monitoring clinic, with data from more than 2000 clinical recordings, has convinced the author that definitive therapeutic decisions can be made on the basis of Vitalog home cardiorespiratory monitoring, without requiring supervised overnight EEG/polysomnography, for most (but not all) patients with obstructive sleep apnea.

A QUALITY-CONTROL /CLINICAL-DECISION-MAKING PROGRAM

One way of addressing many of these issues is to involve users in a regular quality-control/clinical-decision-making program. In a scheme recently initiated by the Clinical Monitoring Center, a single record was distributed to registered users of HMS-3000 systems, together with a clinical background and sleep diary. The users not only scored the record, but a physician associated with each user also provided a severity estimate, requested other tests, and made a therapeutic disposition. The data was compared with corresponding information obtained by multiple scoring of a simultaneously-recorded EEG-polysomnographic recording.

An example of an analysis of the first 37 Vitalog scorings of an unusually difficult record (subject "MarchTest") is shown in Figure 5. This shows that the Apnea + Hypopnea Duration Index (AHDI) (Mean 18 $\pm$ 4.2 minutes per hour) was a more reproducible measure than the Apnea + Hypopnea Index (AHI) (Mean 33 $\pm$ 8.3 events per hour).

After reviewing the clinical material and the independently scored record, 75% of the physicians gave a severity rating of 2 or 3 (mild/moderate or moderate). A trial of CPAP was the most often recommended additional test; Holter monitoring was requested 14 times, and EEG-polysomnography 13 times. The most recommended therapeutic disposition was "sleeping position modification" (22 physicians), followed by "reassurance/weight-loss/later-reassessment" (20 physicians), "nasal CPAP" (16 physicians), and "medication" (14 physicians). Uvulo-

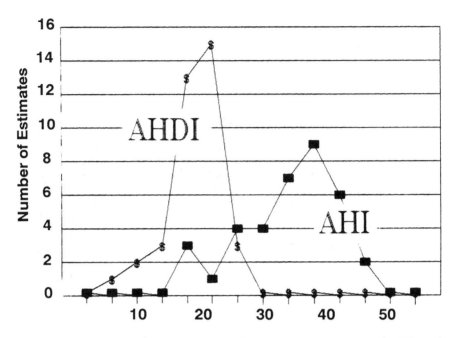

FIG. 5. Frequency histogram of Apnea+Hypopnea Index (AHI) and Apnea+Hypopnea Duration Index (AHDI) as estimated from 37 independent scorings of Vitalog HMS-3000 sleep recording of subject "MarchTest".

palatopharyngoplasty was recommended 6 times. Most of the recommended medications related to treatment of nasal allergies.

At this time, the "MarchTest" EEG-polysomnographic record has not been scored often enough for meaningful comparison with the Vitalog data; but there is also a substantial variation in the scoring and clinical opinions.

This quality-control, technical-validation, clinical-decision-making study, is proposed as a model for the ongoing evaluation of diagnostic procedures *and* the individuals who use them.

SUMMARY

Previous consensus conferences involving both sleep disorders and pulmonary medicine organizations, have concluded that while home monitoring techniques have potential, there was not enough data on which to base a recommendation that such portable home monitoring devices be used for the diagnosis of obstructive sleep apnea (4).

In most other areas of biology and medicine there is no such ambivalence; and cost-effective physiological monitoring and clinical evaluation in the home and work environment is perceived, not as a threat, but as an imminent revolution in health care delivery.

The technical-validation, clinical-decision-making study described in this chapter, is proposed as a model for justification and on-going quality control.

REFERENCES

1. Barr Taylor C., Kraemer, H.C., Bragg, D.H., Miles, L.E., Rule, B., Savin, M., DeBusk, R.F. (1982): A New System for Long Term Recording and Processing of Heart Rate and Physical Activity in Outpatients. *Computers and Biomedical Research* 15:7-17.

2. Bliwise, D., Bliwise, N., Kraemer, H., Dement, W. (1983): Error of Measurement of Respiratory Disturbance During Sleep. *Sleep Research* 12:343.

3. Gyulay, S., Gould, D., Sawyer, B., Pond, D., Mant, A., Saunders, N. (1987): Evaluation of a Microprocessor-Based Portable Home Monitoring System to Measure Breathing During Sleep. *Sleep* 10:130-142.

4. Indications and Standards for Cardiopulmonary Sleep Studies. (ACCP/ASDC committee) (1985): *Sleep* 8:369-379.

5. Miles, L.E., Rule, R.B. (1982): In: *Long Term Monitoring of Multiple Physiological Parameters Using a Programmable Portable Microcomputer,* edited by F.D. Stott et al. pp.249-257. Academic Press Inc. London.

6. Miles, L.E. (1988): A Battery-Operated Device for Home Monitoring of Oximetry, Heart Rate, Respiration, Eye Movements, Sleeping Position, and Body Movement in Patients with Snoring and Sleep Apnea. In: *Chronic Rhonchopathy, Proceedings of the First International Congress on Chronic Rhonchopathy*, edited by C.H. Chouard, pp. 149-151.

7. Miles, L.E., Herekar, B.V., Rule, R.B.. (1986): An Improved Sensor for Recording Respiration by Inductive Plethysmography. *Sleep Research,* 15:249.

8. Miles, L.E. (1988): A "Lunch-Box" Version of the Vitalog Home Cardiorespiratory Monitor. *J. Polysomn. Technol.,* pp. 37-41.

9. Miles, L.E. (1987): Optimization of Nasal-CPAP Airflow Pressure by Use of Home Oximetry Recordings. *Sleep Research,* 16:568.

10. Miles, L.E. (1988): Body Sleeping Position and Sleep Apnea in the Home Environment. *Sleep Research,* 17:218.

11. Nino-Murcia, G., Bliwise, D., Keenan, S., McGregor, P., Foster, R., Butkov, N., Hutchinson, D., Slegel, D., Kraemer, H., Sink, V., Dement, W., Miles, L. (1985): Respiration Monitoring in Sleep: Comparison of Judgements Based on Conventional Polysomnography (PSG) and an Ambulatory Microprocessor-Derived Recording (AMR). *Sleep Research,* 14:274.

12. Nino-Murcia, G., Bliwise, D., Keenan, S., Dement, W. (1986): Inter-Rater Reliabilities of Respiratory Disturbance Variables Using Two Recording Systems. *Sleep Research,* 15:251.

Medical Monitoring in the Home and Work Environment,
edited by Laughton E. Miles and Roger J. Broughton.
Raven Press, New York © 1990.

BIOTELEMETRY SYSTEMS

Michael R. Neuman and Ante Santic*

Departments of Obstetrics and Gynecology
and Biomedical Engineering
Cleveland Metropolitan General Hospital
Case Western Reserve University
3395 Scranton Road
Cleveland, Ohio 44109
*Department of Electrical Engineering
University of Zagreb
Unska 17, Zagreb 41000 Yugoslavia

INTRODUCTION

Telemetry is a process of making a measurement at a distance from the source. Biotelemetry is a subfield of biomedical instrumentation concerned with making biomedical measurements remotely from the signal source. Most people who make use of biotelemetry consider it to be limited to wireless methods of signal transmission, but the International Society on Biotelemetry includes methods of transmitting measured information over wires for long distances and storing information for retrieval at another location in the field of biotelemetry as well. Thus, there are several different ways that biomedical measurements can be telemetered to receiving sites. Table I lists the most common of these.

In active wireless telemetry systems such as radio, the transmitter generates the carrier signal and it must have its own power supply. Passive telemetry transmitters utilize energy beamed to the telemetry device from a remote power source. Some of this energy is converted into a carrier signal, or the load perceived by the external power source is varied to transmit the measured information. Just about every measurement made using electronic systems would fall in the category of telemetry if we use the strict definition, since the signal from the sensor making the measurement is carried by wires to another location where the result of the measurement is displayed. Instead, wired telemetry systems are considered to be special systems which transmit biomedical measurements over long distances using some sort of carrier signal on a directly connected network such as the telephone system. Signals can also be transmitted over the power lines but usually not over as long a distance or with as much fidelity as can be done using the telephone network. In the case of storage telemetry, signals are placed in a memory device which is then transported to the receiving site where the signal is retrieved at a later time. This type of ambulatory monitoring is not always considered to be biotelemetry, and

TABLE 1. Types of biotelemetry systems

Radio
   Very low frequency through microwave
      electromagnetic radiation
Light
   Visible
   Infrared
Sonic
   Audible
   Ultrasound
Passive
   Coupled coils (inductance)
   Variable load
Wired
   Telephone carrier
   Power line carrier
Storage
   Portable, miniature magnetic recorders
   Semiconductor memory devices

applications of it will be reported elsewhere in this volume. A basic biotelemetry system consists of three major components, the transmitter, the communications medium and the receiver. The transmitter takes the information that is gained from the biologic measurement and places it on another signal known as the carrier by the process of carrier modulation. The carrier is able to be propagated through the communications medium, and it can be sensed at a receiver. The receiver then separates the information from the carrier and provides this information in a form suitable for its interpretation.

APPLICATIONS OF BIOTELEMETRY

Biotelemetry systems have been used as a part of instrumentation systems employed in various biological, basic medical science and clinical medicine applications.

Clinical medicine uses of biotelemetry have been reported since the middle of this century. A major application has been in the area of remote patient monitoring with the patient either confined to bed or ambulatory over a limited area. This monitoring has generally been by wireless systems, although the use of patient monitors in patients' homes has increased the use of wired and storage telemetry in clinical care. Most patient monitoring is carried out using noninvasive instrumentation, that is sensors located on the skin surface, and external telemetry devices. Telemetry systems which incorporate indwelling or implantable transmitters have also been developed and applied. In the former case, the transmitters are structured such that they can fit in natural body cavities such as the urinary bladder, the intestinal tract, vagina, etc. Implantable transmitters, on the other hand, reside in cavities that are surgically produced. Examples of these types of devices include transmitters implanted in the chest or abdomen to monitor various hemodynamic variables in experimental animals (11), subcutaneous intracranial pressure monitoring transmitters (3) and transmitters implanted in the bladder to monitor intravesical pressure (2).

Other more recent applications of biotelemetry in medicine include the use of a telemetry link to communicate with an implantable device. Coupled inductance coil telemetry systems are used for reprogramming implanted cardiac pacemakers (4). Telestimulation is a special case where biotelemetry is used to control an implantable electrical stimulator used in functional neurologic stimulation systems (13). In some cases, the stimulator consists of a passive receiver that converts the transmitted signal into the actual stimulus pulse while in others the signal is used just to control an implanted stimulator. Telemetry systems have been employed in health care facilities to help locate ambulatory patients and to detect when they stray from the area to which they are limited (15). This same technique has been employed to monitor low security prisoners who are confined to home.

Non-Medical Human Studies

Biotelemetry is a valuable tool in studying human activities because measurements can be made without limiting the mobility or the activities of the subject. Thus, telemetry devices have been useful in sports medicine for studying the behavior of athletes and in making measurements that can help them to improve their performance (14). Miniature wireless devices can be worn by athletes and measure various biomechanical and/or physiologic factors that can be sent to a remote receiver where the particular activity can be evaluated. The information can be then returned to the athlete to help optimize his or her performance. The same approach can be taken in studying human performance in the workplace (6). Ergonomic performance of factory workers, heavy machinery operators and office workers can be studied to optimize their efficiency and to ascertain the effects of environmental conditions on their work.

Other Applications

Telemetry is a useful tool in non-human biological applications as well. The application of telemetry to study wildlife behavior and physiology has been important in understanding animals on land, in the air and in the sea (1). Not only can the locations of groups of animals be tracked for extended periods of time, but it is also possible to monitor bodily functions such as heart rate, activity, temperature, etc. Today, it is even possible to track and monitor wild animals over an entire continent using navigation satellites (14).

Even more extensive physiological monitoring of animals can be carried out in the laboratory or other confined spaces using biotelemetry. External and implantable systems that can be worn by an experimental animal can be used to monitor various physiologic functions in the unrestrained animal. Agriculture has also benefited from the use of biotelemetry. Times of ovulation and estrus can be identified in farm animals for artificial insemination, animals can be identified through telemetry devices and pregnant animals can be confined and observed when they go into labor to minimize complications.

ADVANTAGES AND LIMITATIONS OF BIOTELEMETRY

The principal advantage of biotelemetry over other measurement methods is that it is possible to make remote observations. Therefore much of the measurement process can be separated from the organism being studied. This means that it is possible to observe the subject in a more natural state. For example, a group of animals may behave differently when an observer is in the same room with them than they would if the observer was not present. A patient whose blood pressure is monitored over a telephone line from home may have lower, more representational values in this environment compared to the anxiety-laden environment of a physician's office.

Biotelemetry allows subjects to have greater mobility than would be possible with direct connection to the instrumentation. Patients who do not feel tethered to a clinical monitor can feel better about their medical progress than those who must have the direct connection to the instrument. The advantage of free ranging animal studies over those where the animal is tethered is obvious. The use of telemetry for ambulatory monitoring allows patients to be watched without undue constraints on their activities.

There are also technical advantages to the use of biotelemetry. Since telemetry transmitters have their own power source, they can be completely isolated from the electrical power mains and from other sources of electrical fields. This means that it is not necessary to "ground" the subject and that interference from these sources can be smaller than seen with wired systems. Since common mode signals, those signals common to both inputs of a telemetry device, are not a problem with an isolated transmitter, the common mode rejection ratio can be very high for biotelemetry systems. This helps to keep sources of external interference to a minimum.

There are also limitations associated with the application of biotelemetry. Biotelemetry systems are generally more complex than the equivalent direct-wired instrumentation systems, and this means that they can be more difficult to use. They are often more expensive. Although highly reliable telemetry systems can be developed, there are additional limitations to reliability that are not seen in direct wire systems. In wireless systems, there may be small regions within the range of the telemetry where accurate transmission is not possible due to constraints of the communications medium. Noise can be introduced into the telemetry system that would not be present in a direct wire connection. Self-contained power sources are necessary for telemetry transmitters except those in passive systems. Often, in miniature telemetry devices, the power source takes up as much or more volume and mass as the actual telemetry electronic circuit.

Finally, some forms of wireless telemetry are regulated by the governments of the countries in which they are applied. In some countries, this is limited to longer range, higher power radio systems, while in others, this applies to all forms of wireless transmission regardless of power.

TELEMETRY SYSTEMS

The actual configuration of a telemetry system is dependent upon the variables being measured and how the system is applied. Most telemetry systems have a similar general configuration as shown in Figure 1. The transmitter is located at the biologic system being measured and is made up of several functional blocks. The measurements of the various biologic variables are carried out by sensors that convert these variables into electrical signals. These signals usually must be processed before they can be transmitted over the telemetry link. The signal processor associated with each sensor can carry out functions such as amplification, filtering, digitization, threshold detection or compression. A single channel telemetry system has only one sensor and signal processor block while multiple channel transmitters have a sensor and signal processor for each channel. The output of the signal processor can go directly to the carrier

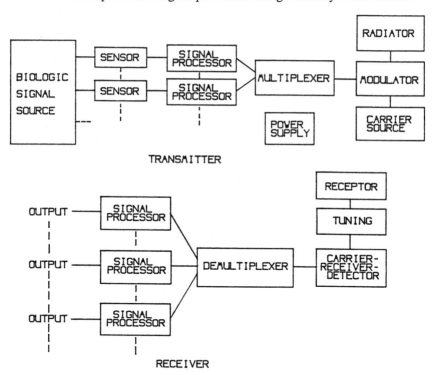

FIG. 1. General telemetry system block diagram.

modulator block in single channel systems, while multiple channel systems must have a multiplexer block to combine the individual signals in some known way before they are applied to the carrier. The multiplexer can be simply a selector switch which samples each signal (time division multiplexing), or it can place each signal on its own subcarrier and add all the subcarriers together so that their signals do not overlap and they can be separated at the receiver (frequency division multiplexing). A subcarrier is sometimes used even with a single channel telemetry system because it can improve signal transmission and baseline stability especially over a noisy communications medium.

The output from either the signal processor in single channel systems or the multiplexer in multichannel systems is then fed to a modulator. This takes the carrier signal necessary for transmission over the communications medium that was generated by the carrier source and varies it in a known way with respect to the signal(s). The two most common types of modulation are amplitude modulation (AM) and frequency modulation (FM). In the former case, the amplitude of the carrier signal is varied according to the amplitude of the signal. For example, amplitude modulation of a carrier by an electrocardiographic signal would mean that the carrier at the output of the modulator would be strongest during the QRS complex and weakest during baseline portions of the waveform.

Frequency modulation utilizes a carrier signal that would have a constant frequency were it not for the modulator. The carrier frequency is varied according to the amplitude of the measured signal by the modulator. Thus, in the example of the electrocardiogram, the frequency of the carrier will be different during the R-wave from what it was during the P-wave.

The modulated carrier wave is introduced into the communications medium by the radiator. In radio telemetry systems, the radiator is the transmitting antenna. This can be as simple as a coil built into the structure of the transmitter itself or it can be an external device such as the whip antenna on a walkie talkie or cellular telephone. In light telemetry systems, the carrier source, modulator and radiator can all be the same component. For example, with an infrared transmitter, infrared light emitting diodes are used to create the infrared carrier, to modulate the intensity of that carrier and to radiate the light in free space.

In an active transmitter system, there must be an internal source of power to operate the various power consuming components of the system. Frequently this consists of an internal electrochemical primary or secondary battery. In some cases it is not possible to have access to the battery to change it when it weakens, and the size constraints forbid using large batteries with long lifetimes. As an alternative, energy can be obtained from photovoltaic sources such as solar cells, time varying magnetic induction from an external power source coil or detection of electromagnetic energy beamed into the transmitter from an external source.

Power sources are crucial for implanted transmitter systems since these generally have to be as small as possible. As stated earlier, the power source can easily take up as much or more space than the actual circuit. Clearly for long-term implantable biotelemetry systems, small, low-mass, high efficiency, long-lasting power sources are needed.

Another major requirement for implantable systems that has not been completely met is a package that can effectively protect the transmitter system from the biologic environment. It must not impede the radiation of the communication signal or consume a major portion of the volume.

Communications Medium

The signal from the transmitter is sent to the receiver over the communications medium. Wireless signals include electromagnetic radiation in the form of radio waves or light and pressure waves in a fluid medium such as sound or ultrasound. Media can also consist of wire links or storage devices. The transmitter determines how the carrier is sent through the communications medium. It is usually desirable in wireless systems that the signal be broadcast isotropically. This often is difficult to achieve with radio communication, due to the inherent directionality of the transmitting antenna. Infrared telemetry systems also have this problem because most infrared light emitting diodes emit infrared energy over a relatively narrow solid angle. Thus, for isotropic coverage, multiple infrared radiators each aimed in a different direction are required. Even so, shadows in the room in which the telemetry system is used can create a problem. Fortunately, this is not a serious problem if the walls and ceiling of the room consist of materials that reflect infrared energy. Often one can get nearly isotropic coverage in a room the size of a hospital room due to multiple reflections from these surfaces.

Receiving System

The receiving system collects the carrier signal from the communications medium. In radio systems, this is done by the receiving antenna, and various types of photodetectors are used for telemetry systems that communicate using light. Signals from this carrier receptor go to the carrier receiver circuit where they are detected (demodulated) to obtain the original signal in the case of single channel systems and the multiplexed signal for multiple channel devices. In this latter case, the original signals must be recovered by a process known as demultiplexing. Each individual signal is identified and sent through a signal processor to its appropriate output. Signal processors carry out similar functions to what they did in the transmitter system.

Receivers require power as do the transmitters. Frequently, the receiver is located at a fixed site and can receive its power from a central source such as the power mains or the power system of a vehicle. Only remote, miniature, portable receiving equipment experience the same power supply problems as do the transmitters.

When multiple telemetry systems are used to send signals over the same communications medium, problems can occur if the signal from one system interferes with that of another. This problem can be minimized by using different carriers for different systems. This is easily achieved with radio telemetry because the wave length of the carrier can be different for each telemetry system. It is then possible to select the desired carrier at the receiver by means of tuning. Although the available spectrum is much broader for optical telemetry systems, unfortunately only very little of the spectrum can be practically utilized due to the limited wavelengths of infrared and visible light emitting diodes. Therefore, there are only a few practical communication channels, and creative approaches need to be developed to separate the signals from multiple transmitters operating on the same communications channel. One approach to this is to use low duty cycle pulses and for each transmitter to transmit pulses with their own particular identification code (10). One can also have two-way communication systems where a transmitter waits to be interrogated by a signal transmitted from the receiver before it responds (5). Although this system is complex, it ensures that only one transmitter is broadcasting at a time.

EXAMPLES OF BIOTELEMETRY SYSTEMS

Biotelemetry systems can be realized in many different ways, and each application helps to define the telemetry systems that are most appropriate for it. Two examples of telemetry systems developed by the authors are briefly presented on the following pages. Additional information can be obtained from the references.

Dual Channel Telemetry Systems for Fetal Cardiotocography

Fetal heart rate and uterine contractions are routinely monitored during labor in the care of the high risk obstetrical patient. Commercially available monitoring equipment involves an electronic monitor that is located near the patient. It provides continuous recordings of these variables. Sensors placed on the mother and fetus are connected to the monitor by cables which can be inconvenient and impede the rapid transport of the patient to the delivery room.

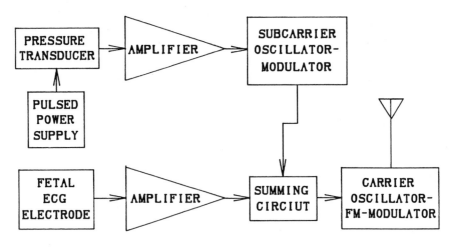

FIG. 2. Fetal cardiotocogram two-channel transmitter.

A block diagram of the two-channel transmitter is shown in Figure 2. The fetal electrocardiogram is obtained from a fetal scalp electrode, and the signal is amplified. It contains frequency components ranging from about 0.1 to 150 Hz. Uterine contractions are sensed by a pressure transducer in the uterine cavity. The signals are amplified and used to frequency modulate a 3 kHz subcarrier oscillator. The pressure transducer used was a silicon piezoresistive strain gauge bridge which consumed a relatively large amount of power when operated continuously. Since uterine pressure varies slowly over time, it is not necessary to operate this sensor continuously. For this reason, a switch pulsed the pressure transducer power supply at the subcarrier frequency. This low duty cycle pulse allowed the sensor to sample the intrauterine pressure while conserving energy from the limited battery power supply.

The relatively low frequency electrocardiogram signal and the uterine contraction signal centered around the subcarrier frequency were added together in the summing circuit and used to frequency modulate a 110 MHz carrier oscillator that produced the radio frequency carrier signal. The oscillator coil served as the antenna in a hybrid microelectronic version of the transmitter (7), and a radio frequency amplifier was interspersed between the carrier oscillator and the coil antenna in a miniature, discrete component version of the transmitter (9). The microelectronic version of the transmitter contained its own miniature 1.35 V battery and was sufficiently small to be placed intravaginally so that there were no external connections between the patient and the receiving system. The discrete component version was larger and was strapped to the patient's leg in place of the conventional monitor's leg plate.

The receiving system was similar to that shown in Figure 1. A conventional FM receiver tuned to the carrier frequency picked up the signal and provided the sum of the subcarrier and the fetal ECG at its output. The demultiplexer which separated these signals consisted of a low pass filter to extract the fetal ECG and a band pass filter centered at the subcarrier frequency to extract the uterine contraction subcarrier. The subcarrier was demodulated, and the fetal ECG and uterine contractions were then fed to their respective inputs of a conventional fetal monitor. The system was evaluated at several centers and found to give equivalent information to that obtained by conventional direct-wired fetal monitoring (8).

Low Power Single Channel Infrared Telemetry System

A simple, single channel telemetry system which can be operated reliably over the limited range of a room using infrared radiation is illustrated in Figure 3. The transmitter produces a series of very low-duty cycle pulses of near infrared light from an array of infrared emitting diodes. Pulses are generated by an oscillator/modulator circuit consisting of a voltage-to-frequency converter that is adjusted to give pulses with durations that are much less than their interval. These electrical pulses need only to be amplified to drive the infrared emitting diodes. Input signals for the telemetry system can come from one of several sources including a variable resistance sensor such as a thermistor for measuring temperature, a variable voltage output sensor such as a microphone, or biopotential electrodes such as used for obtaining the electrocardiogram. Signals from these sensors are processed and used to modulate the frequency of the train of low-duty cycle infrared pulses.

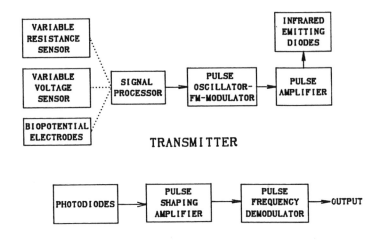

TRANSMITTER

RECEIVER

FIG. 3. Single-channel infrared pulse frequency modulated telemetry system

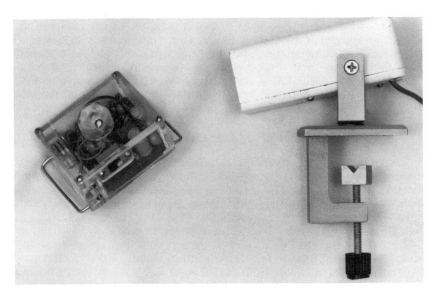

FIG. 4. Infrared telemetry system with transmitter on left and receiver on right.

The receiver is much simpler than the equivalent radio frequency circuit. The infrared receptor function is carried out by one or more photodiodes. The signals are amplified and formed into sharp pulses that are then fed to the pulse frequency demodulator to obtain the original signal. An infrared system such as this can operate reliably in a closed environment such as a hospital room where multiple reflections of the infrared signal from the walls and ceiling will give a nearly isotropic radiation pattern. By using low-duty cycle pulses in the range of from 1 to 10 s, much lower power than is usually required for infrared telemetry systems is needed (10).

The system has been employed in our laboratory for remote continuous monitoring of neonatal heart rate (12). An example of a transmitter realized in miniature, discrete component form is shown in Figure 4 with a receiver module containing four photodiodes. The receiver diodes are recessed in a nonreflective housing so that there is minimal interference from stray infrared radiation in the room.

SUMMARY

Biotelemetry offers the opportunity to make physiologic measurements under more natural conditions and thereby make these measurements more representative of the system under study. New technologies offer smaller size, lower power, and more reliable systems. New communications channels in addition to traditional radio frequency electromagnetic fields are opening new opportunities for biotelemetry. These include infrared radiation, ultrasound, use of the telephone network and storage devices. Telemetry offers many opportunities for more efficacious ambulatory monitoring in clinical care facilities, the home and the workplace.

ACKNOWLEDGEMENT

Supported in part by NIH Grant Nos. M01 RR00210-25 and 2P41RR02024-04.

REFERENCES

1. Amlaner, C.J. and MacDonald, D.W. (1980): *A Handbook on Biotelemetry and Radio Tracking*, Pergamon, Oxford.

2. Delaere, K.P.J., Kimmich, H.P., van Waalwijk, E.S.C., and Debruyne, F.M.J. (1984): In: *Biotelemetry VIII*, edited by H.P. Kimmich and H.J. Klewe, pp. 313-318. ISOB, Nijmegen.

3. Fryer, T.P., Corbin, S.D., Silverberg, G.D., Schmidt, E.V. and Ream, A.K. (1978): *Biotelemetry and Patient Monitoring*, 5:88-112.

4. Gold, R.D. (1984): *Medical Instrumentation*, 18:15-21.

5. Kimmich, H.P. (1975): *Biotelemetry*, 2:207-255.

6. Meyer, H. and Schrader, J. (1982): *Zentralbl. Arbeitsmed. Arbeitsschut. Prophyl. Ergonomie*, 32:434-437.

7. Neuman, M.R., Picconnatto, J. and Roux, J.F. (1970): *Gynecol. Invest.*, 1:92.

8. Neuman, M.R., Roux, J.F., Patrick, J.E., Munro, M.G., Cudmore, D.W., Owen, S.M., Angel, E., Fox, H.E. and Pessel, D. (1979): *Obstet. & Gynecol.*, 54:249-254.

9. Neuman, M.R. and O'Connor, E. (1980): *Biotelemetry and Patient Monitoring*, 7:104-121.

10. Neuman, M.R. and Santic, A. (1984): In: *Medical Telemetry, European Economic Community Report EUR 9158 EN*, edited by H.P. Kimmich and M. Bornhausen, pp. 251-275.

11. Rader, R., Meehan, J. and Henriksen, J. (1973): *IEEE Trans. on Biomed. Engrg.*, BME-20:37-43.

12. Santic, A. and Neuman, M.R. (1984): In: *Biotelemetry VIII*, edited by H.P. Kimmich and H.-J. Klewe, pp.147-150. ISOB, Nijmegen.

13. Smith, B., Peckham, P.H., Keith, M.W. and Roscoe, D.D. (1987): *IEEE Trans. on Biomed. Engrg.*, 34:499-508.

14. Soma, M., Nakamura, A. and Tsutsumi, M. (1987): In: *Biotelemetry IX*, edited by H.P. Kimmich and M.R. Neuman, pp. 319-322. ISOB, Braunschweig.

15. Vos, J.A.J. (1987): In: *Biotelemetry IX*, edited by H.P. Kimmich and M.R. Neuman, pp. 259-264. ISOB, Braunschweig.

16. Weller, C. (1978): In: *Biotelemetry IV*, edited by H.-J. Klewe and H.P. Kimmich, pp. 227-230. ISOB, Braunschweig.

Medical Monitoring in the Home and Work Environment,
edited by Laughton E. Miles and Roger J. Broughton.
Raven Press, New York © 1990.

ACTIVE REMOTE PHYSIOLOGICAL MONITORING USING MICROWAVES

Kun-Mu Chen

Department of Electrical Engineering
Michigan State University
East Lansing, Michigan 48824

INTRODUCTION

Electromagnetic (EM) radiation has been applied in various medical fields including diathermy treatments for relief of muscle spasms and reduction of tissue inflammations, EM hyperthermia treatments for tumors, and nuclear magnetic resonance (NMR) imaging. Recently, EM radiation has found another application in remote and noninvasive sensing of body movements associated with vascular and respiratory systems.

During the last decade, microwave radiation of between 2.5 GHz and 30 GHz has been utilized to detect the heart and respiratory movements (2,5,6). Using the Doppler effect, microwaves have also been employed to investigate the wall properties and pressure pulse characteristics at a variety of arterial sites (4,9). Some investigators have also used the transmission and reflection properties of microwaves at the chest to detect pulmonary diseases [6]. However, all these investigations and applications have been conducted at a short distance of a few centimeters from the human subject.

The feasibility of the remote physiological sensing using microwave radiation a!t a distance of a meter to a hundred meters from the human subject was demonstrated only recently (1,8). In this paper, we will describe two microwave life-detection systems (1) developed by our group at Michigan State University. The first system is an X-band (10 GHz) microwave life-detection system which is capable of detecting the breathing and heartbeats of a human subject lying on the ground at a distance of 30 meters or sitting behind a wall of about 6 inches thick. The second system is a L-band (2 GHz) microwave life-detection system which was specially designed for detecting the body movements, including the breathing and heartbeats, of human subjects located behind a very thick wall (up to a meter thick). Although these system were originally developed for military and security purposes, they should find some medical applications, especially in the remote physiological sensing area.

The principle on which the systems can be developed is straightforward. We illuminate the subject with a low-intensity (much lower than the safety standard) microwave beam. The small amplitude body movements associated with heartbeat and breathing of the human subject will modulate the backscattered wave, producing a signal from which information of the heart and breathing rates can be extracted using phase detection in the microwave receiving system.

PHYSICAL PRINCIPLES

Some relevant physical principles involved in a physiological sensing system using microwaves are discussed here.

Doppler Effect and Phase Modulation of Microwave Signals

It is well known that when a beam of EM wave is aimed at a moving target, the reflected EM wave form the target will display a frequency shift due to the Doppler effect. The frequency shift is given approximately by

$$\Delta f = f(v/c)$$

where Δf is the frequency shift, f is the frequency of EM wave, v is the velocity of the target relative to the EM wave source, and c is the velocity of light.

The backscattered EM wave can be expressed approximately as

$$E_s = A \cos [2\pi f(1\pm v/c)t] \qquad (1)$$

where the positive (negative) sign is used when the target moves toward (away from) the EM source. For example, a police radar gun using a 10 GHz microwave beam can detect a frequency shift of about 1 KHz in the reflected wave from a car traveling at a speed of 60 miles per hour. This frequency shift is sufficiently large to be measured by a conventional frequency detection system such as a heterodyne system.

When an EM wave is to be used to detect a very slow movement of a target, such as the body movement associated with heartbeat and breathing, it is impractical to use the Doppler effect, because the frequency shift is extremely small due to an extremely small value of (v/c). For this type of application, it is much more efficient to measure the phase shift in the reflected wave from the slowing moving target. Our microwave life-detection system is based on the detection of the phase modulation in the reflected wave from the human body.

When a microwave beam is incident upon a slowly moving target, the phase angle of the reflected wave will be modulated (or perturbed) by the target's movement. Mathematically, the reflected wave can be expressed as

$$E_s = A(t) \cos (2\pi ft + \Delta\phi u(t)) \qquad (2)$$

where $\Delta\phi$ is the magnitude of the phase shift and $u(t)$ is a time function which describes the phase variation due to the target's movement. $A(t)$ is the amplitude of the reflected wave and it may also be a function of time due to the target's movement. If a microwave beam is used to detect the body movement due to heartbeat and breathing, the phase shift term $(\Delta\phi u(t))$, is very small compared with the leading term $(2\pi ft)$. However, with a phase detection device, such as our microwave life-detection system, this small phase shift can be accurately measured.

A rough relation between the phase shift and the corresponding frequency shift can be given by

$$\Delta f = \frac{\Delta\phi}{2\pi} \frac{\partial u(t)}{\partial t}$$

This relation implies that for body movement due to the heartbeat of 1 Hz, the fundamental frequency shift in the reflected wave of 10 GHz is in the order of 1 Hz, because both $(\partial u(t) / \partial t)$ and $(\Delta\phi/2\pi)$ terms are in the order of unity. Obviously, it will be extremely difficult to detect a frequency shift of 1 Hz in a microwave signal of 10 GHz.

Mathematical Formulation of the Phase Modulation of a Reflected EM wave from a Moving Target

To understand how the phase angle of the reflected EM wave is perturbed by the slow movement of the human body, we will analyze the backscattered EM wave from the body when it is illuminated by a plane EM wave. To simplify the problem we model the body as a sphere of complex permittivity. The backscattered field from the sphere is well known (3). Using the coordinate system shown in Fig. 1, the expression for the backscattered electric field may be constructed as

$$\vec{E}_{BS} = \hat{x}\,\frac{-E_0}{2k_0 r}\sum_{n=1}^{\infty} j^n(2n+1)\,[-d_n\hat{H}_n^{(2)}(K_0 r) + je_n\hat{H}_n^{(2)\prime}(K_0 r)] \quad (3)$$

where

$$d_n = \frac{\sqrt{\epsilon_r}\,\hat{J}_n'(ka)\,\hat{J}_n(k_0 a) - \hat{J}_n'(k_0 a)\,\hat{J}_n(ka)}{\hat{H}_n^{(2)\prime}(k_0 a)\,\hat{J}_n(ka) - \sqrt{\epsilon_r}\,\hat{J}_n'(ka)\,\hat{H}_n^{(2)}(K_0 a)} \quad (4)$$

$$e_n = \frac{\hat{J}_n(k_0 a)\,\hat{J}_n'(ka) - \sqrt{\epsilon_r}\,\hat{J}_n'(k_0 a)\,\hat{J}_n(ka)}{\sqrt{\epsilon_r}\,\hat{H}_n^{(2)\prime}(k_0 a)\,\hat{J}_n(ka) - \hat{H}_n^{(2)}(k_0 a)\hat{J}_n'(ka)} \quad (5)$$

$$\hat{J}_n(x) = \sqrt{\frac{\pi x}{2}} \; J_{n+1/2}(x) \tag{6}$$

$$\hat{H}_n^{(2)}(x) = \sqrt{\frac{\pi x}{2}} \; H_{n+1/2}^{(2)}(x). \tag{7}$$

ϵ_r is the complex permittivity of the sphere, a is its radius, k and k_0 represent wavenumbers inside and outside the sphere, respectively, and usual notations for Bessel functions and their derivatives are employed. E_0 is the amplitude of the incident plane wave and $\hat{x}$ is the unit vector along the x axis.

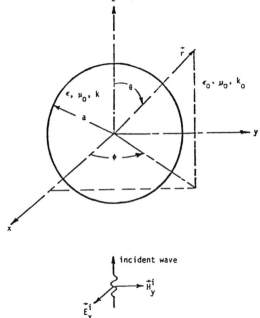

FIG. 1. A conducting sphere illuminated by an incident EM wave.

The phase and the square of the magnitude of the backscattered electric field $\vec{E}_{BS}$ from a sphere of relatively permittivity 39.9 and conductivity 10.3 S/m are depicted in Fig. 2 as functions of the radius multiplied by the wavenumber k_0 of the medium. The frequency of the microwave radiation is assumed to be 10 HGz, and the sphere is situated 30.48 m (100 ft) from the transceiver. Breathing and heartbeat produce small vibrations of the spherical surface due to changes in its radius. From Fig. 2, we conclude that these vibrations will produce a linear change in the phase and a relatively smaller linear change in the amplitude squared of the

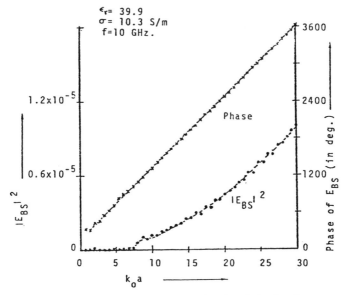

FIG. 2. Phase and square of the magnitude of the back scattered field E_{BS} from a sphere as a function of $k_o a$ at 10 GHz at a distance of 30.48 m.

backscattered field. Similar results were obtained when the body was modeled as an infinitely long cylinder of complex permittivity, illuminated by a TM-polarized plane EM wave.

These simplified models show that there will be, in general, amplitude as well as phase modulation of the incident wave as it is backscattered by the body. However, since the phase variation is more linear and it is easier to detect the phase variation from the viewpoint of the signal/noise ratio, we used the phase modulation of the backscattered wave to find the vibrations of the body surface caused by the heartbeat and breathing.

AN X-BAND MICROWAVE LIFE-DETECTION SYSTEM

In this section, the circuit diagram and operation principle of an X-band (10 GHz) microwave life-detection system, developed by our group, will be described. Typical results on the measurement of heart and breathing signals will also be given.

Circuit Diagram and Operation Principle

The schematic diagram of the X-band life-detection system is shown in Fig. 3. A phase-locked oscillator at 10 GHz produces a stable output of about 20 mW. This output is amplified by a low-noise microwave amplifier to an power level of about 200 mW. The output of the amplifier is fed through a 6 dB directional coupler, a variable attenuator, a circulator, and then to a horn antenna. The 6 dB directional coupler branches out 1/4 of the amplified output to provide a reference signal for clutter cancellation

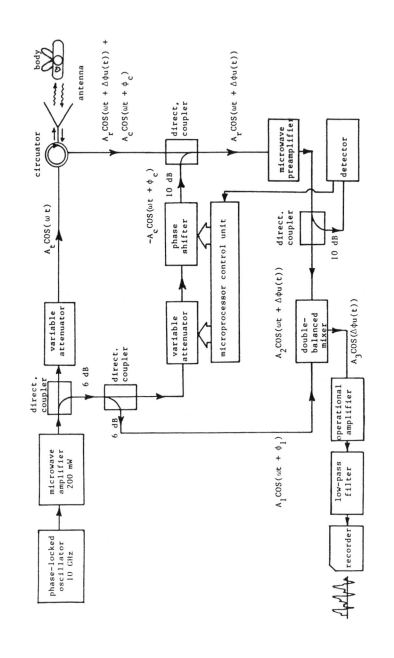

FIG. 3. Circuit diagram of the microwave life-detection system.

and another reference signal for the mixer. The variable attenuator controls the power level of the microwave signal to be radiated by the antenna. Usually, the radiated power is kept at a level of about 10-20 mW. The horn antenna radiates a microwave beam of about 15° beam-width aimed at the human subjects to be monitored. The signal received by the antenna consists of a large clutter and a weak return signal scattered from the body. To be able to detect the weak signal modulated by the body movement, the large background clutter needs to be cancelled. This is accomplished by an automatic clutter cancellation circuit which consists of a variable phase-shifter, a variable attenuator and a microprocessor unit which digitally controls the former two components. This automatic clutter cancellation circuit provides an optimal reference signal which is mixed with the received signal by the antenna in a 10dB directional coupler for the purpose of cancelling the clutter. The output of the 10 dB directional coupler now contains mainly the weak scattered signal from the body. This body scattered signal is a 10GHz CW microwave modulated by breathing and heartbeat. This signal is then amplified by a low-noise microwave preamplifier (30 dB) and then mixed with another reference signal in a double-balanced mixer. Between the microwave preamplifier and the double-balanced mixer, a 10 dB directional coupler is inserted to take out a small portion of the amplified signal for providing an input to the microprocessor unit which controls the phase-shifter and the attenuator. The optimal settings for the phase-shifter and the attenuator are determined by this input to the microprocessor unit. The mixing of the amplified, bodyscattered signal and a reference signal (7-10 mW) in the double-balanced mixer produced low-frequency signals resulting from motion due to breathing and heart motion within the body. This output from the mixer is amplified by an operational amplifier and then passed through a low-pass filter (4 Hz cutoff) before reaching a recorder.

Measured Heart and Breathing Signals

Recordings of the heart and breathing signals of several persons were taken under different conditions. However, only a few of them are presented here for illustration. Fig. 4 shows the measured heart and breathing signals of a human subject lying on the ground at a distance of 30 m with a 4.5 mW, 10 GHz microwave beam aimed at him. The top graph in Fig. 4 shows the breathing signal superimposed upon the heart signal when the human subject was lying on the ground in a face-up position with the body perpendicular to the microwave beam. The middle graph in Fig. 4 shows only the heart signal when the subject was holding his breath. The bottom graph in Fig. 4 shows the background noise. The results of Fig. 4 indicate satisfactory performance of the system in detecting the heart and breathing signals of human subject lying on the ground at a distance of 30 m or farther.

We have also studied the effect of clothing on the system performance by repeating the experiment with different clothing on the subject, e.g., up to four layers of very thick jackets. The effect of the clothing over the sensitivity of the system was found to be insignificant. Furthermore, the polarization effect of the microwave signal on the system performance was also investigated. When circular, linear-vertical, and linear-horizontal

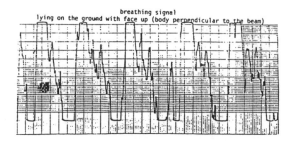

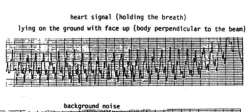

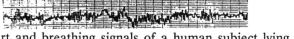

FIG 4. Heart and breathing signals of a human subject lying on the ground at a distance of 30 m measured with a 4.5 mW, 10 GHz microwave beam.

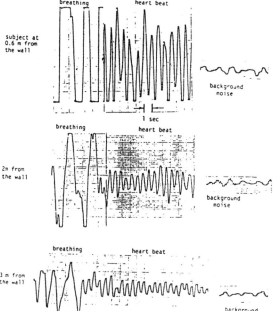

FIG. 5. Measured breathing and heart signals from a human subject sitting behind a cinder block wall (15.24 cm thick) at various distances. The antenna was located on the other side of the wall, and it radiated at a power of about 20 mW at 10 GHz.

polarization were employed, the system sensitivity was found to be of the same order in all three cases.

We have also used this system to detect the heart and breathing signals of a human subject located behind a barrier with success. Fig. 5 shows the measured heart and breathing signals of a human subject sitting behind a dry 15.24 cm (6 in) cinder block wall at a distance of 0.6, 2, or 3 m. The antenna was placed closed to the other side of the wall and energized to radiate 20 mW at 10 GHz. It is observed from Fig. 5 that the heart and breathing signals were clearly detected at all three distances. The background noise in each case is also shown in the figure. The results of Fig. 5 indicate that the microwave beam can penetrate the wall and a satisfactory detection of the heart and breathing signals of human subjects behind the wall is possible. We have repeated the experiment by moving both the system and the human subject away from the wall. It was found that the system could perform satisfactorily even when the human subject was 5 m away from the wall while the antenna on the other side was about 3 m from the wall. If the antenna was moved further from the wall, system performance was affected by movement of the system operator.

This life-detection system can be easily modified to produce a device for monitoring the breathing and heartbeat of a patient in a clinic. To conduct such an experiment, a metallic wire-mesh chamber with the dimensions of 2.5 x 1 x 0.8 m was constructed as shown in Fig. 6. The antenna of the system was replaced by an open-ended waveguide which was mounted on a wall of the chamber. A microwave signal of 100 uW at 10 GHz was radiated into the chamber through the waveguide. A human subject was lying inside the chamber in various positions, face up, or lying on his right or left shoulder. The measured heart and breathing signals of the subject lying in these three positions are shown in Fig. 6. It is observed that a clear detection of the heart and breathing signals can be achieved. It is noted that since the microwave field is confined inside a metallic chamber and the environmental noise is minimal, only very low power microwave radiation is needed for this purpose.

AN L-BAND MICROWAVE LIFE-DETECTION SYSTEM

As described in the preceding section, the X-band microwave life-detection system can be used to detect breathing and heartbeat of a human subject located behind a brick wall of about 15 cm. However, if the wall became thicker, the detection became difficult with the X-band system. An L-band (2 GHz) system was specially designed for the purpose of detecting breathing and heartbeat of a human subject who was located behind a very thick wall or buried under a thick layer of rubble.

The L-band system has the essentially same circuit arrangement as that of the X-band system, with the exception that all the components are larger because of the lower operation frequency. Since the L-band system operates at a much lower frequency than that of the X-band system, its microwave beam is more penetrating.

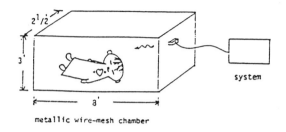

metallic wire-mesh chamber

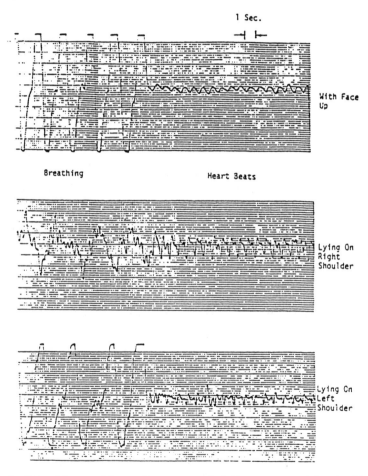

FIG. 6. Breathing and heart beats recorded for a person lying inside a metallic wire-mesh chamber with dimensions 2.5 x 1.0 x 0.8 m. The body was parallel to the radiation beam, with the head away from the antenna. Transmitted power was about 100 uW.

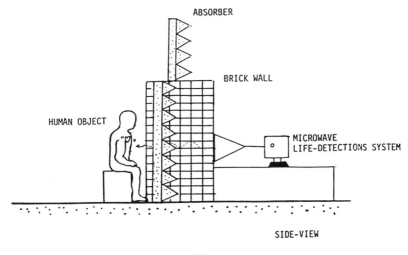

(a)

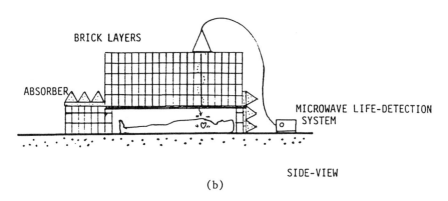

(b)

FIG. 7. Experimental setups for the measurement of heart and breathing signals of a human subject located behind or under a thick layer of bricks using the L-band (2 GHz) microwave life-detection system.

2-GHz Life-Detection System

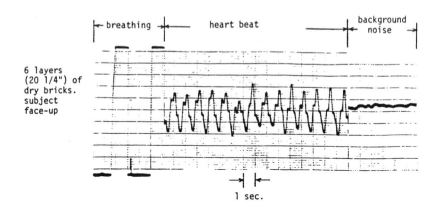

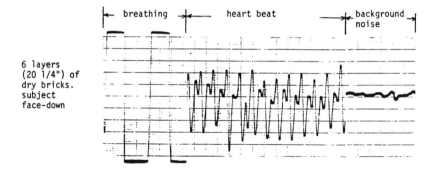

FIG. 8. Heart and breathing signals of a human subject, lying with face-up or face-down position under 6 layers of bricks, measured by the 2-GHz life- detection system.

To test the performance of the L-band life-detection system, two experimental setups depicted in Fig. 7 have been used. The first setup shown in Fig. 7a consisted of a brick wall (1 m wide and 1.4 m high) of various thicknesses lined with microwave absorbers along the edge. A human subject sat behind the brick wall within a distance of 0.3 to 0.6 m. The antenna of the life-detection system was placed close to the other side of the brick wall. The second setup shown in Fig. 7b simulated a situation where a human subject was trapped under a thick layer of rubble. In this setup, various layers of bricks were laid on a wooden frame which formed a cavity for a human subject to lie down in it. Microwave absorbers were used to line the sides of this structure to prevent the microwave scattering through the sides of the brick structure. The antenna of the life-detection system was placed on the top of the brick structure aiming at the human subject under the bricks.

Typical measured results on the heart and breathing signals of a human subject behind or under a thick layer of barrier are shown in Fig. 8. This figure shows the heart and breathing signals of a human subject lying with face-up or face-down position under six layers (52 cm) of dry bricks measured by the 2-HGz life-detection system. In these recorded graphs, the breathing signal, the heart signal (the subject holding his breath) and the background noise were included. It is observed that both the heart and breathing signals were clearly detected. These results demonstrate the feasibility of monitoring the physiological signs of human subjects through a thick barrier with an EM radiation with a frequency in the L-band or lower range.

CONCLUSION

We have shown that it is feasible to use EM radiation, especially in the microwave range, for remote physiological sensing or monitoring. The technology is available for further developments to meet requirements for various medical applications. A low-intensity microwave radiation (much lower than the safety standard) should be employed to minimize the concerns on potential health hazards due to EM radiation.

REFERENCES

1. Chen, K.M., Misra, D., Wang, H., Chuang, H.R. and Postow, E. (1986): An X-band Microwave Life-Detection System, *IEEE Trans. on Biomedical Engineering*, Vol. 33, pp. 697-701.

2. Griffin, D.W. (1978): MW Interferometers for Biological Studies. *Microwave Journal*, Vol. 21, pp. 69-72.

3. Harrington, R.F. (1961): Time Harmonic Electromagnetic Fields. McGraw-Hill Book Co., New York

4. Lee, J.Y. and Lin, J.C. (1985): A Microprocessor-Based Noninvasive Arterial Pulse Wave Analyzer, *IEEE Trans. on Biomedical Engineering*, Vol. 32, pp. 451-455.

5. Lin, J.C. (1986): Microwave Propagation in Biological Dielectric With Application to Cardiopulmonary Interrogation, *Medical Application of Microwave Imaging*, L. Larson and J. Jacobi (Eds.), IEEE Press, N.Y.

6. Lin, L.C., Kiernicki, J., Kiernicki, M. and Wollschlaeger, P.B. (1979): Microwave Apexcardiography, *IEEE Trans. on Microwave Theory and Techniques*, Vol. MTT-27, pp. 618-620.

7. Pedersen, P.C., Johnson, C.C., Durney, H. and Bragg, D.G. (1976): An Investigation of the Use of Microwave Radiation for Pulmonary Diagnostics, *IEEE Trans. on Biomedical Engineering,* Vol. 23, pp. 410-412.

8. Seal, J., Sharpe, S.M., Schaefer, D.J. and Studwell, M.L. (1983): A 35-GHz FM-CW System for Long-Range Detection of Respiration in Battlefield Casualties, *Abstract of the Bioelectromagnetics Society Meeting,* p. 35.

9. Stuchly, S.S., Smith, A., Goldberg, M., Thansandote, A. and Menard, A. (1980): A Microwave Device for Arterial Wall Motion Analysis, *Proc. 33rd Annual Conference Eng. Medical Biology,* 22: 27.

Medical Monitoring in the Home and Work Environment,
edited by Laughton E. Miles and Roger J. Broughton.
Raven Press, New York © 1990.

THE SPHYGMOCHRON FOR BLOOD PRESSURE AND

HEART RATE ASSESSMENT: A CHRONOBIOLOGIC

APPROACH

Franz Halberg, Germaine Cornelissen, *Julia Halberg, **Earl Bakken,
**Patrick Delmore, +Wu Jinyi, Salvador Sanchez de la Pena and Erna
Halberg

Chronobiology Laboratories, University of Minnesota Minneapolis,
Minnesota 55455
*St.Paul-Ramsey Medical Center, St. Paul, Minnesota
**Medtronic Inc., Minneapolis, Minnesota, USA
+Chengdu College of Traditional Chinese Medicine Chengdu, Sichuan,
People's Republic of China

INTRODUCTION

Throughout biology and medicine, time-unspecified measurements have been the rule rather than the exception (2,19), and are associated with a substantial number of false-positive and false-negative conclusions. However, by reference to the chronobiology of blood pressure (9,11,12), a case can be made that improvements in clinical practice and clinical research are possible.

Chronobiology is the study (logos) of time (chronos) in the fabric of life (bios), and is characterized by rhythms, defined as algorithmically validated, with reproducibly recurring dynamics. A broad (mathematical) spectrum of rhythms with different frequencies has been found to characterize every biologic function measured thus far with sufficient density and for sufficient length. Many of these body functions can be self-assessed by methods learned in early public education. Modern technology, however, brings us to the threshold of a revolution in diagnosis and treatment, based on the combination of several emerging technologies, including chronobiologic understanding of the health effect of rhythms; the availability of portable, personal, long-term ambulatory monitors of biologic variables such as blood pressure, the ECG, or EEG, which undergo changes that recur spontaneously and as responses; availability of database systems to acquire and analyze volumes of data obtained from personal monitors availability of statistical procedures to analyze and model the biologic rhythms and from them to devise optimal dosage time patterns for specific individuals; and availability of portable, programmed prosthetic devices to administer therapy, e.g., by physiologic rate-adjusted cardiac pacemakers or drug pumps.

These developments represent an exciting potential for the employment of chronobiologic methods in routine medical screening, diagnosis, prognosis, treatment and, most important, disease prevention (11,12).

Status Quo Concerning Blood Pressure Measurement

The usual way of measuring and interpreting blood pressure is far from acceptable. A diagnosis based on `casual' blood pressure readings can be incorrect. In interpreting blood pressure, a conventional approach seeks to separate values that are too high or too low from acceptable ones, but using arbitrary consensus-based time-unspecified reference standards, such as 140/90 mm Hg (systolic/diastolic), as dividing lines between health and disease. These casual spotchecks are made without taking time into consideration. Since one or a few measurements taken on one or a few occasions can be unusually high or low for the individual being screened, false positive and false negative diagnoses can occur. Some individuals who are treated but do not need treatment pay for such errors in terms of well-being, economics and social stigma; conversely, people who do need treatment are lulled into a false feeling of safety. We therefore suggest using fully automatic ambulatory blood pressure monitors that can be programmed to take measurements at present intervals. These blood pressure measurements are stored on memory cassettes, and these in turn can be directly transferred to computers for data analysis. When automatic monitors are unavailable, multiple measurements covering the day and night are more difficult to obtain, and (if they must be made by a physician or nurse) are too costly. For a long time, self-measurement has been the only way to get sufficient data; for many it remains the only choice. But whether the data are systematically self-measured or automatically monitored, special methods for the interpretation ofthe variations of blood pressure are needed. The computer has given us not only a better way to collect the measurements, even during sleep, when self-measurements are not possible, but also an easy way to analyze and interpret blood pressure variations once they have been measured.

Ambulatory Monitoring and Self-Measurement

Self measurements (2,9,19) taken at intervals of 15 minutes (or eg. beat-to-beat HR) for 48 hours or longer, if need be, automatically (5,15-18,21) or hourly during wakefulness, with only one interruption of midsleep, on only one night, represent an advance. The full gain available from new tools and the concepts of chronobiology is not realized, however, as long as one relies upon the inspection only of a graph for the determination of the peak and the nadir and a comparison with time-unspecified reference standards. By the same token, the computation only of the conventional means (for 24 hours, and separately for the day and night spans) and possibly of standard deviations and coefficients of variation, offers only a partial interpretation of the data at hand. Similar limitations apply to the percentage of values lying above the consensus-derived (yet arbitrarily fixed) limit of 140/90 mm Hg for the systolic and diastolic blood pressure, respectively (16,21).

Chronobiology

Chronobiologic methods (3,4,6,8,10-12) improve the interpretation of both single and serial measurements by the introduction of reference standards that take into account variations with time. Whether one deals with self-measurements or preferably with data obtained by the use of modern automatic ambulatory instrumentation, the computer resolution of rhythms lead to new endpoints and reference standards. Some of these standards are characteristics of rhythms or rhythm parameters. They are defined and shown in Figure 1. In addition to these parametric estimates, based on inferential statistical assumptions, chronobiologists also proceed without any assumptions to directly estimate blood pressure and heart rate excess and/or deficit. This approach, called nonparametric, yields the endpoints shown in the third section of the sphygmochron (Figure 2) for blood pressure, heart rate and the SBP x HR product. The specific endpoints are the percentage of 24 hours associated with excess, timing of the excess, extent of excess during 24 h and ten-year projection of cumulative excess. Chronobiologists then interpret the parametric and nonparametric results according to facts concerning the body's dynamics, a time structure made up of the rhythms that computers resolve for applications in medical practice as well as for research. For instance, the circadian amplitude and/or acrophase, defined in Figure 1, can serve to identify individuals or groups at risk of developing diseases associated with high blood pressure. Computer programs even provide estimates of the uncertainties involved in the assessment of parameters and their comparison between different risk groups (8,10). Moreover, these endpoints work in detecting blood pressure and heart rate behavior that deviates from a personal or peer-group reference standard (11,12), even when the mean values, based on the same extensive data base, fail to separate the same different risk groups.

MATERIALS AND METHODS

The Sphygmochron

There are charts called the short and long form of the `sphygmochron' (sfig * mo * kron) - [See Figures 2 and 3]. *"Sphygm"* denotes a relation to the circulation-a sphygmomanometer is the device used to measure blood pressure-and *"chron"* (from chronos) refers to a rigorous evaluation over time, which one obtains as an individualized record, based on a comparative computer study of the measurements. The sphygmochron is a comparison of an individual's given `time-lapse' data set with 1) data of clinically healthy peers comparable in terms of gender, age and ethnicity and, in addition, earlier data of the same subject, when available; 2) one or several prior profiles of the given individual. Around-the-clock (preferably 48-hour) blood pressure series from continuing international studies on clinically healthy people are being summarized as reference standards or chronodesms. These time-varying limits allow the interpretation of time-specified single measurements and also serve as ranges for rhythm characteristics or parameters. These ranges for parameters, given as prediction limits for single rhythm characteristics, such as the MESOR,

----

LEGEND to FIG. 1.

Rhythm characteristics and their uncertainty. The computer-yielded time-microscopic estimates of rhythm characteristics such as MESOR, amplitude, acrophase and period can each be given with their uncertainties, shown as small vertical bars for MESOR and amplitude, and as horizontal uncertainties for acrophase and period.

The MESOR is a rhythm-adjusted mean that takes into consideration the period of the rhythm illustrated by the cosine curve. In this graph, the data have been stacked into a single cycle of the rhythm. Means and standard errors have been computed for each of 24 hourly classes spanning this cycle, as shown by the vertical bars. Each dot represents a measurement. This subject's MESOR is 117 mm Hg, with a 95% confidence interval indicated by the small box around the horizontal line representing the MESOR.

The double amplitude is the predictable extent of change around the MESOR. The systolic blood pressure of this subject varies predictably by 50 (2 x 25) mm Hg within each day. The uncertainty for the estimation of the amplitude is indicated by the small box at the trough of the cosine curve fitted to the data. Note that the range between the highest and lowest value by far exceeds the double amplitude.

The acrophase is a measure of the timing of overall high values, measured as a lag from a selected reference time such as midnight to the crest of the cosine curve fitted to the data. The acrophase is expressed in degrees, with 360° equated to the period length. For a rhythm with a period of ⁻24 hours, an acrophase of -217° indicates that the systolic blood pressure reaches its overall highest values around 14:30. The 95% confidence curve for this acrophase is shown as a small box at the crest of the fitted cosine curve.

The period of the rhythm can also be estimated in its own right by nonlinear least-squares techniques. The period of a rhythm is the time elapsed for the pattern to recur. In this case, the rhythm is found to have a period of 24:03 hours. The uncertainty of this estimate is shown as a small box around the horizontal line joining identical rhythm stages on two consecutive cycles to show the uncertainty of the recurrence span of the cosinusoidal pattern.

----

amplitude and acrophase (see legend to Figure 1 for terminology), are chronodesms for parameters, briefly paradesms. These paradesms are given on the short form of a sphygmochron with each characteristic.

The sphygmochron may indicate, instead of a range, the number of standard deviations from the subject's prior estimate and/or a peer-group's mean. The paradesm for the amplitude-acrophase pair estimated concomitantly is described by an elliptical prediction region for a directed line (a vector), the length of which describes amplitude and the direction of

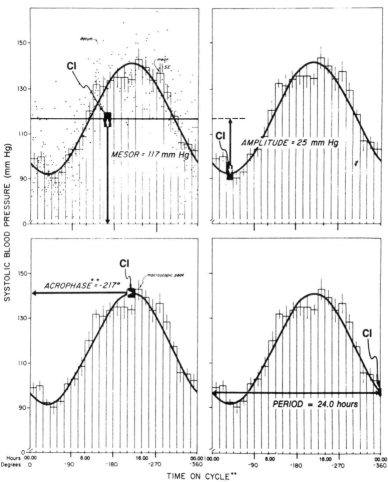

HYPOTHESIS TESTING AND *ESTIMATION* OF
CIRCADIAN PARAMETERS OF SYSTOLIC BLOOD PRESSURE
ESTIMATED BY NON-LINEAR LEAST-SQUARES FIT
OF COSINE CURVE TO 7 DAYS OF DATA (summarized by plexogram)

* From healthy women 60 yrs of age

** Zero-time = 00°° clock hours

If amplitude's confidence interval does not overlap midline of cosine curve (i.e., zero amplitude), rhythm can be considered statistically significant; confidence intervals (95% CI) can then be given for each parameter (MESOR), Ampliltude (Acrophase); confidence interval estimates approximate since serial correlation in time series not assessed.

FIG. 1. Rhythm characteristics and their uncertainty.

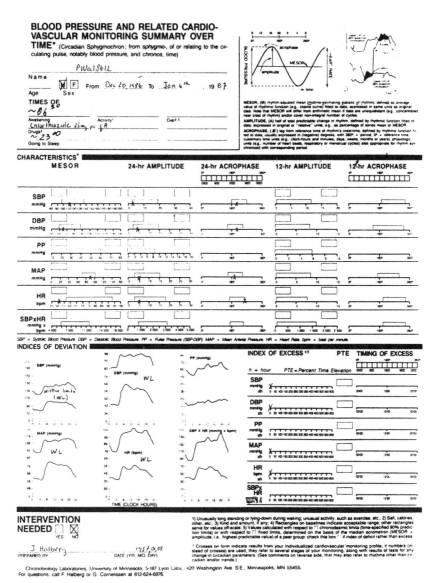

FIG. 2. Long form of the sphygmochron. The middle section serves to show characteristics of 24-hour and 12-hour components of variation. Analyses based on harmonics other than the 24- and 12-h harmonics, if they are informative, are summarized on the back of the form. Time-varying limits (chronodesms) are shown below on the left and the nonparametric indices of deviation below on the right, including excess, can be given numerically in mm Hg x h (BP) or bpm x h (HR), with the percentage of the total time during which excess occurs (PTE) and the timing of excess. Abstract hyperbaric and hypobaric indices are introduced in the upper right-hand corner as back areas; these areas quantify excess or deficit.

SPHYGMOCHRON™-S (short form)

MONITORING PROFILE OVER TIME; COMPUTER COMPARISON WITH PEER GROUP LIMITS

BLOOD PRESSURE (BP) AND RELATED CARDIOVASCULAR SUMMARY.

(Circadian Sphygmochron; from *sphygmo-*, of or relating to the circulation, notably blood pressure, as well as pulse and *chronos*, time)

Name _____ Patient # _____ No. of Profiles _____

Age _____ Sex [M] [F] Monitoring From _____ To _____ 19 ___

TIME OF AWAKENING (A) _____ (_____) **FALLING ASLEEP (S)** _____ (_____)
Day of Profile   (Habitually)   Day of Profile   (Habitually)

R$_X$: _____

COMMENTS[1,2] _____

CHRONOBIOLOGIC CHARACTERISTICS

	SYSTOLIC BP (mmHg)		DIASTOLIC BP (mmHg)		HEART RATE (bpm)	
	PATIENT VALUE	NUMBER OF SD' FROM PEER GROUP MEAN	PATIENT VALUE	NUMBER OF SD' FROM PEER GROUP MEAN	PATIENT VALUE	NUMBER OF SD' FROM PEER GROUP MEAN
ADJUSTED 24-h MEAN (MESOR)						
PREDICTABLE CHANGE (DOUBLE AMPLITUDE)						
TIMING OF OVERALL HIGH VALUES (ACROPHASE) (hr:min)**						

'SD = STANDARD DEVIATION; '' L MEANS LATER, E EARLIER

PERCENT TIME OF ELEVATION			
TIMING OF EXCESS	(hr:min)	(hr:min)	(hr:min)
EXTENT OF EXCESS DURING 24 HOURS	(mmHg x hour)	(mmHg x hour)	(bpm x hour)
10-YEAR CUMULATIVE EXCESS	(mmHg x hour) (in 1,000's units)	(mmHg x hour) (in 1,000's units)	(bpm x hour) (in 1,000's units)

INTERVENTION NEEDED

☐ No
☐ Yes ☐ Drug ☐ Non-Drug

MORE MONITORING NEEDED

☐ Annually
☐ As soon as possible
☐ Other specify_____

PREPARED BY _____ DATE ___ / ___ / ___

1) Unusually long standing or lying-down during waking, unusual activity, such as exercise, emotional loads, or schedule changes, e.g., shiftwork, etc. 2) Salt, calories, kind and amount, other, etc.

Chronobiology Laboratories, University of Minnesota, 5-187 Lyon Labs., 420 Washington Ave. S.E., Minneapolis, MN 55455
For questions, call F. Halberg or G. Cornelissen at 612-624-6976

FIG. 3. Short form of the sphygmochron.

which describes acrophase, as gauges of the predictable extent and timing of change, respectively. Once obtained, the set of chronodesms, shown for single rhythm characteristics on both sphygmochrons, can be used for interpretation of whole profiles from a given individual. The single time-specified values can be interpreted in the light of time-qualified chronodesms, shown on the long-form of the sphygmochron, Figure 2. The initial analyses on a given data set provide the individualized reference standard that serves to interpret the corresponding characteristics in follow-up profiles.

Parametric And Nonparametric Estimates

Some of the chronobiologic characteristics, e.g., the inferential statistical parameter described in Figure 1, are given in a section called Characteristics on the long form (in Figure 2) and also in a section of the short form of the sphymochron (see Figure 3). The reference standards for comparisons of a person's blood pressure and heart rate characteristics have to be age- and gender-specified. Standards are needed for the amplitude and acrophase at the about-24-hour (circadian) period and for a set of harmonic components of this period in the blood pressure spectrum. These harmonics (e.g., 24/2 hr = 12 hr; 24/3 hr = 8 hr, etc.) in conjunction with the fundamental period (e.g., 24 hours) may represent the nonsinusoidal waveform. This ultradian aspect of the spectrum, i.e., the components with frequencies higher than one cycle in 20 h, gradually increases in prominence with age (1). Chrono-biologists thus quantify the waveform as a set of harmonics included with a given fundamental period corresponding to a given rhythm (such as the circadian one).

In addition to the MESOR and the circadian and ultradian amplitudes and acrophases, chronobiologists resolve a number of other endpoints, that require longer-than-48-h records. The 48-h span, however, serves for a tentative estimate of the circadian period, as a guage of gross time structure alteration, indicated by a 95% confidence interval not overlapping 24 h or altogether by a lack of circadian rhythmicity that prompts continued monitoring for an exploration of free-running, intermodulation or data quality.

A Better-Than-Conventional Mean: MESOR

Parametric indices include a midline-estimating statistic of rhythm, the MESOR, which is superior to the arithmetic mean as a location index when measurements are unequally spaced. For equally-spaced measurements, the MESOR is identical to the mean. The MESOR is characterized by a smaller standard error (uncertainty), as compared to that of the arithmetic mean when the data are equidistant, cover an integral number of cycles and are rhythmic, and hence a (non-zero) amplitude and an acrophase are also computed. For this reason, as an example, the effect of a treatment may be rigorously validated for a given individual by a MESOR test with a $P < 0.05$, when a comparison of means of the identical data by a t-test may fail to achieve this task ($P > 0.05$) (12).

Harbingers

Changes in rhythm characteristics such as circadian amplitude or acrophase usually precede an elevation of the MESOR outside acceptable limits. Thus, rhythm alterations can be harbingers of problems to come that should be prevented by timely intervention (11,12). The need for intervention may be indicated by a chronobiologic examination summarized as a sphygmochron.

RESULTS

Screening

Various kinds of chronobiologic characteristics can be routinely computed from blood pressure and heart rate data, and can be quite useful in signaling risk, prior to overt disease (9,11). Their use for risk assessment on the pregnant woman and her baby is the topic of ongoing research. A different timing of high values, e.g., with peaking by night rather than day, called circadian blood pressure ecphasia, is not uncommon in pregnancy and may characterize preeclampsia (14). Other examples of rhythm alteration are an increase of the circadian amplitude beyond peer group limits. Thus, a circadian amplitude-elevation (CAE) may occur without a MESOR increase; or the hyperbaric index (HBI, a measure of excess, may exceed the 90% peer-derived upper limit of 50 mm Hg x h in 24 hours. In either case, hygienic measures and further monitoring are indicated as a start. Drug therapy may become necessary if non-drug intervention fails to eliminate CAE or the HBI $\geq$ 50 mm Hg x hr for 24 hours.

Diagnosis

A series of values outside chronodesms (time-qualified reference intervals) may be found at odd times and may underlie an estimate of the amount of time and the extent to which an individual's blood pressure or heart rate will be deviant, increasing the risk of health problems. These `odd-time hyper-tensives' might have appeared normotensive with the conventional approach to blood pressure evaluation involving only casual, time-unspecified blood pressure readings during regular office hours. Conversely, individuals who on the basis of single blood pressure measurements at three office visits are diagnosed as hypertensive can show acceptable values in around-the-clock profiles obtained by ambulatory monitors under ordinary conditions. These represent false positive diagnoses, the white-coat or office hypertensives (12,15).

Treatment

On an individualized basis, the sphygmochron serves to ascertain that blood pressure is, most of the time, within peer group limits and that the hyperbaric index is reduced (to below 50 mm Hg x h in 24 hrs for systolic blood pressure) or normal. If this is not the case, i.e., if parametric and/or non-parametric endpoints are deviant, such findings in the sphygmochron should prompt interventions in order to achieve acceptable endpoints.

On an individualized basis, the sphygmochron can tell whether, for the given case examined, a reduction of dietary sodium intake is useful, indifferent or possibly undesirable (since, in some individuals, blood pressure rises when dietary sodium is withheld or reduced). The effect of a reduction in dietary calories can also be ascertained in a sphygmochron on an individualized basis with statistical inference (P-value) (11,12). Once a certain extent of calorie restriction is achieved, a statistically significant lowering of the blood pressure MESOR is often seen (12,13).

The sphygmochron can help the physician prescribe medication to lower blood pressure or heart rate only at times when the individual would have high values. This timing of treatment not only makes the medication more effective, but helps avoid lowering the blood pressure at times when it may already be low, and thus avoid the dizziness people may experience when taking antihypertensive medication. A follow-up sphygmochron can be carried-out while on medication. This follow-up, in conjunction with objective tests of any inter-profile changes (20), allow the physician to observe and, if necessary, improve drug treatment by changing the dose and/or timing of medication, thus helping prevent undesirable or harmful side-effects (7,12). Insufficient treatment while reducing the MESOR enlarges the circadian amplitude (12), a condition that must be recognized so that treatment by drugs or by diet is readjusted to alleviate or eliminate this problem.

When Should A Sphygmochron Be Used?

The sphygmochron should be used routinely for every new patient examined in apparent health and for follow-up physical examinations, rather than only in special cases. When an automated monitor is unavailable, systematic self-measurement may be used as a substitute. Thus, diagnoses and treatment will be proved. A patient might appear to be well-treated, while there exists (undetected) undesirably high pressure or fast heart rate at odd times. By the same token, a patient may be overtreated because of isolated high readings in a physicians' office as an emotional response. A sphygmochron will be helpful in avoiding labeling a person as well-treated or insufficiently treated when neither is the case. Moreover, use of the sphygmochron may save medication and reduce side effects, since a lesser amount of drug is needed, when treatment is given at the right time, as indicated by the sphygmochron. The use of a sphygmochron differs from the conventional approach of 24-hour ambulatory monitoring as well as from casual measurements for 4 reasons: 1. the monitoring is started early in life, preferably at birth; 2. the recording is started in all individuals including those who would not otherwise be monitored or interviewed; 3. the minimal recording span at the outset is of 48 hours or longer, rather than of 24 hours; 4. the interpretation of the record is chronobiologic, with parametric and nonparametric analyses.

A 48-hour recording span using automatic ambulatory measurement is advocated since two consecutive 24-hour profiles can differ considerably from each other, notably if the analysis focuses upon dynamic parameters, including the period of rhythms. Differences among different days of monitoring are also found more readily when comparing MESORs instead of arithmetic means, because the arithmetic means usually have a larger standard error.

A sphygmochron, based on a 48-hour profile, should be part of a first physical examination at any age. It should optimally be prepared for every newborn and should constitute an integral aspect of late primary and secondary education, as part of chronobiologic computer literacy. If a first sphygmochron is not deviant, it may be repeated at 5- or 10-year intervals thereafter, with consideration of medical history and age. The inter-profile interval chosen should depend on the absence or presence of any deviation, e.g., increase, and in the latter case on the kind and extent of deviation. General use of the sphygmochron, interpreted in the light of time-varying rather than arbitrary fixed limits, cannot fail to help the individual and those in health care to work together to prevent the serious health problems related to by high blood pressure.

DISCUSSION

Choices we face:

Nonchronobiologic alternatives:
1) Current recommendations of the World Health Organization, based on casual samples interpreted in the light of arbitrary limits, e.g., 140/90 mm Hg;
2) 24-hour ambulatory monitoring, also relying on the same arbitrary limits rather than time-specified limits and on mean values, without assessment of rhythm characteristics; or

Chronobiologic alternative:
3) The sphygmochron: a chronobiologic blood pressure and related cardiovascular summary; a computer comparison with time-specified data from peers and the individual's personalized standard, if earlier data are available.

We need no longer ask whether one should rely on the conventional casual manual blood pressure measurement or upon an automatic ambulatory 24-hour monitor. Currently, the only argument for the choice between methods for measuring blood pressure confronting health care personnel is the cost-effectiveness of assessing the systolic and/or the diastolic blood pressure or the mean of several repeated casual or automatic 24-hour measurements. This ill-formulated alternative must be rephrased. The real issue is the need to retrieve information contained in the predictable variations of blood pressure. The choice is between conventional and chronobiologic blood pressure and heart rate assessment, whether the measurements are taken as self-measurements, or automatically. The patient willing, the physician recommends ambulatory monitoring and then examines the sphygmochron. Nurses or technicians prepare and standardize the instruments, test them, instruct the patient, collect the monitors, transfer and analyze the data, and fill out the sphygmochron. If self-measurements are recommended for the first time at an adult age, many will find that they are too cumbersome; this limitation can be overcome by education in chronobiology within the context of late primary and secondary schooling. While ambulatory equipment is expensive, it will be much cheaper if appropriate large markets are opened, and will become cost-effective if used chronobiologically.

New equipment, coupled with education, can reduce or eliminate the enormous cost both of unjustified medication in the many cases of false positive diagnoses of high blood pressure and of `after-the-fact' health care which, in 1987 in the U.S. alone for conditions associated with high blood pressure, has been estimated to have totaled $55.4 billion by Dr. Gerald Payne (Associated Director for Scientific Programs, Division of Epidemiology and Clinical Applications, NHLBI, Bethesda, MD 20892) and Dr. Duane Alexander (Director, National Institute for Child Health and Human Development, NIH, Bethesda, MD 20205).

SUMMARY

There is a need for chronobiologic monitoring because it offers advantages over other approaches.

1) The reliability of the average is enhanced by computing it with a smaller standard error as the MESOR of equidistant data of a rhythm.

2) Characteristics of variation such as amplitudes and acrophases, computed on the basis of all data, can provide new information, e.g., of risk, when the best mean, computed from the same data, is not informative.

3) The description of excess or deficit relates the individual's blood pressure profile to realistic time-varying prior individualized and/or peer group limits.

4) The foregoing approaches may improve the sensitivity of screening, and the reliability of diagnosis.

5) The prognosis may be more accurate once the sphygmochron provides a 10-year projection of cumulative excess as a first tentative approximation of a harm function.

6) The timing and efficacy of treatment can be placed chronobiologically on an individualized basis and effects can be assessed for statistical as well as biologic significance. In addition to this obvious merit, research much continue on

7) the prevention of deviant (high or low) blood pressure, extending, to intervention trials, the scope of current international cooperation on pregnant women and their babies.

ACKNOWLEDGEMENTS

Supported by U.S. Public Health Service (GM-13981 and HL-40650); Colin Medical Instruments (South Plainfield, New Jersey); Medtronic Inc. (Minneapolis, MN); Dr. Earl Bakken and Dr. Betty Sullivan Funds.

This paper is based on a newsletter prepared for Dialogue in Hypertension by one of us (FH). Most of the evidence for the statements made herein is found in reference 12.

REFERENCES

1. Anderson S., Cornelissen G., Halberg F., Scarpelli P.T., Germano G., Livi R., Scarpelli L., Cagnoni M. and Holte J. (1988): Ultradian components as a function of age and gender in the human blood

pressure spectrum - Abstract, *1st international Conference of Chronobiology and Chronomedicine*, Chengdu, People's Republic of China, pp. 9-10,

2. Canadian Coalition for High Blood Pressure Prevention and Control, (1988): Recomendations on self-measurement of blood pressure. *CMAJ* 138: 1093-1096.

3. Carandente F., Halberg F. (eds.) (1987): Chronobiology of Blood Pressure in 1985. *Chronobiologia* 11, #3. (152 pp). (See esp. Halberg F., Drayer J.I.M., Cornelissen G., Weber M.A.: Cardiovascular reference data base for recognizing circadian mesor-and amplitude-hypertension in apparently healthy men. Chronobiolgia 11:275-298, 1984; Halberg F., Scheving L.E., Lucas E., Cornelissen G., Sothern R.B., Halberg E., Halberg J., Halberg Francine, Carter J., Straub K.D., Redmond D.P.: Chronobiology of human blood pressure in the light of static (room-restricted) automatic monitoring. Chronobiologia 11:217-247, 1984; Halberg F., Ahlgren A., Haus E.: Circadian systolic and diastolic hyperbaric indices of high school and college students. Chronobiologia 11:299-309, 1984).

4. Carandente F. (1987): Circadian rhythms and hypertension. *Dialogue in Hypertension* 2 (4): 1-3.

5. Cheung D.G., Weber M.A. (1988): Circadian changes in blood pressure: clinical significance. IM: *Internal Medicine for the Specialist, Special Supplement: Circadian Rhythms and Cardiovascular Disease*. June 1988, pp. 18-28.

6. Cornelissen G., (1987): Instrumentation and data analysis methods needed for blood pressure monitoring in chronobiology. In: *Chronobiotechnology and Chronobiological Engineering*, edited by L.E. Scheving, F. Halberg, C.F. Ehret; Martinus Nijhoff, Dordrecht, The Netherlands, pp. 241-261 (see also pp. 262-269,270-277, 278-281, 282-288, 289-298, 299-303, 304-309, and 310-317).

7. Gullner H.G., Bartter F.C., Halberg F. (1979): Timing antihypertensive medication. *The Lancet*, September 8, p. 527.

8. Halberg F., (1969): Chronobiology. *Ann. Rev. Physiol.* 31:675-725, 1969.

9. Halberg F., Johnson E.A., Nelson W., Runge W., Sothern R. (1972): Autorhythmometry-procedures for physiologic self-measurements and their analysis. *Physiol. Tchr.* 1:1-11.

10 Halberg F. (1980): Chronobiology: methodological problems. *Acta med. rom.* 18:399-440.

11. Halberg F., Bakken E., Cornelissen G., Halberg J., Halberg E., Delmore P., (1988): Blood pressure assessment with a cardiovascular summary, the sphymochron, in broad chronobiologic perspective. In: *Heart &*

Brain, Brain & Heart, edited by Refsum H., Sulg J.A., & Rasmussen K., Springer-Yerlag, Berlin, (in press).

12. Halberg F., Cornelissen G., Halberg E., Halberg J., Delmore P., Bakken E., Shinoda M. (1988): Chronobiology of human blood pressure. *Medtronic Continuing Medical Education Seminars,* (4th ed.), 242 pp.

13. Lee J.Y., Gillum R.F., Cornelissen G., Koga Y., Halberg F., (1982): Individualized assessment of circadian rhythm characteristics of human blood pressure and pulse after moderate salt and weight restriction. In: *Toward Chronopharmacology, Proc. 8th IUPHAR Cong. and Sat. Symposia,* Nagasaki, 1981, edited by R. Takahashi, F. Halberg and C. Walker, Pergamon Press, Oxford/New York, pp. 375-390.

14. Miyamoto S., Shimokawa H., Sumioki H., Touno A., Nakano H. (1988): Circadian rhythm of plasma atrial natriuretic peptide, aldosterone, and blood pressure during the third trimester in normal and preeclamptic pregnancies. *Am. J. Ob. Gyn.* 158:393-399.

15. Pickering T.G. (1988): White coat hypertension. *Proc. III Meeting on `Conflicting aspects in the clinical approach to hypertension',* Monte Cassino, Oct. 21-22.

16. Weber M.A. (1988): Automated blood pressure monitoring: a new dimension in diagnosis. *Mayo Clinc. Proc.* 63: 1151-1153.

17. White W.B., (1988): Average daily blood pressure not office blood pressure determines left ventricular function in patients with hypertension. *Proc. III Meeting on `Conflicting aspects in the clinical approach to hypertension',* Monte Cassino, Oct. 21-22, 1988, unpaginated (2 pp.).

18. White W.B., Schulman P., McCabe E.J., Dey H.M., (1989): Average daily blood pressure, not office blood pressure, determines cardiac function in patients with hypertension. *JAMA* 261: 873-877.

19. World Hypertension League (1988): Self-measurement of blood pressure. *Bull. WHO,* 66:155-159.

20. Wu J., Halberg F., Nomura T., Yamaguchi M., Iwata N., Weber M., Drayer J.I.M., Shinoda M., (1988): Intraindividual comparison for novelty effect of two `ambulatory' 24-hour blood pressure and heart rate profiles in healthy human adults. *Abstract, 1st International Conference of Chronobiology and Chronomedicine,* Chengdu, People's Republic of China, October 2-7, pp. 21-23.

21. Zachariah P.K., Sheps S.G., Ilstrup D.M., Long C.R., Bailey K.R., Wiltgen C.M., Carlson C.A., (1988): Blood pressure load--a better determinant of hypertension. *Mayo Clinc. Proc.* 63:1085-1091.

Medical Monitoring in the Home and Work Environment,
edited by Laughton E. Miles and Roger J. Broughton.
Raven Press, New York © 1990.

AUTORHYTHMOMETRY: A USEFUL CONCEPT FOR TEACHING HEALTH EDUCATION

Lawrence E. Scheving

University of Arkansas for Medical Sciences
Department of Antomy #510
4301 W. Markham
Little Rock, AR   72205

INTRODUCTION

It has been recognized that individuals respond differently to an identical stimulus given at different times along a 24-hr time scale. Vigilance, sensory acuity, memory and the ability to learn, as as well as response to drugs and physical agents are all influenced by biological time-of-day.   Metabolic and physiological functions also undergo rhythmic changes. Thus rhythms are ubiquitous at all levels of organization and in all forms of life.   These rhythms are not impressed from without as are conditioned reflexes; instead they are generated from within, but are capable of being synchronized to the 24-hr geophysical cycle, and in the case of man social routine also may influence synchronization (17).

Chronobiologists who study time structure and rhythmic variation in physiological and psychological functions recognize rhythmicity as a fundamental property of life which offers new insight into the physical, emotional and social health of the individual.   Moreover, there is even evidence that rhythms are altered in disease.   If humans are constantly experiencing cyclic variation in their mental and physical capacities, are they adequately educated if they are unaware of the influence of these variations?   With jet travel now so common, can a person be considered "health educated" if he or she is not informed of the great influence that biological "clocks" during travel can have on physical, mental and social performance?   Is the supervisor responsible for scheduling shift workers acting in their best interest if he does not understand problems associated with shifting body rhythms?   Are we now scheduling important examinations, which have impact on a persons future, at the best time for optimal performance? Are those in charge of making important decisions, such as diplomats and military commanders, at a disadvantage if they ignore or fail to understand the temporal variation that characterizes ability to function optimally in decision making?

It has been suggested that self-measurement of body rhythms should be a skill developed no later than in high school. Ideally, each individual and his or her physician should be aware of this unique temporal organization.

The question asked is, can chronobiology and its implications for human health behavior be conceptualized by the typical high-school student?

It was Professor Franz Halberg of the Chronobiology Laboratories at the University of Minnesota School of Medicine who first advanced the concept of teaching students early in life ways in which they could monitor their own health in a chronobiological manner (7). He and his colleagues put together a series of measurements for vital signs such as oral temperature, pulse rate, blood pressure and pulmonary functions. They also selected or developed several performance tests; among which were short-term memory, long-term memory, and random addition as well as tests designed to measure eye-hand coordination and physical strength, the response of which may change along the 24-hour time scale.

Individuals can be taught to make these measurements accurately; and then, after the learning process, they do them repeatedly while they are awake for at least 72 hours. Thus they come to appreciate the tremendous amount of variation that can be documented not only in their blood pressure, but in every other function they measure including their ability to perform mental and physical tasks. If they make measurements during what would normally be sleep time, the degree of variations are even greater.

Most of these rhythms are "silent" to all of us; they only become overt when they are systematically measure over a span of time: and this of course explains why so many rhythmic events have been overlooked for so long. The concept of making such measurements on oneself is commonly called autorhythmometry (self-measurement of rhythms).

With the above as background, three Little Rock public high schools agreed to introduce such a program into their biology curriculum for a one year feasibility study. It shall be the objectives of this chapter to: a) describe each of the measurements that the student learned to make; b) explain the rationale for doing each of them, when it may be apparent; and c) comment on the problems encountered. We emphasize that in this particular study the primary objective was educative and not simply to gather experimental data. Earlier we have used these same tests to gather scientific data on several populations including healthy young soldiers, patients with leprosy, and aging populations.

DESCRIPTION OF TESTS

The name selected for our high school program was "Operation Heartbeat". The following test procedures are explained in the sequence in which the subject performed them, and are presented here in the same form in which they were given to the students.

General Instructions

1) **Preparation.** The first thing to do is to find a spot where you can sit down and take the measurements without being disturbed; a table or desk is best. Avoid distraction or noise. Remember measurements should be made at least 20 min. before taking anything that would affect oral temperature, such as hot or cold drinks, strenuous exercise, singing, being in a sauna or out in the cold. On the data sheet provided (Table 1), record

FIG. 1. shows the instruments used to make the various measurements along with the bag in which the student carried the instruments.

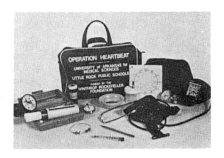

your school, name, age, sex, race, month and sheet number. Then record the day, hour and minute. Time is recorded according to the 24-hour system with local midnight equal to 0000 hours, local noon to 1200 hours, 1:00 p.m. to 1300 hours, etc. For example, 1 minute past midnight would be written 0001, 30 minutes past would be 0030, 8:20 a.m. would be 0820, and 8:20 p.m. would be 2020. Moreover, data should always be recorded as Standard Time (Central Standard Time if you live in Arkansas), not as Daylight Savings Time; this simply is a convention of science. Of course, if you travel to another time zone while carrying out your series of studies, time would be recorded according to the new zone. The next step is to record the time you got up this morning and then the time of the first measurement under the column headed "now". It also is important to remember to record the time of retiring each night.

Table I

CHRONOBIOLOGY LABORATORIES, DEPARTMENT OF ANATOMY, UNIVERSITY OF ARKANSAS, AND LITTLE ROCK PUBLIC HIGH SCHOOLS

High School_____ Name_____ Subject Code_____ Age_____ Sex____ Race_____ Month_____ Sheet____

Day	Time Zone	Time: Arise	Retire	Now	M	V	Time Est.	Pls Min	Blood Press. Syst./Diast.	Eye-Hand :kill	Ring Test	Fing. C'tg.	Randm # Add	Randm # Mem	Oral Temp	Strength Rt	Left	Peak Flow I	II	Comments*

*Strenuous exercise (E), Anxiety (AX), Consumption of Alcohol (AL), Anger (AG)

2) Oral temperature. Pick up the thermometer and shake the mercury column to below the $96^{\circ}F$ mark. Be careful not to strike it against some object and break it. Place the bulb as far back under your tongue as is comfortable and leave it there for at least three minutes; five minutes is even better. Record the value on the data sheet to the nearest 0.1 degree.

3) Mood and vigor rating. While taking your temperature you should also record mood and vigor ratings. Both of these use the 1-7 point scale listed below.

MOOD

Depressed, "blue"	1
Somewhat depressed	2
Slightly less cheerful than usual	3
Usual state	4
Slightly more cheerful than usual	5
Quite cheerful	6
Happy, elated	7

PHYSICAL VIGOR

Inactive,tired	1
Somewhat tired	2
Slightly less active than usual	3
Usual state	4
Slightly more active than usual	5
Quite active	6
Active (full of pep)	7

4) Minute estimation. Start the stop watch and estimate one minute. Look away from the dial and wait for what seems like exactly one min. to go by (you may count from 1 to 60 at a nearly steady pace if you wish). Stop the watch when you believe a min. has passed and record the actual number of seconds.

5) Pulse (heart rate). Place two fingers firmly over the radial artery in your wrist (close to the base of the thumb). Do not take this measurement with the thumb, because it has a pulse of its own. Count the number of beats for a full min. and record this value. Do not use the short-cut method of counting for only a half or a quarter of a min. and then multiplying; this will reduce your accuracy considerably.

6) Blood pressure. Open the exhaust valve of the blood pressure cuff and deflate it. Wrap the cuff firmly around the biceps of your upper right arm (or upper left arm, if you are left handed, in which case note under "comments" on sheet one). Your forearm should rest on the table at the level of your heart. Tighten the cuff and close the exhaust valve. Pump the bulb until the dial reads about 160 mm Hg (or at least 20 mm above your highest previously recorded pressure). The purpose of this is to put enough pressure on the radial artery so that the blood flow through it stops. Carefully place the stethoscope diaphragm on the antecubital fossa (front of the elbow joint) and listen for beats. If beats are heard immediately, deflate the cuff and inflate it again to a pressure at least 30 mm higher than originally. If beats are no longer heard, partially release the exhaust valve so that the pressure drops very slowly (about 2 mm per second). As the needle moves slowly, record the dial reading when the first pulse beat is heard (systolic pressure) and when the pulse beat disappears or drops considerably in volume (diastolic pressure). Always use the opposite hand to squeeze the bulb. If you have the thermometer in your mouth while making the blood pressure measurement, be careful that you do not knock it out with the stethoscope or bite it while wrapping the cuff around your arm or when you are squeezing the bulb of the sphygmomanometer.

7) Eye-hand skill (E-H skill). Remove the small tube from the coordinometer and screw it onto the top of the case. wipe your hands free of sweat and transfer all 35 beads to the standard bead bowl. Place the coordinometer on the left. (Note: the table should be at a comfortable height). Hold the stop watch in your left hand, face down. Do not hold the coordinometer. Start the stop watch and simultaneously begin transferring beads into the tube and counting them one by one as fast as possible, using the right hand under visual control. After 30 beads have been placed in the tube, stop the watch and record the elapsed time to the nearest 0.2 seconds. (The arrangement of the coordinometer, bead-bowl and stop watch should be reversed for a left-handed subject.)

8) Nut-threading ring test. The ring test of eye-hand coordination should be carried out in a standardized sitting position. You should hold your shoulders upright and back, heels touching, chin up and look forward. The thumb and first two fingers of the left hand should be placed around the left side of the ring and the last two fingers below the ring, with the hand grasping the ring at a 90° angle to the left of the thread, which should be at the top of the ring at eye level (left handed subjects should reverse the sequence). The nuts at the bottom of the ring should be so arranged that the colored nut is the first in the sequence. Once the ring is firmly in the hand, start the stop watch with your free hand and begin to thread the four nuts, one at a time, through the threads as fast as possible with the free hand. Once the nut is properly in line on the thread (use your eyes), a twirling motion to speed up the threading may be used. After the last nut is completely through the threads, stop the watch and record the elapsed time.

9) Finger counting (fngr.cntg.). Hold the stopwatch in your left hand. Raise your right hand, palm upward, elbow flexed to a horizontal position; allow for good separation of fingers. start the watch, touch the thumb to the index finger and silently count "1"; then move the thumb to middle finger and count "2". Continue moving the thumb to the fourth and fifth fingers, and then go back to the index finger, as fast as possible, until the count of "25" is reach. On the 25th count, the thumb should touch the index finger. If the count is not correct, start over. Immediately repeat the count to 25 as above, and stop the watch after the second count of "25". Record the elapsed time to the nearest second.

10) Random number addition (r-number-add). Refer to the random number tables (Table 2). Enter your name, school and the consecutive sheet number in the spaces provided on the top of each table. Place the stopwatch face down on the table, start it and as quickly as possible accurately add consecutive pairs of digits in a single column of random digits (entering each pair-sum to the right of the column, between digits). For example, for a column with digits 7,1,5,2,9, etc., the first sum would be 7 plus 1 equals 8, the second sum 5 plus 2 equals 7, etc.

11) Short term memory. 7-digit random numbers (Table 3). Enter your name, the year, month and consecutive sheet number in the spaces provided at the top of each SHORT TERM MEMORY sheet.

Record the day and the reference time zone, hour and min. of both reference (indicate) and local time zones, in boxes provided at left of each row of numbers. Hold stopwatch in left hand, with face down. Start stopwatch, look at the first 7 digit number, cover it with bottom p[art of stopwatch and write the number in the space provided. Proceed with the next number in the same manner. After the last 7 digit numb in the row has been written down, stop the watch and record the elapsed time to the nearest 0.1 second in the space provided under "Sec" at right of the sheet. Also record the total number of incorrect digits under "Err". Each digit in the written number should be compared with the respective digit in the printed number. If 8175945 was written 8179545, two errors were made.

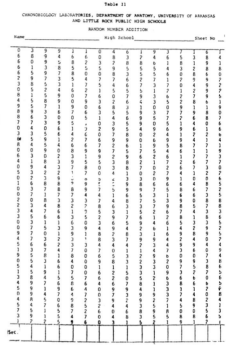

Table II

CHRONOBIOLOGY LABORATORIES, DEPARTMENT OF ANATOMY, UNIVERSITY OF ARKANSAS AND LITTLE ROCK PUBLIC HIGH SCHOOLS

RANDOM NUMBER ADDITION

Name_____ High School_____ Sheet No _____

Table III

CHRONOBIOLOGY LABORATORIES, DEPARTMENT OF ANATOMY, UNIVERSITY OF ARKANSAS, AND LITTLE ROCK PUBLIC HIGH SCHOOLS

SHORT-TERM MEMORY: 7-DIGIT RANDOM NUMBERS

Day	Local Time	Name_____			Year____ Month____				Sheet_____		Sec	Err
		7410888	2228857	0740152	5704910	3501755	1475048	9683860	3628808	7873951	6059221		
		2230490	3147287	7173343	9283051	4911748	1210280	5804186	7177105	9621065	5407850		
		7395079	4431794	4056006	0478033	4325852	5890558	2163961	8498659	9326660	6742792		
		9504352	6804678	0564870	9971594	8137006	2218564	2449103	0455477	0818598	4996169		
		4592165	7874171	7198309	4557589	3173257	2604767	0076544	6376253	6694746	4958069		
		1703740	3869959	0307943	0471803	2683505	5111245	9913140	8345889	7535941	8577108		
		1055998	7871122	1476157	2776743	5848530	1889772	9490697	1473035	4120774	6990931		
		0130251	4338540	6615243	4772466	7334743	1439053	1048566	9980217	3629298	5252433		

12) Dynamometer readings. Turn the needle follower to zero before making each test. Stand up and assume a military stance (eyes forward, shoulders back, with feet about a foot apart). With the dynamometer held comfortably in the right hand, extend your arm downward at about a 30° angle from the body and squeeze. Record the value indicated by the needle follower. Repeat with your left hand.

13) Peak expiratory flow (PEF). The peak flow meter should be held in both hands with the dial facing vertically. Make sure the indicator is on zero. Inhale as deeply as possible, put the mouthpiece to your lips and exhale as hard as you can a short, sharp blast. Record the indicator reading as accurately as possible.

14) Record any comments that might have affected any of the tests.

COMMENTS RELATIVE TO THE TESTS

Mood and Physical Vigor: Psychologists believe that a rather objective measure of a person's mood or physical vigor can be obtained by simply having a check list consisting of short phrases designed to suggest an attitude or a condition. Our sequence of tests has such a check list for evaluating mood and vigor. The subject is asked to respond to a series of short phrases using a numerical scale of 1-7. We have used such tests on several different categories of subjects including young healthy soldiers (9) patients with leprosy (16) and elderly subjects (15). It has been our experience that this seemingly subjective evaluation works, that one can reproduce data from one day to the next, and that all groups seem to have essentially the same phasing. Figure 2 (H-I) illustrates the variation in mood and physical vigor that was self-measured along a 24-hour time scale by a group of young healthy soldiers. Figure 3 shows the results of another vigor evaluation done on a group of blinded individuals of varying ages, all living under a similar social routine (14). Note the similarity of the phasing of the vigor rhythms in the two groups (compare Figure 2-I with Figure 3). Clearly, mood as well as physical vigor appear to vary in a circadian manner, with "best" mood and vigor associated with wakefulness and reaching a peak about mid-afternoon.

Pulse Rate: The average heart rate for a young adult is slightly over 70 beats per minute during wakefulness but may drop to a lower rate at night, even though he or she might not go to bed. It has been recognized for a long time that heart rate also is related to body temperature. For every 1oF rise in temperature, the heart rate increases 10 or 15 beats per min. Figure 2 illustrates the heart rate (B) and temperature (A) rhythms plotted side by side for a group of subjects. Of course the heart rate is easily perturbed; and the post-prandial (after eating) increase is especially prominent when on monitors heart rate repeatedly along the 24-hour time scale. Therefore the pulse should be taken before eating.

Blood Pressure: The rhythm in blood pressure may have a very high amplitude in some individuals. About mid-sleep, a rise in diastolic pressure may precede that in systolic blood pressure, pulse and activity. The sequence of changes is preparatory to awakening and is not simply secondary to the sleep and wakefulness cycle, because blood pressure will begin to rise even though the subject remains up and active during the night. Figure 4 illustrates the pattern of fluctuation in both systolic and diastolic blood pressure for a group of 20 untreated hypertensive patients compared with pattern for a group of five normal subjects (normotensive). Clearly normal readings for many of the hypertensive patients were obtained at certain times of the day.

Figure 5 illustrates a record of 17 days (around the clock) of a 61-year-old man hospitalized for study at the National Institutes of Health. By conventional standards, it readily can be seen that this patient was normotensive every morning; but the blood pressure determined in the late afternoon provides equally convincing evidence that the patient was hypertensive.

Figure 6 shows the variations in systolic and diastolic blood pressure of a 53-year old executive who was, at the time of making his self measurements, on medication to control his blood pressure. Clearly the rhythm persists even while one is taking medications.

It is interesting to note that the highest peak in systolic blood pressure occurred on a day (11-5-79) when this man was conducting an all day executive meeting, thus demonstrating the effect of stress (6). Note that on the abscissa the dark bar indicates what he reported as his sleep or rest time during the monitoring span. Since no measurements were taken during the sleep time, it is quite likely that the trough each night fell much lower than is indicated on the graph.

Performance Test: It is well documented that eye-hand coordination varies considerably along the 24-hour time span. This can be demonstrated with the test which involved dropping beads into a container and with the simple finger counting exercise. With such tests it is not uncommon to see as much as a 30% to 50% circadian variation in individuals, even after the learning period. Figure 2 demonstrates that the best eye-hand coordination (C) occurs about the time of peak body temperature (A). (Note that the peak of this and other performance rhythms actually represent the slowest or "worst" time, and the troughs represent the fastest or "best" time.) It has been disconcerting to pilots of

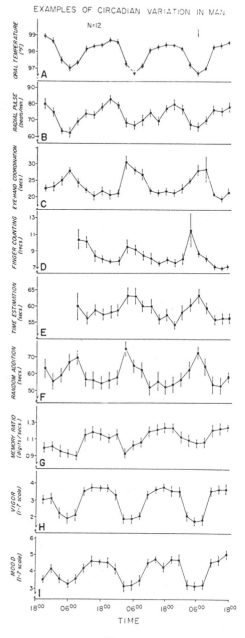

Figure 2.
Rhythmic variation in diverse variables in a group of 12 presumably healthy young men over a 72-hour period (sampled at 3-hour intervals). Note that the time of poorest performance in C, D and F represents the crest of the rhythm. Meal times: 0615, 1215 and 1630 hours; rest or sleep time: 2100-0600, however subjects were awakened for sampling at 2400 and 0300 (Scheving, 1978).

transoceanic jetliners to learn
that from the time they take off
from New York in the evening
until they land several hours later
in Europe, their eye-hand
coordination may deteriorate
continually. There has been a
great deal of interest in variation
of performance. We frequently
have heard the statement that
efficiency is impaired at night
and that this follows the drop in
body temperature. This
statement is correct based upon
evidence from a number of
studies.

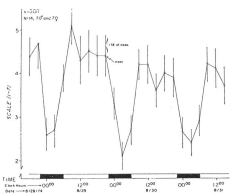

Figure 3.
The individuals gave a subjective rating for vigor on a scale of 1 to 7. The population tested consisted of 7 male and 7 female blinded individuals (Pauly, et al., 1975).

As early as 1934, Freeman and Holvand (4) reviewed much of the evidence available and concluded: "The balance of evidence apparently favors an afternoon superiority for sensitivity and motor performance." This relationship is seen by comparing the rhythms of eye-hand coordination (C) and finger counting (D) with temperature (A) in Figure 2.

The question as to when is the best time for optimum performance must take into consideration the type of task to be performed. The reader is referred to a review of chronobiological performance, which amplifies on this, by Folkard (3).

Peak expiratory flow and Grip Strength both vary rather dramatically. Figure 7 is an example of variation in peak expiratory flow in a group of blind individuals all living under similar circumstances (14).

CONCLUSIONS

As might be expected a number of problems arose in carrying out the high school project "Operation Heartbeat" for the one semester span. Approximately 492 students from three high schools gathered data. Most of them did a good job; but some (the minority) were careless in collecting data that otherwise would have been useful in evaluating for circadian variation. However, we believe that even those individuals must have learned a good deal about their own body physiological variation.

Some equipment was stolen or damaged. Instruments sometimes malfunctioned, but remained in better shape than had been predicted by some at the beginning. For the future we recommend a sphygmomanometer cuff that is easier for the student to put on: these are now available. Of course, the program resulted in additional work for those teachers who took the study seriously, and they are to be complimented.

One major problem was that the battery of measurements required more time to complete than the original estimation of three min. When measurements made during school hours required more than the five min. between class periods, some teachers from non-biological disciplines complained about the infringement on their class time. Another problem involved scheduling the measurements so that minimum class disruption occurred. When students attempted to adhere to a rigid interval of three

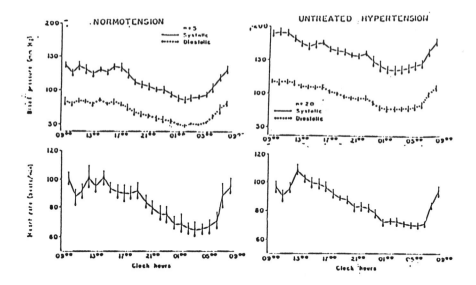

FIG. 4. Hourly mean systolic and diastolic blood pressure in untreated hypertension (20 patients) and in normotensives (5 patients). Also illustrated is mean heart ratio (Miller-Craig, 1977).

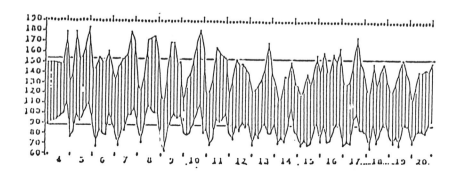

FIG. 5. Blood pressure measurements taken six times each day for 17 days in a 61-year-old patient. By conventional standards, this patient was normotensive every morning; yet, the blood pressure determined each day at 6 p.m. provides equally convincing evidence that he was hypertensive (Bartter, 1974).

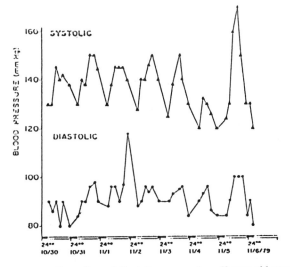

FIG. 6. Self-measurement of systolic and diastolic pressure by a 53-year-old executive. He was on medication at the time for hypertension. On the last day, he was chairman of an all-day meeting, which may account for the rather high peak in systolic and diastolic blood pressure on this day (Glasgow et al., 1982).

hours between measurements, the test frequently had to be done in the middle of a class period. Teachers who were not as fully informed as they might have been about "Operation Heartbeat" sometimes objected to the interruptions. These problems were solved later in the school year with the help of the high school principals by reducing the number of tests per session during the school week,

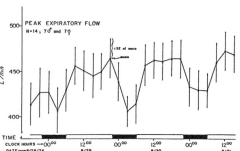

Figure 7

informing all teachers about the program, and requesting that the last five min. of class time be set aside for students to make their measurements.

Several recommendations are being made should this program be adopted. One is that students carry out the entire battery of measurements only on weekends and continue the reduced number during weekdays. The emphasis could be on vital signs such as oral temperature and blood pressure. Another recommendation is that biology teachers participating in "Operation Heartbeat" spend some time during and in-service meeting sharing ideas about implementation of the program. Some teachers had successful methods for minimizing equipment loss; other teachers had unique procedures for teaching students to make the measurements and record the data. Sharing these ideas will help all teachers do a better job if the program is to be officially implemented.

In general, it is the opinion of the author that the program went quite well considering it was the first year; certainly in the future, should the program be implemented, the logistics of conducting the tests should improve.

REFERENCES

1. Bartter, F. (1974): Periodicity and medicine. In: *Chronobiology,* edited by L.E. Scheving, F. Halberg and J.E. Pauly, pp. 6-13. Igaku Shion, Ltd., Tokyo.

2. Colquhoun, W.P. (1971): In: *Biological Rhythms and Human Performance,* edited by W.P. Colquhoun. Academic Press, London.

3. Folkard, S. (1980): In: *Chronobiology, Principles and Applications to Shifts in Schedules,* edited by L.E. Scheving and F. Halberg, pp. 293-306. Sijthoff and Noordhoff, The Netherlands.

4. Freeman, G.L. and Hovland, C.I. (1934): *Psychol. Bull.,* 31:777-138.

5. Gates, A.I. (1916) Univ. Calif. Pubs. In: *Psychology,* 21:1-156. Berkeley, California.

6. Glasgow, D.R., Scheving, L.E., Pauly, J.E. and Bruce, T.A. (1982): *J. Ark. Med. Soc.,* pp. 1-11.

7. Halberg, L.F., Johnson, E.A., Nelson, W., Runge, W. and Sothern, R. (1972): *Physiol. Teacher,* 1:1-11.

8. Halberg, F., Haus, E., Ahlgren, A., Halberg, F., Strobel, H., Angellar, A., Kuhl, J., Lucas, R., Gedgaudas, E. and Leong, J. (1974): In: *Chronobiology,* edited by L.E. Scheving, F. Halberg and J.E. Pauly, pp. 372-378. Igaku Shoin, Ltd., Tokyo.

9. Kanabrocki, E.L., Scheving, L.E., Halberg, F., Brewer, R.L. and Bird, T.L. (1973): *Space Life Sciences,* :258-270.

10. Kleitman, N. (1939): In: *Sleep and Wakefulness.* Univ. of Chicago Press. Chicago, Illinois.

11. Luce, G. (1970): In: *Biological Rhythms in Psychiatry and Medicine.* Public Health Service Publication, No. 2088, Supt. of Documents, U.S. Government Printing Office, Washington D.C. 20402.

12. Miller-Craig, M.W., Bishop, C. and Raftery, E.B. (1977) In: *Proceedings of 2nd Ints. Symposium on Ambulatory Monitoring,* edited by F.D. Stott, E.B. Raftery, P. Sleight and L. Goulding, pp. 133-141. Academic Press, Inc., London.

13. Palmer, J.D. (1976) In: *Introduction to Biological Rhythms.* pp. 137-138. Academic Press, Inc., New York.

14. Pauly, J.E., Scheving, L.E., Burns, E.R., Landon, J. and Stone, J.E. (1977) In: *The Int. Soc. Chronobiology XII International Conference Proceedings.* "Il Ponte", Milano, pp. 19-28.

15. Scheving, L.E., Roig, C. III, Halberg, F., Pauly, J.E. and Hand, E.A. (1974) In: *Chronobiology,* edited by L.E. Scheving, F. Halberg and J.E. Paul, pp. 353-357. Igaku Shion, Ltd., Tokyo.

16. Scheving, L.E., Enna, C.C., Halberg, F., Jacobsen, R.R., Mather, A. and Pauly, J.E. (1975): *Int. J. Leprosy,* 43:364-377.

17. Scheving, L.E. (1976): *Endeavor,* 35:66-72.

18. Scheving, L.E. (1978) In: *Proceedings of the 11th Collegium International Neuro-Psycho-Pharmacologicum (C.I.N.P.). Congress,* edited by B. Saletu, pp. 629-642. Pergamom Press Ltd., Oxford. Vienna, Austria.

Medical Monitoring in the Home and Work Environment,
edited by Laughton E. Miles and Roger J. Broughton.
Raven Press, New York © 1990.

BEHAVIORAL MONITORING WITH FEEDBACK
INTERVENTION

Kent F. Burnett and *C. Barr Taylor

Department of Counseling Psychology
University of Wisconsin-Madison
Madison, Wisconsin 53706
*Laboratory for the Study of Behavioral Medicine
Stanford University School of Medicine
Stanford, California 94305

INTRODUCTION

Behavioral scientists have established a number of behavior change principles that have been widely adopted for promoting positive changes in health-related behavior (1). These principles include: (a) reinforcement, (b) feedback, (c) goal-setting, and (d) contracting. Researchers have repeatedly demonstrated that interventions based on these principles are enhanced by the use of short-term goals, as opposed to distant goals, and by the use of immediate feedback mechanisms, as opposed to delayed feedback mechanisms (2,3,5). The recent availability of interactive ambulatory microcomputers has provided behavioral health counselors and behavioral medicine specialists with an opportunity to better integrate these behavior change principles with long-term monitoring of behavior in the natural environment. In this chapter, we review the efforts made by our group to develop long-term behavioral monitoring and feedback procedures that incorporate these behavior change principles.

LONG-TERM BEHAVIORAL MONITORING WITHOUT FEEDBACK

Our first goal was to develop methods for long-term monitoring of measures that are relevant to behavioral interventions. Our efforts focused on measuring sleep, physical activity and exercise, adherence to therapeutic regimens, and self-report.

Sleep Monitoring

All-night, laboratory-based polysomnography is the standard method used to evaluate persons experiencing sleep difficulties such as chronic insomnia. While polysomnography is without doubt the gold standard for sleep evaluation, the procedure is expensive and requires the patient to sleep in an unfamiliar setting under less than ideal conditions. As an alternative to laboratory-based polysomnography, home-based monitoring procedures have been developed which utilize a remote transmitting device, located in the patient's home, to send polysomnographic signals over the telephones lines back to the clinic. Home-based monitoring has the advantage of allowing the patient to sleep in familiar surroundings; however, the procedure is still very costly, requiring skilled technicians, not only in the laboratory, but also to travel to the home setting each night and morning to attach and unattach electrodes.

Research conducted using various methods for ambulatory recording of physical activity level has demonstrated the promise of activity monitoring as a less costly and less obtrusive method for evaluating the total sleep time of insomniacs (7). Although less accurate than polysomnography, many behavioral researchers believe that a less precise measure is acceptable for certain purposes, including documenting the process of therapeutic change in insomniacs participating in behavioral interventions.

In the late 1970's, cardiac rehabilitation and sleep researchers at Stanford explored the use of the "Vitalog"[1] for long-term monitoring of exercise, anxiety, sleep and "normal activity". The Vitalog is a microprocessor-based ambulatory solid-state device capable of continuously recording heart rate and physical activity level, as well as other physiological parameters, for periods of up to several weeks. The recorded data can be quickly transferred into a desktop microcomputer for data storage and analysis.

Burnett, et al. (6) determined the validity of the Vitalog, compared to polysomnographic recordings, for measuring sleep parameters. Nine insomniacs and two normal sleepers wore Vitalog devices continuously for a 60-hour period, during which time two consecutive all-night home polysomnographic recordings also were made. Heart rate and physical activity data collected using the Vitalog recordings were compared to the polysomnographic recordings using two methods. First, subjective ratings of sleep onset, wake-after-sleep onset, and final wake times were made by visual inspection of computer-generated histograms. Second, completely computer-generated estimates of sleep onset and final wake times were made using a software program called "VSTAT". The VSTAT program used a linear regression model to evaluate heart rate and physical activity level and to place each 5-minute data segment into one of four categories:

1. Exercise (high heart rate, high activity level)
2. Anxiety (high heart rate, low activity level)
3. Sleep or "Downtime" (low heart rate, low activity)
4. Normal activity

The mean absolute difference between sleep onset times judged by visual inspection of the heart rate and physical activity data and sleep onset times judged from the polysomnographic records was 10.6 minutes (SD = 8.8). The mean absolute difference between final wakes times as judged using these two methods was 7.5 minutes (SD = 7.4). The mean absolute difference between total wake-after-sleep-onset (WASO) times as judged using these two methods was 33 minutes (SD = 42.1). Although not

---

[1] "Vitalog" is a registered trademark of Vitalog Monitoring Inc., 643 Bair Island Road, Redwood City, California, 94063.

sufficiently precise for many sleep research applications, the sleep estimates made from visual inspection of the heart rate and physical activity level data appear to be within acceptable limits for the purposes of many behavior therapists. Clearly, the accuracy of the WASO estimates needs to be improved however.

The sleep estimates that were automatically computer-generated by the VSTAT program were within acceptable limits only for measuring final wake time (mean absolute difference 8.9 minutes, SD = 10.9). The VSTAT measures for sleep onset had a mean absolute difference of 16.4 minutes (SD = 25.3) when compared to the polysomnographic sleep onset estimates.

While subjective judgements based on visual inspection of the heart rate and physical activity level data proved superior to the completely computer-generated estimates made using VSTAT, we consider the results promising. Potentially, the algorithms used in the VSTAT program can be refined until acceptable levels of validity are achieved. In theory, the Vitalog could be used to measure WASO and total sleep time in remote locations for many nights of sleep.

Exercise Monitoring

Exercise physiologists have a long-standing interest in monitoring exercise in naturalistic settings. Ambulatory monitoring allows: (a) heart rate profiles to be evaluated and (b) patterns of adherence to exercise to be evaluated. A comparison of heart rate to activity, recorded and displayed in real time, allows meaningful evaluation of exercise sessions (8).

One specific interest has been to compare the physiological effects of various exercise regimens to determine if the same total caloric expenditure achieved at different exercise intensities reliably results in similar physiological changes. In one study, subjects were prescribed exercise sessions designed to elicit an energy expenditure of approximately 4 kcal/kg per session (9). This level of energy expenditure is associated with a reduced risk of mortality from coronary heart disease. Based on the heart rate-oxygen uptake relation during treadmill exercise testing, the time required to expend 4 kcal/kg at 65% of peak heart rate was calculated. For example, a subject whose oxygen uptake during treadmill testing was 20 ml/kg/min at 65% of peak heart rate would require 41 minutes of training time to expend 4 kcal/kg body weight.

Using the Vitalog for recording, we obtained nine days of ambulatory heart rate and physical activity recordings from each subject: three days at baseline, three days at 12 weeks into the exercise program, and three days at 24 weeks into the program. We found that the adherence to individually prescribed exercise training sessions, expressed by the integral of exercise intensity and duration was 108% in men and 90% in women. On average for men, heart rates exceeded prescribed limits for 9% of the prescribed period.

We are now using these monitoring techniques in a large community-based study involving over 340 men and women randomized to one of four exercise regimens. The sample will be followed for two years. We assume that there will be sufficient variance in adherence to use the sample to determine dose-effects of exercise.

Adherence to Therapeutic Regimens

The previous section illustrated the use of ambulatory microcomputers to monitor adherence to exercise in a research setting. Microcomputers also can be used to monitor adherence to other research and therapeutic regimens.

For example to determine the adherence to relaxation practice, 23 hypertensive patients receiving relaxation training were given tape recorders and a relaxation tape and were told to listen to the tape five or more times a week (10). Unbeknown to subjects, the tape recorder contained electronics designed to measure for up to 1 month when one of the tapes was turned on and off. From the outside, the tape recorders looked like standard portable cassette tape recorders. Inside, a microelectronic solid-state printed CMOS circuit with a clock, event counter, and memory had been placed. A microphone noted the beginning and ending of any 60 HZ sounds. The relaxation tapes were recorded with a superimposed 60 HZ sound which is inaudible to humans. Although self-report and computer-monitoring were significantly correlated, particularly during weeks 1-4 of therapy, subjects systematically overreported their practice in the next four weeks. The relationship between self-reported and computer-monitored frequency of practice sessions is illustrated in Figure 1.

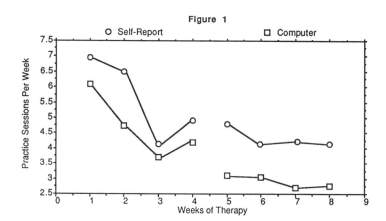

Figure 1

To determine a patients's adherence to medication usage, we developed a device which recorded the time that medication was taken from a dispenser. In one application, the device was used to establish that a patient had taken her medication as prescribed. Previous to this data collection, her physicians had doubted that she had been taking the medication. Influenced by the adherence data, and the apparent refractoriness of her hypertension in the face of the use of powerful antihypertensive medications, specific causes for her hypertension were reexplored and she was found to have renovascular hypertension. Surgical correction of her arteries resulted in normalization of her blood pressure.

Self-Report Data

Ambulatory self-report devices permit collection of self-report data in real time. In one application designed to study the phenomenology of panic attacks, we used a small hand-held computer to "beep" subjects on the hour. Subjects were then asked a series of questions related to their experience of anxiety; branching procedures were employed to determine the exact series of questions asked. The time of each response was stored along with the response itself continuously for one week. The data was then downloaded into a desk top computer for data storage and analysis[2]. In another application, we tied making self-reports to the occurrence of ischemic episodes noted on an ambulatory solid-state ST-segment monitoring device which the subjects were wearing. Subjects responded to a variety of questions about their activity, emotions, and psychological response to the device and symptoms.

REAL-TIME MONITORING PLUS SIMPLE FEEDBACK

In addition to using ambulatory computers to reliably monitor behavior, we also have explored the uses of ambulatory computers for providing feedback to the user. As part of our exercise studies, for instance, we programmed the Vitalog to provide feedback on the subject's heart rate range while exercising: exceeding the upper heart rate limit resulting in one tone; dropping below the heart rate range resulting in another tone. Devices employing simple feedback also can prompt client behavior in other ways. For instance, a pill dispensing device could indicate to the patient that medication has not been taken.

INTERACTIVE COMPUTER-ASSISTED THERAPY

Devices capable of real-time monitoring plus feedback, controlled by artifical intelligence programming, provide therapeutic tools capable of facilitating complex behavior change. In this section, we review the development of a diet and exercise training program, one of several interactive ambulatory computer-assisted therapy programs currently under development by our group.

Diet and Exercise Training: LBM-102 and CADET I

In 1981 behavioral scientists at Stanford University began development of a completely interactive ambulatory microcomputer system. The hardware that was developed weighed approximately two pounds and was capable of operating for up to 45 days without changing batteries. The system had a two-line liquid crystal screen, as well as an auditory signalling device, for providing feedback to the client. It also contained a keyboard for client input of self-observational data, and an eight channel analog-to-digital conversion chip, capable of sampling physiological indices. Because the system contained a real-time clock, all self-report and physiological data

---

[2] The program, called "Diary", is available from Behavioral Science Products, Inc., 451 Chaucer Street, Palo Alto, California 94301.

could be stored in memory together with the actual time and date of recording. These data could then be automatically transferred to a desktop microcomputer or scrolled across the screen of the ambulatory computer. The ambulatory computer was dubbed the "LBM-102", after the Laboratory for the Study of Behavioral Medicine at Stanford, which funded its development.

The LBM-102's debut came in 1983, when it was used to implement the "CADET I: Computer-Assisted Diet and Exercise Training"[3] program. The CADET I software was designed to aid obese clients in modifying their eating and physical activity patterns. The software permitted clients to enter codes and portion sizes for each food consumed throughout the day and to enter exercise codes along with the duration of each activity. Originally, a piezoelectric ceramic crystal transducer, an "accelerometer", had been developed for use in automatically monitoring exercise level; however, the LBM-102 prototype proved to be too bulky to use during exercise. As a result, a self-monitoring scheme was developed and validated against heart rate and physical activity data collected from subjects who wore Vitalog ambulatory monitors.

After a baseline monitoring period, the client using CADET I and the LBM-102 device was able to interactively set daily caloric intake limits and exercise goals. During this treatment phase, CADET I displayed both quantitative and qualitative feedback on goal attainment level following each client report. Feedback also could be obtained "on demand" by pressing the appropriate key on the computer keyboard.

Qualitative feedback consisted of personalized, reinforcing messages displayed on the screen following client self-reports that indicated controlled eating or progress toward exercise goals. Positively-worded, corrective instructions were displayed whenever self-reports indicated a pattern of eating that would be unlikely to result in goal attainment. The algorithms that governed the display of messages were based on expert opinion regarding the type of feedback that a therapist might provide--if it were feasible to "tag along" with the client 24 hours per day.

Because clients often forget to make self-reports after engaging in target behaviors, the LBM-102 was programmed to emit an audible signal (a "beep") every fours throughout the day and early evening hours to prompt the client to enter any eating and exercise data that had not already been entered. Although initially some clients found the audible prompt objectionable, almost all clients came to greatly rely on the prompting system to help them remember their therapeutic goals. One client stated that she kept the LBM-102 in her office drawer during work hours, but could still plainly hear the signal just prior to lunch. The signal became a reminder not only to make reports, but to carefully plan a healthful, low-calorie lunch. Another client reported that while watching television in the evening, she often had thoughts of having ice cream as a snack. After hearing the signal from the computer, she would instead select a low-calorie snack.

---

[3] "CADET" versions I-III and "CADET: Computer-Assisted Diet and Exercise Training" are registered trademarks of Behavioral Science Products, Inc., 451 Chaucer Street, Palo Alto, California 94301.

In a preliminary investigation (5), the short-term weight change of six obese female subjects who used CADET I was compared to the weight change of six matched subjects who attempted to lose weight using traditional paper-and-pencil self-monitoring and goal-setting procedures. During eight postbaseline study weeks, the mean weight loss for the CADET I subjects was 8.1 pounds (SD = 2.7) compared with 3.3 pounds (SD = 3.2) for the control subjects t(5) = 2.62, p < .05. The mean weight loss at eight months posttreatment for the CADET I subjects was 17.7 pounds (SD = 13.8) compared with 2.3 pounds (SD = 7.3) for the control subjects, t(5) = 3.80, p < .01. The outcome data are illustrated in Figure 2.

Figure 2

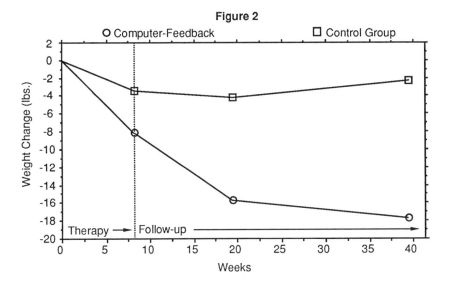

The mean short-term weight loss of 1 pound per week for the CADET I subjects was comparable to that achieved in other research using clinic-based behavioral interventions conducted by human therapists. Perhaps even more important was the fact that subjects who participated in the CADET I program continued to lose weight during the eight months after their computers were returned to the clinic. This suggests that the intensive daily feedback provided by CADET I helped them to learn important self-control skills that were well-maintained despite the absence of continued computer feedback.

CADET II

Development of the "CADET II: Computer-Assisted Diet and Exercise Training" program was completed in 1985. CADET II was designed to run on a commercially-available hand-held computer (Casio PB-700). The PB-700 weighed only 11-ounces and featured a four-line-by-20 character liquid crystal display and 16K of random access memory. This compared favorably to the two-line display, 12K memory, and heavier weight of the LBM-102 prototype devices used for the CADET I program. Several program features were included in the CADET II program that simply were not feasible given the limited memory of the earlier hardware.

One added feature permitted the user to ask "What if..." questions such as "What will my snack calorie total be if I consume this slice of chocolate cake?". In fact, the entire day's menu and exercise agenda could be strategically planned each morning using this feature. The CADET II program also had a "Slim Thoughts" feature that permitted the user to develop, edit, and display a series of motivational statements. The software was accompanied by a printed instruction manual and an audiotaped guided tour that included models for how to create positive motivational statements.

Another new feature was the "Pacer", a software clock, that was designed to help the user avoid rushing through meals. The Pacer could be set to begin counting down from any desired interval. Relaxation instructions and the "time remaining" were intermittently displayed on the screen until a signal was sounded when the countdown ended. Finally, the CADET II program was capable of utilizing its screen to depict the most recent 14 days of food, exercise, and bodyweight data. This data could be displayed either as a series of line graphs or in tabular format.

Currently, the CADET II program is being tested with several hundred subjects in research projects located at both Stanford University and the University of Wisconsin-Madison. Various monitoring schedules and levels of auxiliary therapeutic support are being systematically evaluated. Preliminary data analyses indicate that the program is most effective when subjects are instructed to monitor seven days per week as opposed to only four days per week or four-to-seven days per week. Auxiliary group support does not appear to be necessary for individuals to succeed in the program.

In addition, a subsample of the research subjects used a modified version of the program that was designed to transparently track and store the frequency of use of each program feature selected by the subject. These data are now being evaluated using regression analyses to determine which program features are most associated with positive outcomes. The use of an ambulatory microcomputer for program delivery has enabled researchers for the first time to evaluate actual behavioral predictors of therapeutic outcome. Previous research has had to rely primarily upon self-report measures regarding level of usage of specific treatment components.

The Future of the CADET Approach

Based upon our experience with CADET I and II, as well as technological advances in hardware, work recently has been completed on CADET III[4]. The CADET III program features an on-line food item dictionary that includes both calorie and fat values for each food item. Previous versions of the CADET program required the user to manually look-up and enter either calorie values or food code numbers. The CADET III program also includes a greatly enhanced library of positive feedback and corrective instruction statements and a much more elaborate set of rules governing their display. The program also is considerably more

---

[4] The CADET III program is available from Behavioral Science Products, Inc., 451 Chaucer Street, Palo Alto, California 94301.

intelligent. Users who do not make satisfactory progress at one level of the program are automatically shifted to a different set of contingencies.

The CADET approach also has been suggested as appropriate for the treatment of overweight persons suffering from non-insulin dependent diabetes (4). Although the current versions of the CADET program can be used for this purpose, a future version of the CADET program is planned that will incorporate American Dietetic Association food exchange information for each food item.

SUMMARY

Monitoring of client/patient behavior in real-life settings is a commonly used clinical evaluation technique employed by behavioral health counselors and behavioral medicine specialists. We have found that ambulatory microcomputers can be used to efficiently and relatively unobtrusively aid in the monitoring process, both in the long-term collection of physiological data and in gathering self-report information from clients/patients regarding their thoughts, feelings, and actions. In addition to these clinical monitoring functions, the use of interactive ambulatory computers to provide immediate, goal-related feedback to clients/patients during the course of their normal daily routines is viewed as a major advance in behavioral intervention methodology.

REFERENCES

1. Agras, W.S. (1987): So Where Do We Go From Here? *Behavior Therapy*, 18:203-217.

2. Bandura, A. (1969): *Principles of Behavior Modification.* Holt, Rhinehart and Winston, New York.

3. Bandura, A. and Simon, K.M. (1977): The Role of Proximal Intentions in Self-Regulation of Refractory Behavior. *Cognitive Therapy and Research*, 1:177-193.

4. Burnett, K.F. Taylor, C.B., and Agras, W.S. (1987): Computer-Assisted, Management of Weight, Diet, and Exercise in the Treatment of Type II Diabetes. *The Diabetes Educator*, 13:234-236.

5. Burnett, K.F., Taylor, C.B., and Agras, W.S. (1985): Ambulatory Computer-Assisted Therapy for Obesity: A New Frontier for Behavior Therapy. *J. Consult. Clin. Psychol.*, 53:698-703.

6. Burnett, K.F., Taylor, C.B, Thoresen, C.E., Rosekind, M.R., Miles, L. and DeBusk, R.F. (1985): Toward Computerized Scoring of Sleep Using Ambulatory Recordings of Heart Rate and Physical Activity. *Behav. Assess.*, 7:261-271.

7. Kripke, D.F., Mullaney, D.J., Messin, S. and Wyborney, V.G. (1978): Wrist Actigraphic Measures of Sleep and Rhythms. *Electroenceph. Clin. Neurophysiol.*, 44:674-676.

8. Mueller, K.J., Gossard, D., Adams, F.R., Taylor, C.B, Haskell, W.L., Kraemer, H.C., Ahn, D.K., Burnett, K.F. and DeBusk, R.F. (1986): Assessment of Prescribed Increases in Physical Activity: Application of a New Method for Microprocessor Analysis of Heart Rate. *Amer. J. Cardiol.*, 57:441-445.

9. Rogers, F., Juneau, M. Taylor, C.B., Haskell, W.L. Kraemer, H.C., Ahn, D.K. and DeBusk. R.F. (1987): Assessment by a Microprocessor of Adherence to Home-Based Moderate-Intensity Exercise Training in Healthy, Sedentary Middle-Aged Men and Women. *Amer. J. Cardiol.*, 60:71-75.

10. Taylor, C.B., Agras, W.S., Schneider, J.A. and Allen, R.A. (1983): Adherence to Instructions to Practice Relaxation Exercises. *J. Consult. Clin. Psychol.*, 51:952-953.

Medical Monitoring in the Home and Work Environment,
edited by Laughton E. Miles and Roger J. Broughton.
Raven Press, New York © 1990.

HOME MODIFICATION OF SLEEP POSITION
FOR SLEEP APNEA CONTROL

Rosalind D. Cartwright

Rush-Presbyterian-St. Luke's Medical Center
1653 West Congress Parkway
Chicago, Illinois   60615

INTRODUCTION

That sleep in an all-night monitoring laboratory may not be a good representative sample of home sleep has long been recognized. This was first noted in the research literature as a "first night" effect (1). This term referred to the observation that sleep onset was often longer, and sleep efficiency lower on the first than on subsequent nights of recorded sleep. Assuming that this was the result of some anxiety associated with the unfamiliar environment, it became a standard procedure to allow a night of adaptation preceeding nights of any serious data collection. This caution has been generally abandoned in clinical sleep recordings. In clinical studies the issue is more often the presence and frequency of some abnormal events, such as apneic pauses in respiration or muscle twitching of the legs that are calculated on a per hour of sleep basis. It has been assumed that the delayed onset or lowered sleep efficiency would not interfere with a good estimate of these events as experienced at home. In the case of sleep apnea, the commonest of the disorders seen in the clinical sleep services, this assumption can be very misleading.

In a survey of 184 sleep apnea patients recorded for one night in our laboratory, diagnosed by the standard procedure (2), 111 or 60% were found to be sleep position sensitive (4). This designation is given to any patient whose rate of apneic plus hypopneic events per hour of supine sleep is two or more times the rate when they are sleeping in the lateral position. Repeated nights have confirmed that, over a one month period, this is a stable patient characteristic (3). Given this finding, a majority of apnea patients are more severely affected when they sleep on their backs, and given the constraints on free movement many experience in the laboratory due to the monitoring electrodes, sleep in the supine position is often over represented. This can seriously inflate the overall apnea+hypopnea index (A+HI), with respect to the patient's usual home sleep.

There are several ways this problem could be approached: 1) Reassure the patient about their freedom of movement prior to sleep and record their time in each major sleep position. Calculate apneic indicies for lateral and supine sleep separately. 2) Require patients to spend multiple nights in the laboratory to adapt them before diagnosing the severity of their disorder. 3) Have patients sleep half the night supine and half in the lateral position by waking them to request a position change if they have remained supine. 4) Monitor patients at home using a position monitor that accumulates time by position and adjust the severity estimate obtained in the laboratory on the basis of these data. The first of these is the simplest and the one all laboratories can do with no further equipment and at no further expense or inconvenience for the patient. This procedure has been standard in our laboratory for many years. Sleep position can be recorded manually on the record by the technician observing via a video monitor, or automatically through a position sensitive device worn by the patient on the chest. This is interfaced with the polygraph to activate an event marker which registers, by a coded signal, the period of time in supine, prone, right and left lateral positions.

Once it is established that the patient has a significant increase in the rate of respiratory events when sleeping in the supine position, the possibility of reducing his apnea through home training to avoid this position becomes viable. This has been done by introducing an alarm into the posture monitor which sounds whenever the patient assumes the back position for more than 15 seconds. By adding a digital counter that sums the total number of times the alarm was activated during the night, a home sleep position trainer is available for testing. Patients then can record their own progress in learning to sleep from side to side by logging their number of alarms each morning before resetting the counter to zero for the next night. Patients are then restudied in the laboratory for two nights. On night one, the patient is recorded with the alarm activated to compare the number of signals needed to avoid supine sleep in the laboratory to the home log. This tells whether the training has generalized to other sleep environments. On a second night without the alarm, it can be shown whether the training has been completed or if the patient still needs the reinforcement of the signal to avoid supine sleep. The data from both nights can help determine if the apnea has been significantly reduced by this training.

PATIENT STUDY OF SLEEP POSITION TRAINING

Recently twenty male patients diagnosed as having mild to severe apnea (A+HI 12-75) on an all night basis, who met the positional criterion, agreed to use the posture alarm for eight weeks at home every night, to log their number of alarms, and return to the laboratory to be restudied for two nights of polysomnography, one with the alarm activated and one with the alarm silent. Table 1 gives the number of minutes of sleep recorded in the supine position for the three laboratory nights (one the diagnostic, and two after eight weeks of home treatment), the number of alarms recorded at home averaged for week one and week eight, and the number of alarms recorded in the laboratory during the signal "on" night. Table 2 gives the A+HI on an all night basis and separately for time in the side and back sleep position on the diagnostic night and the all night rate after training (prone sleep time was rare and deleted for the sake of comparability).

TABLE 1. <u>Minutes of Supine Sleep Before and Following Home Training</u>

Subject	Minutes Night 1	Signal "On"	Signal "Off"	Average Home Wk 1	Signals Wk 8	N Lab Signals "On"
1	202.5	0.0	0.0	0.3	0.4	0.0
2	115.5	0.0	0.0	1.7	0.3	0.0
3	230.0	1.0	57.0	30.0	16.8	3.0
4	112.5	0.0	0.0	3.0	1.0	0.0
5	45.0	0.0	29.0	9.8	4.0	5.0
6	181.0	0.0	110.5	5.5	2.1	0.0
7	61.5	0.0	58.5	8.4	11.2	1.0
8	108.0	0.0	0.0	4.0	0.6	0.0
9	50.5	4.0	0.5	7.0	0.0	0.0
10	137.5	0.0	30.5	6.6	2.2	0.0
11	26.5	0.0	0.0	1.0	0.4	0.0
12	120.0	0.0	0.0	3.0	0.6	0.0
13	114.0	0.0	11.5	6.9	1.0	1.0
14	138.0	0.0	18.0	18.6	15.0	3.0
15	62.0	1.0	0.0	25.8	0.3	1.0
16	325.5	0.0	3.5	0.5	0.7	1.0
17	107.5	0.0	172.0	19.0	25.2	0.0
18	37.0	0.0	55.0	6.8	11.4	0.0
19	44.0	0.0	0.0	8.1	6.8	5.0
20	43.0	0.0	0.0	1.7	0.1	0.0
Mean	113.08	0.30	27.30	8.39	5.01	1.00
S.D.	75.92	0.92	45.20	8.45	7.15	1.65

After home training, supine sleep time is significantly reduced even on the night without the signal. All patients had less than five minutes of supine sleep with the signal on and without it, 11 patients had less than five minutes of supine sleep. Looking at the average number of signals recorded at home on week one and week eight, showed learning did occur. The group seems to divide naturally into those who learned rapidly, a group of slow learners, and those who continued to have high signal counts throughout the eight weeks of training (See Table 3).

Turning to the nights of laboratory recording following training we find that all the rapid learners at home also had low signal counts their night with the signal "On." Some who were slow to learn at home showed that they had mastered side sleeping in the laboratory where they may have been responsive to the positive reinforcement of the expectation to perform well. Even those who did not learn at home had much lower signal counts in the laboratory. These patients were also the most clinically severe.

TABLE 2. <u>**A+HI All Night and By Position for Diagnostic and Post Training Nights**</u>

	Diagnostic Night 1			Night 2 Total "On" A+HI	Night 3 Total "Off" A+HI
	Total A+HI	Back A+HI	Side A+HI		
1	22.2	43.5	0.0	0.3	0.2
2	12.5	35.8	1.3	0.0	0.0
3	74.5	101.5	12.6	7.3	36.4
4	15.0	27.7	8.7	57.4	43.2
5	16.7	98.7	1.0	0.2	7.0
6	19.7	31.2	5.6	6.4	14.1
7	52.9	96.6	37.1	38.3	25.0
8	16.6	35.0	16.6	5.0	2.7
9	15.5	35.9	11.5	5.3	1.1
10	21.9	34.0	3.4	1.1	17.1
11	23.5	67.9	13.8	2.6	23.7
12	46.8	72.0	4.2	0.0	0.0
13	29.4	60.0	16.5	4.3	30.0
14	37.9	83.5	7.3	36.4	8.7
15	44.8	106.5	32.1	36.2	59.4
16	19.6	23.2	0.0	2.1	2.1
17	65.4	103.8	45.1	2.2	11.5
18	19.7	61.6	14.2	3.2	13.5
19	61.6	170.5	35.9	16.7	20.7
20	18.8	87.9	5.4	7.6	4.3
Mean	31.75	68.84	13.62	11.63	16.04
S.D.	19.16	37.55	13.52	16.53	16.31

TABLE 3. <u>**Speed of Home Learning: Number of Lab Signals, and A+HI on "Off" Signal Night**</u>

Rapid Learners			Slow Learners			Did Not Learn		
Pt No	Lab Sig	A+HI "Off"	Pt No	Lab Sig	A+HI "Off"	Pt No	Lab Sig	A+HI "Off"
1	0	.2	3	3	36.4	7	1	25.0
2	0	2.2	5	5	7.0	14	3	8.7
4	0	43.2	6	0	14.1	17	0	11.5
11	0	23.7	8	0	2.7	18	0	13.5
12	0	0.0	9	0	1.1	19	5	20.7
16	1	2.1	10	0	17.1			
20	0	4.3	13	1	30.0			
			15	1	59.4			

DOES THE HOME TRAINING HELP TO REDUCE SLEEP APNEA?

When patients sleep without the alarm in the laboratory, the A+HI of five of seven rapid learners was within normal limits. Two of the eight slow learners were within normal limits; but none of those who failed to improve their signal count at home reached this level of control in the laboratory without the help of the alarm. Eleven patients reduced their apnea index 50% or more on both post-treatment nights,and five more reached this level only with the continued help of the signal. This suggests that further home training might be helpful to bring them under control. Of the four patients who were not improved by home position training, numbers 4, 7, 15, and 19, two were massively obese (over 350 pounds), and two had some difficulty hearing the signal.

CONCLUSIONS

In many patients sleep apnea is positional, with two or more times the rate of respiratory difficulties when they sleep supine. Some laboratories may be over-diagnosing these patients due to the patients feeling constrained to remain supine by the monitoring equipment. After eight weeks of home training, eleven of 20 positional patients had less than five minutes of supine sleep without the help of the position signal. Sixteen reduced their A+HI by at least 50% with no other treatment, and eleven reached this level of success without the signal being turned on. Some patients learned to avoid the signal more rapidly than others, and had a more complete remission of sleep symptoms. Two factors lead to a poor response: massive obesity and difficulty hearing the signal. If these factors are introduced into the selection of patients for position training, most apneic patients who are more severely affected in the supine position can learn to sleep from side to side and so reduce their respiratory disorder to acceptable levels. Home training of sleep posture is a simple, rapid option for reducing the number of apneic events in those that are posture sensitive.

Learning to sleep only in the lateral position with the posture alarm at home appears to depend largely upon avoidance conditioning. The feedback cue of the buzzer is aversive. Once sleeping from side to side has been learned there is also the positive reinforcement of feeling better in the morning to help sustain it. Home learning of this skill does not predict laboratory performance since even those patients who did not do well at home performed well during the signal "on" night. The laboratory is a very different learning environment than the home. Here, not only does the avoidance conditioning come into play, but also the pre-sleep social expectations that the subjects will perform well. These seem to heighten the patients ability to monitor their sleep position throughout the night. In the absence of these added social cues at home not all patients did perform as well.

Just as there is a first night effect creating differences between laboratory and "natural" home sleep, the learning situation in the laboratory is unlike the home situation. This underlines the need for the testing of learned behaviors to be done under the same circumstances that the performance must be carried out: at home.

ACKNOWLEDGMENTS

This study was supported by a grant from the National Institutes of Health, # HLB HL36252.

REFERENCES

1. Agnew, H., Webb, W., and Williams, R. (1966): The First Night Effect: An EEG Study of Sleep. *Psychophysiology*, 2:263-266.

2. Bornstein, S. (1982): Respiratory Monitoring During Sleep: Polysomnography In: *Sleeping and Waking Disorders: Indications and Techniques.* edited by Guilleminault, C., pp. 183-212. Addison-Wesley. Menlo Park, California.

3. Cartwright, R. (1984): Effect of Sleep Position on Sleep Apnea Severity. *Sleep*, 7:110-114.

4. Lloyd, S. and Cartwright, R. (1987): Physiologic Basis of Therapy for Sleep Apnea. Letter to the editor. *American Review of Respiratory Disease,* 136:525-526.

Medical Monitoring in the Home and Work Environment,
edited by Laughton E. Miles and Roger J. Broughton.
Raven Press, New York © 1990.

CONTINUOUS MONITORING OF SLEEPINESS

Torbjorn Akerstedt

IPM and Karolinska Institute
Box 60205, S-10401 Stockholm, Sweden

INTRODUCTION

The concept of sleepiness has recently received considerable attention in relation to various sleep/wake disorders and accident risk (2). This has brought about the need for methods of objective measurement of sleepiness, particularly in normal life situations with subjects being able to move about freely, at work and at home. This paper will review some techniques in this area.

SLEEPINESS

The concept of sleepiness is not very clearly defined. Normally, however, it seems to refer to signs that indicate a tendency towards sleep (13). At moderate levels of sleepiness these signs may include a feeling of slowing down, of reduced activity, or of a need to yawn (19). Higher levels may include itching of the eyes, an inability to concentrate, some difficulty remaining awake or in keeping one's eyes open, etc. At the end of the scale, sleep intrudes and purposeful interaction with the environment ceases. This common sense conception involves subjective as well as behavioral and physiological components. Thus, whereas many would associate "sleepiness" with a subjective state, it still seems reasonable to include also physiology and behavior in the definition.

Most of the existing knowledge about sleepiness has been based on self-rating techniques. Such techniques do, however, have limitations with respect to validity and with respect to the possibility to capture moment to moment fluctuations. Performance measures present similar problems and can hardly be said to indicate sleepiness *per se* (although certainly the consequences of it). Other, more physiologically oriented techniques may be evoked potentials, pupillography and critical flicker fusion. None of these, however, can easily be used to monitor sleepiness continuously. In our opinion the only technique that objectively does that would be the polysomnographic methods used to monitor sleep. This will be discussed further below.

POLYSOMNOGRAPHY

Sleep and wakefulness are mainly defined by polysomnographic parameters. These include brain waves (EEG), eye movements (EOG) and muscle tonus (EMG) in the chin (35). Frequently also body movements, breathing and other parameters are recorded. The main parameter, however, is always the EEG. Traditionally, the recording instrument has been the EEG machine or the polygraph, often combined with a tape recorder. This equipment is bulky and has for a long time tied the user of the polysomnographic method to the laboratory and kept him away from many real life issues. The telemetric technique made it possible to move outside the laboratory but it still makes heavy demands on resources for obtaining the signal from the subject. Recent developments of subject worn recorders have, however, made it possible to obtain data without any supervision at all. This has made it feasible to begin to answer questions about sleep and wakefulness in real life settings.

The traditional analysis of sleep and wakefulness is done visually, based on one or two EEG derivations (35). The EEG content is divided into epochs and classified into sleep stages 0-4 and REM (rapid eye movement sleep). Stages 0-4 represent a continuous scale from wakefulness to deep sleep. The visual method has provided large amounts of data on sleep and wakefulness. Nevertheless, the method is crude and the human being is unable to make use of more than a fraction of the variability of the EEG. The alternative is automatic (computer) analysis (36). Several methods exist and are often highly correlated. Here we will focus on spectral analysis.

Spectral analysis divides the EEG pattern into its component frequencies, usually by application of the fast Fourier transform (FFT). The resulting spectrum (amplitude or power) may be integrated across the frequencies of interest - for example, into 1-Hertz bands or into the delta, theta, etc. bands. The major advantage of the automatic methods is that they quantify (background) EEG activity much faster and with enormously greater amounts of information than what is possible by visual analysis. The output may be used to obtain a continuous scale of EEG activity instead of the six (or seven) stages of traditional sleep/wake analysis.

In our own studies we use portable recording equipment with miniature preamplifiers close to the electrodes. This make it possible to record the EEG/EOG of individuals in their normal daily activities. We often record for 24 hour periods and afterwards subject the EEG to spectral analysis (FFT) in 7.5 second intervals (39). This is done at 30 times the recording speed which makes it feasible to analyze a 24 hour recording in less than one hour.

RATIONALE

The first EEG descriptions of the process of falling asleep were reported by Loomis et al. (27-29). They showed that relaxed subjects lying with closed eyes showed a predominant alpha (8-12Hz) activity and responded to environmental stimuli. When alpha started to break up, however, the subjects ceased to respond. Further progression showed that the EEG frequency decreased into the theta (2-8Hz) and, later, the delta

(0-2Hz) range, i.e., into sleep proper. In other studies it has been shown that the disappearance of alpha "downwards" towards the theta range coincides with the loss of muscle tonus (7) and with a feeling of "drifting away" (11). Similar results have been obtained by Simon and Emmons (38), Kamiya (21), Kuhlo and Lehmann (22) and Liberson and Liberson (24).

Not only closure of the eyelids but also the movement of the eye is related to EEG changes, Usually, slow (0.1-0.6 Hz) eye movements (SEMs) start to appear when the alpha activity breaks up and the subject begins to "drift off" (21,22,24,35,38). As sleep is more firmly established the slow eye movements begin to disappear, although they may sometimes remain for a while in Stage 2.

The above results clearly indicate that significant EEG/EOG changes characterize the falling asleep process. This observation has been exploited by Carskadon and Dement (9) who defined sleepiness as the tendency to fall asleep, operationalized as the latency from the intention to sleep until sleep (theta activity-Stage 1) eventually occurs. This sleep latency technique is now an established clinical test of sleepiness; but it does not, however, provide for continuous monitoring of that state. Nevertheless, its rationale - equating sleepiness with some propensity for sleep to occur - may also be applied to continuous monitoring of sleepiness.

Using another approach, Bjerner (5), showed that exceptionally long reaction times were associated with alpha blocking (decrease) towards theta, and interpreted this as "transient phenomena of the same nature as sleep". A similar connection between alpha disappearance and vigilance omissions has been demonstrated by Williams et al. (44), Mirsky and Cardon (30) and Davis and Krkovic (10). Similarly, Guilleminault et al. (16,17) have demonstrated in narcoleptics that inadequate performance was associated with intrusion of theta activity. Other studies have found that the duration of alpha activity after eye closure decreases with increasing sleep loss, fatigue and performance deterioration (3,6,32,37). The disappearing alpha activity is usually replaced by theta activity.

It should be emphasized that the above studies have used relaxed and closed-eyes conditions, in which case the presence of alpha signals alertness. If the eyes are open, however, this is reversed (10). In a rather detailed study of simulated radar watching O'Hanlon and Beatty (33) showed a high correlation between a measure of poor performance ("sweeps" to detect the target) and the % theta, % alpha, and % beta activity in the EEG. The authors particularly emphasize the need to include several EEG bands, since alpha activity may change either upwards or downwards, indicating increase or decrease, indicating increased and arousal, respectively.

In our own work we have tried to demonstrate changes in spectral parameters as a function of dozing off while active (40). In this study the subjects performed a visual vigilance task for 45 minutes. During the session the subject's face was videotaped and all instances of dozing off (closed eyes and a lowering of the head, usually ended by a jerk into wakefulness) were scored. Alpha and theta power increased 6 and 3-fold, respectively, from hit to dozing off. Missed signals fell in between. Slow eye movements also increased strongly prior to dozing off.

In a somewhat different approach eight subjects spent a night in the laboratory from 2300 hr to 1100hr, being awake all the time (2). Every two hours they sat down and focussed on a spot on the wall for 5 minutes. The session in which the subjects reported maximum subjective sleepiness showed 3-fold increases in alpha and theta power compared the baseline alertness. Slow eye movements (with eyes open) were not observed during the alert session, whereas sleepiness caused almost continuous slow eye movements. All three variables correlated highly (intra-individually) between themselves and with rated sleepiness.

The results above indicate that it should be possible to use EEG/EOG indices for continuous measurement of intrusions of sleep or sleep like states. Whether such intrusions should be called sleepiness or not may be debated. If, however, one defines sleepiness as a tendency to fall asleep (13) the sleep intrusions must represent at least *manifest sleepiness*, i.e. the outcome of latent (true) sleepiness on the one hand and situational factors influencing latent sleepiness (physical work load, mental work load, consequences of performance failures, etc.) on the other.

APPLIED STUDIES WITH RESTRICTED SUBJECTS

The laboratory approaches described above have been extended to different worklike situations. As one example, Lecret and Pottier (23) recorded the EEG from eight car drivers. They used a bi-occipital electrode derivation, recording via head-worn amplifiers and a tape recorder. The EEG was band pass filtered for the alpha frequency and yielded an alpha index (time with alpha). On the whole, the amounts of alpha increased with decreasing levels of stimulation, the early part of the drive showing less alpha than later parts, as did city driving as compared to rural driving. Blinkings as monitored by a vertical EOG were fewest during city driving and early in driving.

Caille and Bassano (8) studied four subjects during night driving with different amounts of carbon monoxide. The EEG was recorded telemetrically via frontoparietal and parieto-occipital derivations (also EOG was recorded). The data were analyzed with spectral analysis as well as with other methods. Towards the end of driving, alpha bursts frequently appeared, followed by theta and sometimes sigma waves (apparent microsleep episodes).

O'Hanlon and Kelley (34) carried out one of the rare attempts to correlate continuous performance (night driving) with continuously recorded EEG parameters. They recorded a parieto-occipital derivation with amplification close to the electrodes. The EEG was bandpass filtered into the usual frequency bands. The results showed that mainly poor drivers increased their power in the alpha band over the duration of the drive and for monotonous segments (lane-drifting). The authors also observed several cases of subjects apparently falling asleep while driving. It was also concluded that the alpha band is sensitive to changes in medium alertness while the theta and delta bands are necessary for distinguishing lower ranges of arousal.

Fruhstorfer et al. (14) applied spectral analysis to various EEG derivations from three subjects driving at night. The results (preliminary) showed a clear increase in alpha power during monotonous segments, as well as occasional theta bursts and a 14-18 Hz activity which "was not sleep spindles". Interestingly, blink duration increased and EOG velocity decreased in connection with the increase of alpha. No correlations were presented, however.

In our own studies we have looked at the development of spectral power density over a night of continuous activity in ambulatory subjects (2). Alpha and theta power increased significantly across the night. Furthermore, ratings of sleepiness (two-hourly) correlated highly with both indices.

FIELD STUDIES WITH AMBULATORY MONITORING

The techniques described above have also been brought to actual work situations in which the subjects have been allowed to move around freely. One early study by Adey et al. (1) concerned an astronaut on the Gemini flight GT-7. The data were mainly obtained from a vertex-occipital bipolar derivation and tape recorded. The data were analyzed by various computer techniques. With increasing flight time the power in the theta band increased and it was concluded that the EEG patterns "followed in excellent detail the fine aspects of transiently focussed attention or brief episodes of drowsiness or light sleep".

In a study of our own, we recorded the EEG and EOG of 11 train drivers during a 4.5-hour night or day trip, always along the same route (39). In order to illustrate the role of sleepiness we divided the drivers into those who reported severe sleepiness during the night drive and those who were barely affected. There was no difference between the groups during day driving. During night driving, on the other hand, alpha power rose significantly above day time levels for the sleepy group. This group also exhibited significantly higher night trip alpha power than the alert group. The results were very similar for theta power and slow eye movements. Self-rated fatigue (measured every half hour) paralleled the EEG data and exhibited high mean intra-individual correlations with all three variables. During day trips no significant correlations were found. The results clearly indicate that night work causes increased sleepiness, and that the degree of sleepiness is reflected in the EEG spectral content mainly in the alpha and theta bands as well as in slow eye movements.

In a second study we monitored the EEG and EOG for 24-hour spans in process operators working night and afternoon shifts (41). The results show increased amounts of alpha and theta activity during the night shift, as well as a 20% incidence of (inadvertent) napping during the night shift.

Apart from the studies cited above there is at least one further field study using similar techniques. One concerned helicopter pilots of the Swedish Air Force who exhibited pronounced increases in alpha power towards the end of 3-4 hour mission (26). No attempt, however, was made to relate the data to sleepiness or to performance lapses. In another study air traffic controllers were monitored during shift work (25). The EEGs were evaluated visually but no consistent conclusions could be drawn. In another visually evaluated study, Haslam (18) demonstrated an increase in alpha index in sleep deprived soldiers.

In this context it may also be pertinent to mention 24-hour recordings of clinical groups. De Groen et al. (12) and Zschocke et al. (45) have demonstrated the feasibility of long term monitoring of sleep attacks in narcoleptic and other patients.

FINAL COMMENTS

The EEG/EOG measures were found to be closely related to the indices of perceived sleepiness and performance. Thus, it seems that they should be useful for continuous monitoring of fluctuations of the sleepiness level. Nevertheless, one must bear in mind that one measures the manifest type of sleepiness, i.e. the sleepiness that is allowed expression by the particular conditions of the situation. It is, for example, likely that a sleep-deprived individual, with a high degree of latent sleepiness according to the sleep latency test, may be activated by a subsequent task to the extent that a continuous recording of EEG/EOG parameters during the task will fail to indicate sleepiness. On the other hand, the find of, for example, increased theta or alpha activity together with slow eye movements should be possible to interpret as increased sleepiness. It is, however, not clear to what extent such parameters may be used to quantify sleepiness in absolute terms as is possible with the MSLT.

A very important issue in this context concerns the ability to predict performance lapses using the polygraphic techniques. In particular, it is of interest to be able to predict accident risks. Even if the available data indicate high general correlations between performance and some EEG/EOG parameters, we still lack absolute criteria. We also lack systematic studies of the functional significance of particular EEG patterns. There are also indications that not only EEG patterns during a performance requirement are of importance, but also the patterns preceding it (43). Other problems that need to be addressed are why moderate variations of EEG patterns seem unrelated to performance lapses (42), and how to account for the fact that alpha and theta activity may be increased by arousing stimuli (15).

Another problem concerns individual differences. It seems that at least some alpha poor subjects do increase their alpha content with increasing sleepiness. We do not know, however, if this is a rule and we do not know to what extent comparable changes in alpha or theta activity mean that they are equally sleepy. It is also apparent that different subjects react with different EEG bands to sleepiness.

Nevertheless, irrespective of the interpretative problems long periods of continuous alpha and theta activity will indicate that the individual is asleep or falling asleep. This will clearly be important information in many work situations in which safety of individuals or property may be affected by the actions of an operation. Thus, continuous monitoring of EEG/EOG changes should be of great importance in identifying sleep(iness) inducing work environment factors. Shift work is, very likely, one major such factor. Process monitoring, vibrations, long work hours, infrasound may be others.

REFERENCES

1. Adey, W.R., Kado, R.T. and Walter, D.O. (1967): *Aerospace Med.*, 38:345-359.

2. Akerstedt, T., Torsvall, L. and Gillberg, M. (1985): In: *Sleep 1984*, edited by W.P. Koella, E. Ruther, and H. Schulz, pp. 88-89. Gustav Fischer, Verlag, Stuttgart.

3. Armington, J.C. and Mitnick, L.L. (1959): *J. Appl. Physiol.*, 14:247-250.

4. Aserinsky, E. and Kleitman, N. (1959): *Science*, 118:273-274.

5. Bjerner, B. (1949): *Acta Physiol. Scand.*, 19S:

6. Blake, H. and Gerard, R. (1937): *Am. J. Physiol,* 119:697-703.

7. Blake, H., Gerard, R.W. and Kleitman, N. (1939): *J. Neurophysiol.*, 2:48-60.

8. Caille, E.J. and Bassano, J.L. (1977): In *Vigilance*, edited by Mackie, R.R., pp. 59-72. Plenum Press, New York.

9. Carskadon, M.A. and Dement, W.C. (1982): *Sleep*, 5:567-572.

10. Daniel, R.S. (1967): *Perc. Mot. Skills,* 25:697-703.

11. Davies, D.R. and Krkovic, A. (1965): *Am. J. Psychol.*, 78:304-306.

12. De Groen, J.H.M., Koper, H., Bergs, P.P.E., Verheyen, M.J.N. and Caberg, H.B. (1985): *Electroencephalogr. Clin. Neurophysiol.*, 60:420-422.

13. Dement, W.C. and Carskadon, M.A. (1982): *Sleep*, 5:56-66.

14. Fruhstorfer, H., Langanke, P., Meinzer, K., Peter, J.H. and Pfaff, U. (1977): In: *Vigilance*,. edited by Mackie, R.R., pp. 147-162. Plenum Press, New York.

15. Gale, A. (1977): In: *Vigilance*, edited by Mackie, R.,R., pp. 263-285. Plenum Press, New York.

16. Guilleminault, C., Billiard, M., Montplaisir, J. and Dement, W. (1975): *J. Neurol. Sci.*, 26:377-393.

17. Guilleminault, C., Philips, R. and Dement, W. (1975): *Electroencephalogr. Clin. Neurophysiol.*, 38:403-413.

18. Haslam, D.R. (1982): *Ergonomics*, 25:163-178.

19. Hoddes, E., Zarcone, V., Smythe, H., Phillips, R. and Dement, W. (1973): *Psychophysiology*, 10:431-436.

20. Hori, T. (1982): *Psychophysiology*, 19:668-672.

21. Kamiya, J. (1961): *Functions of Varied Experience,* edited by D.W. Fiske and S.R. Maddi, pp. 145-174. Dorsey, Homewood-Illinois.

22. Kuhlo, W. and Lehmann, D. (1964): *Arch. Psychiat Z ges Neurol.*, 205:687-716.

23. Lecret, F. and Pottier, M. (1971): *Trav. Hum.*, 34:51-68.

24. Liberson, W.T. and Liberson, C.w. (1966): *Proc. Soc. Biol. Psychiat.*, 19:295-302.

25. Lille, F. and Cheliout, F. (1982): *Eur. J. Appl. Physiol.*, 49:319-328.

26. Lofstedt, P. Englund, K., Lindmark, A. and Landstrom, U. (1985): *Arbete och halsa*, 41:5-49.

27. Loomis, A.L., Harvey, E.N. and Hobart, G. (1937): *J. Exp. Psychol.*, 21:127-144.

28. Loomis, A.L., Harvey, E.N. and Hobart, G. (1936): *J. Exp. Psychol.*, 19:249-279.

29. Loomis, A.L., Harvey, E.N. and Hobart, G. (1935): *Science*, 81:597-598.

30. Mirsky, A.F. and Cardon, P.V. (1962): *Electroencephalogr. Clin. Neurophysiol.*, 14:1-10.

31. Mitler, M.M., Carskadon, M.A., Czeisler, C.A., Dement, W.C., Dinges, D.F. and Graeber, R.C. (1988): *Sleep*, 11:100-109.

32. Naitoh, P., Kales, A., Kollar, E.J., Smith, J.C. and Jacobson, A. (1969): *Electroencephalogr. Clin. Neurophysiol.*, 27:2-11.

33. O'Hanlon, J.F. and Beatty, J. (1977): In: *Vigilance*, edited by Mackie, R.R., pp. 189-202. Plenum Press, New York.

34. O'Hanlon, J.F. and Kelley, G.R. (1977): In: *Vigilance*, edited by Mackie, R.R., pp. 189-202. Plenum Press, New York.

35. Rechtschaffen, A. and Kales, A. (1968): A manual of standardized terminology, techniques, and scoring system for sleep stages of human subjects, *Brain Information Service.*

36. Remond, A. (1977): *EEG Informatics,* Elsevier, Amsterdam.

37. Rodin, R.A., Luby, E.D. and Gottlieb, J.S. (1962): *Electroencephalogr. Clinc. Neurophysiol.*, 14:544-551.

38. Simon, C.W. and Emmons, W.H. (1956): *J. Exp. Psychol.*, 51:89-97.

39. Torsvall, L. and Akerstedt, T. (1987): *Electroencephalogr. Clin. Neurophysiol.*, 66:502-511.

40. Torsvall, L. and Akerstedt, T. (1988): *Intern J. Neuroscience,* 38:435-441.

41. Torsvall, L., Akerstedt, T., Gillander, K. and Knutsson, A. (1989): *Psychophysiology,* (in press).

42: Townsend, R. and Johnson, L.C. (1979): *Electroencephalogr. Clin. Neurophysiol.,* 47:272-279.

43. Valley, V. and Broughton, R. (1983): *Electroencephalogr. Clin. Neurophysiol.,* 55:243-251.

44. Williams, H.L., Lubin, A. and Goodnow, J.J. (1959): *Psychological Monogr.*

45. Zschocke, S., Hunger, J. and Alexopoulos, T. (1982): In: *EEG Monitoring,* edited by Stefan, H. and Burr, W., pp. 19-26. Gustav Fischer, Stuttgart.

Medical Monitoring in the Home and Work Environment,
edited by Laughton E. Miles and Roger J. Broughton.
Raven Press, New York © 1990.

AMBULANT MONITORING OF SLEEP-WAKE STATE, CORE BODY TEMPERATURE AND BODY MOVEMENT

Roger J. Broughton, Claudio Stampi, Wayne Dunham and Martin Rivers

Human Neurosciences Research Unit
Ottawa General Hospital, University of Ottawa
Ottawa, Canada K1H8L6

INTRODUCTION

The research laboratories at the Human Neurosciences Research Unit (HNRU), University of Ottawa and the clinical sleep laboratories of the Ottawa General Hospital became involved in ambulatory monitoring in 1974 (1), when practical portable units for sleep-wake monitoring first became available from Oxford Medical Systems (U.K). Since then our laboratories have been continuously using and further developing this technology for both research and diagnostic purposes.

The reasons for adopting the approach were several. Continuous and prolonged sleep-wake recordings are of fundamental importance to our understanding of numerous sleep pathologies such as the hypersomnias and circadian sleep schedule disorders. However, using traditional polysomnography (PSG), such studies required a shiftwork approach typically employing 3 technologists each on an eight hour shift. With the new technology, staff time and overhead could both be reduced greatly while still obtaining essentially identical information. Ambulatory monitoring, moreover, has great usefulness in optimizing the probability of recording various parasomnias. These include the NREM sleep arousal disorders (sleepwalking, sleep terrors, confusional awakenings), which are actually reduced in frequency in laboratory recordings compared to the home (2), and others, such as nocturnal seizures and vascular headaches, which may simply be relatively rare and be very expensive to document by repeated overnight PSG.

Our laboratories' joint experience with ambulatory monitoring is extensive. Over these past 15 years it has involved numerous research projects plus the recording of many hundreds of patients for assessment or diagnosis. Studies have concerned: acquisition of normative data; investigation of patients with narcolepsy - cataplexy, idiopathic CNS hypersomnia, recurrent hypersomnias and epilepsy; use for home MSLT; combined sleep-wake recording with core body temperature monitoring using tympanic ear electrodes;combined sleep-wake recordings with wrist actigraphy; development of an automatic sleep-wake analyser for ambulant data; and applications to chronobiology.

139

Early studies employed the original 4 channel Medilog recorders. Since 1982 the 8 channel (plus one time code channel) Medilog 9000 system has also been used. Paper writeout has been by the high speed Mingograph system (Elema-Schonander, Sweden), usually with playback at 20x recording speed. Other technological aspects are mentioned below and have been described in detail elsewhere (3,4).

SLEEP-WAKE STATE MONITORING

Normative Studies

Normal subjects have been recorded for several purposes. These include the assessment of normal sleep structure using this technique compared to PSG, the gathering of matched control data in research projects such as the study of sleep around the 24 hrs in narcolepsy-cateplexy (5), and in order to create a normative data bank for the development and testing of new hardware such as the laboratory's automatic sleep-wake scorer built a decade ago and for our current work on ambulant core body temperature monitoring.

Our main findings are twofold. Satisfactory overnight and 24 hr recordings can be efficiently obtained. And home sleep-wake patterns are comparable to laboratory recordings with only three main differences. a) The first night effect is minimal or absent. b) Most subjects spend a period of several minutes or dozens of minutes in (usually light) sleep before the overnight sleep period begins [This phenomenon is due to their frequently dozing off while watching TV or while reading, followed by a period in which they reawaken and sleep logs indicate that, if seated, they get up and go to bed or, if already in bed, they turn off the lights and go (back) to sleep]. c) 24 hour studies confirm the quite high frequency of napping (6), almost always in the mid-afternoon and often with slow wave sleep (SWS). Mean data around the 24 hrs in 10 normal adult subjects is shown in Fig. 1 and exemplifies these features.

In the late 1970's some sleep laboratories (such as the late Elliot Weitzman's at Montifiore, personal communication) tried ambulatory sleep-wake monitoring only to abandon the technique, due to frustrations in obtaining reliable and quality recordings. Such labs generally employed the same approach for electrode attachment as in traditional PSG and also used regular EEG or polygraphic apparati for playback. However, satisfactory ambulatory sleep-wake recording demands much more care and some differences in approach. Electrodes must be more solidly attached for all leads; and for EOG and EMG they must be more flexibly attached. Batteries are a major concern. Calibration of the cassette tape should always be performed. The quality of the data must be confirmed before the subject leaves the laboratory. And writeout should employ satisfactory means such as the high speed, high frequency, high resolution Mingograph apparati which jets ink onto the moving paper using oscillographs with a linear frequency response up to 400 Hz real time.

By following a number of technical guidelines our laboratories have had fewer than 5% unsatisfactory recordings for many years. Great care is taken to very solidly anchor EEG electrodes with gauze squares and collodion.

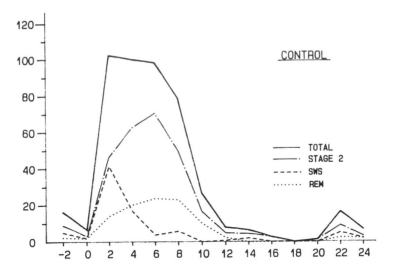

FIG. 1. Sleep-wake state in normals around the 24-hrs in 2 hr blocks and aligned for evening sleep onset. Note the period of sustained overnight sleep, the small amount in the mid-afternoon related to napping, and the increase in the late evening prior to sleep onset.

EOG and submental EMG electrodes are never anchored with guaze-collodion, due to the latter's inflexibility which causes lifting off the skin due to facial movements. Rather they use high quality sticky tape, such as the Micropore surgical type, while also ensuring both that all conductive paste stays in the electrode cup and that the electrode wires are strongly anchored with cross-tapes. Electrode impedances must be initially <3000 ohms. A 100 Hz sinusoidal calibration signal is applied through the system for 2 or more min and recorded on the C-120 cassette. Only high quality cassettes are used, as cheap ones give many problems. In-so-far as possible, batteries are of known shelf life or are ordered directly from the manufacturer. Perhaps most importantly, a short segment of the taped data is always played back prior to the subject leaving the lab in order to ensure initial quality of the data. A sleep log should always be used in conjunction with ambulant sleep-wake monitoring, as it can greatly help in the interpretation of results.

The montage with the 4-channel system has either been C4-A1 (or C3-A2), right eye - left mastoid and left eye - right mastoid EOGs and submental EMG; or C4-A1, O2-A2 (or the contralateral leads), right eye - left eye EOG, and submental EMG. The Medilog 9000's most common montage has been central and occipital referential leads, right and left EOGs, submental EMG, precordial ECG and a further optional lead such as core body temperature.

Sleep Disorder Patients

Sleep-wake monitoring alone over the 24-hrs in patients with narcolepsy-cataplexy compared to matched controls has been accomplished in two studies. The first involved the Ottawa patients in a collaborative study with Dr. Mortimer Mamelak (Sunnybrook Medical Center, Toronto) of the effects of treating the nocturnal sleep of narcoleptics with oral doses of gamma-hydroxy-butyrate. It was found that GHB improved the quality of night sleep by increasing SWS, reducing stage 1, increasing sleep efficiency, and reducing REM sleep fragmentation (7). In the daytime portion, total sleep (excluding stage 1 drowsiness), stage 4 and the number of sleep episodes over 45 min were all reduced. Clinically, there was corresponding subjective improvement of quality of night sleep, as well as reductions in daytime sleep need and in the frequency of cataplexy, sleep paralysis and nightmares, although diurnal drowsiness continued relatively uninfluenced (8). The findings with ambulant recording done in Ottawa were essentially identical with the traditional PSGs recordings done in Toronto in both the patients and controls.

In the second study, sleep patterns in untreated narcoleptics were directly compared to matched controls using 24 hr monitoring with emphasis upon the chronobiological aspects (5). This project added further details by objectifying the significant daytime increase in narcoleptics of stages 1A, 1B, 3, 4 and REM sleep, their greater number of day sleep episodes > 1 and > 10 min in duration, the presence of fewer than 2 sleep episodes per day with a sleep onset REM period (SOREMP), the presence of a circasemidian (2/day) distribution of sleep, the persistence of 2 interposed daily periods of minimal or no sleep reflecting the "forbidden zones" of Lavie (9), a mean interval between the onset of initial SWS and daytime SWS of some 13.6 hr, essentially identical to that in extended sleep in normals (10, 11), and the relative absence under these conditions of a 90-110 min ultradian daytime rhythm of sleep episodes, as appears more evident with studies in the laboratory environment.

Other hypersomnias of interest have been studied in individual patients. In idiopathic CNS hypersomnia (4) the increase in night sleep duration and amount of SWS has been confirmed, as has the propensity to a single long mid-afternoon sleep period (12). Similarly, in a patient with recurrent hypersomnia of the Kleine-Levin type the sleep-wake patterns around the 24 hrs have been documented when both asymptomatic and hypersomnic (4).

A further application has been the development of home multiple sleep latency tests (MSLT). Subjects leave the laboratory with written instructions for the nap schedule, as well as with an alarm clock. Twenty min is allowed for each nap. Just prior to each scheduled "lights out" the subject sets a photographer's clock at 20 min and then presses the event button. Our experience with this cost effective and time saving approach is summarized elsewhere (4). It holds promise of being a useful screening procedure. In studies with short home sleep latencies, the test has given results essentially identical to those in the laboratory. However, long sleep latencies may be due to uncontrolled arousing stimuli at home such as telephone rings. Apparently negative results in a patient with a convincing history of EDS must therefore be repeated in the laboratory setting.

In sum, our experience is that ambulatory home recordings can give satisfactory assessment of sleep-wake patterns either nocturnal, diurnal or both (i.e., around the 24 hrs). We have performed continuous recordings for as long as 120 hrs without significant problems employing daily replacement of cassettes and batteries along with checking of electrode impedences and correction of any electrode problems. In some patients, however, skin problems will develop after the first day and require cessation of the study. As well as the above applications, the technique has also been used in our laboratories for investigation of patients with sleep difficulties related to shift-work, in delayed sleep phase syndrome, and in insomnia. In all instances it has been possible to obtain satisfactory recordings.

CORE BODY TEMPERATURE MONITORING

There is considerable interest in the measurement of core body temperature in association with sleep-wake patterns. Some authors have proposed that temperature is a major determinant of sleep-wake status with low body temperature associated with high probability of sleep (13). Others have shown the major nap in freerunning studies to be most frequently associated with the moment of highest, rather than lowest, core body temperature (14). The body's thermal regulation is largely sleep-dependent with maintenance of waking-type thermoregulation in NREM sleep, but with loss of regulation and consequent poikilothermy in REM sleep. This occurs in most mammals (15), although perhaps not in man (16). Finally, temperature is closely associated with performance capacity in all tests other than perhaps those with a high memory load (17).

Ambulatory core body temperature has typically been assessed by a rectal thermoprobe with an integral memory device. The probes are often rejected by subjects due to considerations of esthetics and convenience. Based on the studies of Berger et al. (18) and others, we have developed a system which combines sleep-wake and core body temperature recording by an readily acceptable tympanic ear electrode using the Medilog 9000 system. The electrode consists of a fine wire disposable thermoprobe (Mon-A-Therm Inc. St. Louis) which is introduced into the external auditory meatis up to the ear drum, pulled back a few mm, and then held in place by a set of collapsible small plastic spokes. The sensor is interfaced to the recorder using a lightweight Mon-A-Therm 400A battery powered adapter to a Medilog AR-90 DC amplifier. The system (Fig. 2) can be calibrated and appears to have few movement artefacts. Temperature can be observed on the play-back screen, be plotted (most clearly at very slow speeds) by the Mingograph or otherwise, and can be A/D converted for further quantitative analyses. To date we have used the technique in both normals and narcoleptics. As well as preliminary test recordings 80 full 24 hour recordings of temperature and sleep-wake status have been gathered in 4 normal subjects following a sleep schedule consisting of 4 hours of anchor sleep and 3 different daytime nap regimes (19). To date only 4 narcoleptics have been so studied with the objective of confirming the phase advance of the circadian temperature rhythm described by Mosko et al. (20) and to analyse the relationships between temperature changes and daytime sleep episodes. Preliminary analysis of selected tapes from these ongoing studies indicates that satisfactory ambulatory core body

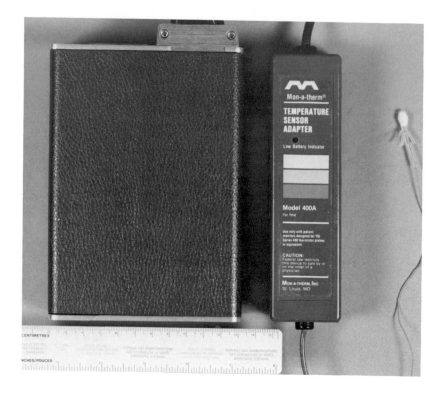

FIG. 2. Oxford 9000 recorder, Mon-a-Therm temperature sensor adaptor, tympanic electrode and 6 inch ruler.

temperature recordings are feasible. We have been able to observe the overall circadian variation in core body temperature, the phasic decrease at nocturnal sleep-onset, and daytime nap-related increases associated with SWS and decreases with REM onsets. Fig. 3 illustrates typical plotted data using the Mingograph at very slow playback speed.

BODY MOVEMENT RECORDING (ACTIGRAPHY)

A further approach to sleep-wake studies employs the recording of body movement by actigraphy. We have employed commercially available actigraphs (A.M.I., Inc, New York) in a number of applications with several objectives. These include assessment of the usefulness of actigraphs to determine sleep-wake status, the analysis of chronobiological aspects of

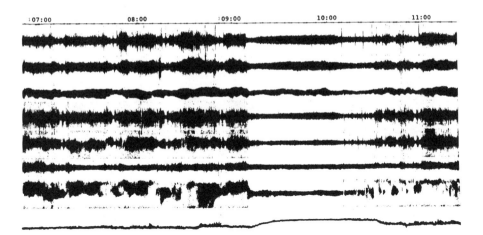

FIG. 3. Sleep-wake state and core body temperature (tympanic electrode) in a normal subject following a napping protocol. A temperature increase is seen during a nap beginning with sleep onset at 0907 hrs. Channels are: time of day, C3-A2, C4-A1, O1-A1, right EOG-A1, left EOG-A2, EKG, submental EMG and temperature.

motricity, and quantification of overall state-dependent movement levels in patient groups versus normals.

Wrist actigraphs were used in a project directed by one of us (C.S.) in combination with sleep logs in transatlantic solo sailors in the 1988 Calsberg sponsored C-Star race from Plymouth, England, to Newport, Rhode Island. Others kindly loaned actigraphs (R.Angus, Toronto; P. Lavie, Israel; and Wm. Gruen of A.M.I., New York). Apart from the loss overboard of 2 actigraphs and irreparable damage of one by submersion in salt water, the monitors gave acceptable recordings similar to those in less hostile environments. Actigraphs were attached both to the wrist (or leg) and to the yacht hulls. Data due to body movement could be distinguished from that due to yacht movement (Fig. 4). The data are being analysed and a preliminary abstract by Stampi and Broughton is in press (21).

Actigraphs were also worn in the multinap study in association with sleep-wake and temperature recording. And either the first two, or all three variables, have been recorded in 8 untreated patients with narcolepsy-cataplexy. An example of combined actigraphic and sleep-wake data is provided in Fig. 5. To date analyses have confirmed the findings of others that actigraphic data is reasonably predictive of sleep-wake state (22).

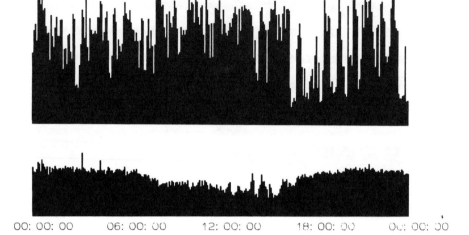

00: 00: 00   06: 00: 00   12: 00: 00   18: 00: 00   00: 00: 00

FIG. 4. Actigraphic data during transatlantic solo race across a 24-hr period with sailor wrist data above and yacht motion below. The repeated brief sailor sleep episodes (also noted in sleep logs) are evident, as is the overall effect of yacht motion on the wrist data.

Moreover, in narcoleptics, the overall activity level has been lower than in matched controls (23), a finding compatible with the lowered amounts in narcoleptics of EEG-polygraphically defined of "active wakefulness" in the home environment during normal activities (5).

AUTOMATIC SLEEP ANALYSIS

Because of the amounts of data in 24 hr ambulant monitoring and the duration, inconsistency and expense of visual scoring, we decided early on to develop our own automatic sleep-wake scoring system. The approach was to employ a hybrid system consisting of hardware devices to detect those PSG events used for visual scoring each giving an all or none output which were led to a microprocessor whose software replicated the Rechtschaffen-Kales guidelines.

This work took over six years and involved numerous colleagues. An alpha rhythm detector and spindle detector were developed in collaboration with a Master's student (D. Green) using a phase locked loop approach (24, 25); a K complex detector by another graduate student (O. Sherif) using a charged couple device (26); slow wave detection used baseline crossing and amplitude measures; EEG artefact detection for both muscle artefacts and preamplifier blocking; REM detection by out of phase plus slope of movement and amplitude detection; and EMG tone by amplitude discrimination in 2 sec mini-epoches (27). Reliability of each event detector was compared to "blind" human visual scoring.

Software was developed for epoque by epoque staging and reliability again assessed. Then further software handled the R-K contingency rules. Each epoque was given a tentative staging and then reassessed according to those of the preceeding and subsequent epoches. Again reliabilty was checked against the consensus of three independent scorers, who re-examined epoches on which they disagreed. The final overall agreement (28) for consensus scored epoches in normal overnight recordings was: WASO 94.1%, stage 1 91.6%, stage 2 98.4%, stage 3 97.7%, stage 4 90.1%, REM sleep 93.1%, and movement time 88.7%. Total sleep time reliability was 99.6%, sleep efficiency 98.1%, delta latency 83.4% and REM latency only 57.4%, due to a number of false detections of SOREMPs. Even for epoches with only 2 concording judges, reliability was over 85% for all sleep stages.

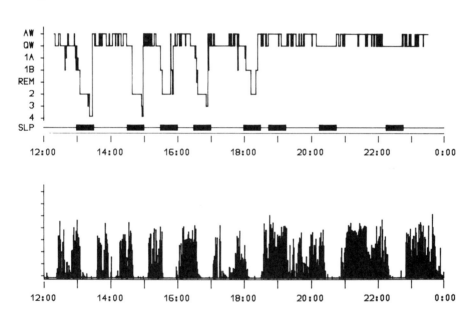

FIG. 5. Sleep-wake status, scheduled naps (black horizontal bars) and actigraph data during 12 hrs of a fragmented sleep study. For the first 5 scheduled naps the subject was able to sleep. Nap 6 was ignored; and quiescence but no sleep occurred for scheduled naps 7 and 8.

The development work was done without commercial intent. The sleep stager was later commercialized under University of Ottawa contract by

Oxford Medical Systems. Our experience with the first commercial model which had several modifications was that it was significantly less reliable than the prototype. The third generation Oxford SS9O-III sleep stager, however, appears equally reliable for normative data (29).

ADVANTAGES AND DISADVANTAGES

Although there is still room for improvement in ambulant sleep-wake recording techniques, our experience indicates that they have come of age for accurate cost effective recordings for at least some applications. There are both advantages and disadvantages which are summarized in Tables I and II.

Table I. Advantages of Ambulant Monitoring over PSG.

1. Low technologist time per study.
2. Reduced number of recording rooms needed.
3. Recordings done in normal home environment.
4. Procedure more convenient to many patients.
5. Easier accumulation of long duration recordings, especially useful for chronobiological studies.
6. Little or no adaptational first recording effect.
7. Probable higher incidence of various parasomnias.
8. Facilitates documentation of daytime sleep.

Table II. Disadvantages of Ambulant Monitoring.

1. Behaviour during recording not documented.
2. Fewer number of channels (currently limited to 8).
3. Technical difficulties not evident until playback.
4. Recording system delicate requiring more care.
5. Large number of movement artefacts in wakefulness.
6. Home recording conditions (activity level, noise) difficult to control.
7. No home medical backup for very ill patients.
8. Higher frequency of repeated tests.

CONCLUSIONS

Although various laboratories are now using ambulatory monitoring to accumulate data on a number of clinical sleep disorders including various hypersomnias, insomnias, sleep-wake schedules disorders and parasomnias, it is still unknown whether such patterns are diagnostic of the specific entities. Sleep apnea represents a particular case. To what extent ambulant screening or actual diagnosis of sleep-related respiratory disease is possible remains to be fully assessed. This is particularly important, as the respiratory conditions are so prevalent and the costs of performing a laboratory study in all patients with snoring or other suggestive symptoms are so significant. Further work also needs to be done concerning the promising area of ambulatory MSLT tests. Due to the advantages in a number of applications, it is apparent that increasing use of ambulatory monitoring will occur in the sleep field in the future.

ACKNOWLEDGMENTS

The research was supported by the Medical Research Council of Canada and the Department of Supplies and Services, Government of Canada.

REFERENCES

1. Healey, T., Maru, J. and Broughton, R. (1975): *Sleep Res.,* 4:254.

2. Broughton, R. (1968): *Science,* 159:1070-1078.

3. Broughton, R. (1989): In: *Textbook of Sleep Medicine,* edited by M. Kryger, T. Roth and W. Dement. Saunders, Philadelphia/London.

4. Broughton, R. (1989): In: *Ambulatory EEG Monitoring,* edited by R. Ebersole. pp. 277-298. Raven, New York.

5. Broughton, R., Dunham, W., Newman, J., Lutley, K., Duchesne, P. and Rivers, M. (1988). *Electroenceph. Clin. Neurophysiol.,* 80:473-481.

6. Evans, F., Cook, M., Cohen, H., Orne, E. and Orne, M. (1977): *Science,* 197:687-689.

7. Broughton, R. and Mamelak, M. (1980): *Can. J. Neurol. Sci.,* 7:23-31.

8. Broughton, R. and Mamelak, M. (1979): *Can. J. Neurol. Sci.,* 6:1-6.

9. Lavie, P. (1986): *Electroenceph. Clin. Neurophysiol.,* 63:414-425.

10. Gagnon, P. and De Koninck, J. (1984): *Electroenceph. Clin. Neurophysiol.,* 58:155-157.

11. Gagnon, P., De Koninck, J. and Broughton, R. (1985): *Sleep,* 8:118-128.

12. Roth, B., Nevsimalova, S. and Rechtschaffen, A. (1972): *Arch. Gen. Psychiat.,* 26:456-462.

13. Kronauer, R., Czeisler, C., Pilato, S., Moore-Ede, M. and Weitzman, E. (1982): *Amer. J. Physiol.,* 242: R3-R17.

14. Zulley, J. and Campbell, S. (1985): *Hum. Neurobiol.,* 4:123-126.

15. Parmiggiani, P.L. (1980): *Experientia,* 36:6-11.

16. Palka, J., Walker, J. and Berger, R. (1986): *J. Appl. Physiol.,* 61:885-892.

17. Folkard, S., Knauth, P., Monk, T. and Rutenfranz, J. (1976): *Ergonomics,* 19:479-488.

18. Berger, R., Palca, J., Walker, J. and Phillips, N. (1988): *Neuroscience Letters,* 86:230-234.

19. Stampi, C. and Broughton, R. (1988): *Sleep Res.,* 17:100.

20. Mosko, S. Holowach, J. and Sassin, J. (1983): *Sleep,* 6:137-146.

21. Stampi, C. and Broughton, R. (1989): *Sleep Res.,* 18:

22. Mullaney, D., Kripke, D. and Messin, S. (1980): *Sleep,* 3:83-92.

23. Newman, J., Stampi, C., Dunham, W. and Broughton, R. (1988): *Sleep Res.,* 17:343.

24. Green, D., Pajurek, B., Healey, T. and Broughton, R. (1975): *Sleep Res.,* 6:185.

25. Broughton, R., Healey, T., Maru, J., Green, D. and Pajurek, B. (1978): *Electroenceph. Clin. Neurophysiol.,* 44:677-680.

26. Sherif, O., Pajurek, B., Mahmoud, S. and Broughton, R. (1977): *Proc. IEEEE. Conf.*

27. Broughton, R., Maru, J., Da Costa, B., Green, D., Sherif, O. and Pajurek, B. (1978): *Sleep Res.,* 7:278.

28. Broughton, R., Roberts, J., Suwalski, W., da Costa, B. and Liddiard, S. (1983): *Sleep Res.,* 12:344.

29. Carskadon, M., Bliwise, D., Keenan, S., Roberts, S. and Davies, W. (1989): *Sleep Res.,* 17:330.

Medical Monitoring in the Home and Work Environment,
edited by Laughton E. Miles and Roger J. Broughton.
Raven Press, New York © 1990.

COMPUTER-BASED MONITORING OF PHYSICAL ACTIVITY

Lawrence F. Van Egeren

Department of Psychiatry
Michigan State University, A227 East Fee Hall
East Lansing, Michigan 48824

INTRODUCTION

Central to clinical ambulatory monitoring is the unimpeded motion of the patient during the period of observation. Diagnostic evaluation may include monitoring the patient's physical activity. Body motility can profoundly affect other physiological parameters that are being monitored and it may be desirable or necessary to take this influence into account explicitly. For example the interpretation of changes in blood pressure is incomplete, without knowledge of the patient's activity at the time of the readings.

Apart from their effects on physiological processes, motor functions themselves may be the clinical focus. Monitoring body motility around the clock may be part of a comprehensive evaluation of motor disturbances of patients with extrapyramidal conditions (Parkinson's disease, Huntington's chorea, motor dysfunctions of psychiatric patients on neuroleptic drugs), neuromuscular disorders, or mobility restrictions accompanying injuries, or biological aging processes. Continuous monitoring of motor activity has been employed to study circadian rhythms in manic-depressive patients (16), recovery in myocardial infarction patients (5), sleep disorders (1,9), antidepressant (6) and hypnotic (4) drug effects, and hyperactivity in children (2,10).

Physical activity is difficult to quantify and define. The biomechanics of displacement and rotation of the body are complex. People vary greatly in free-living body motion, even when performing the same task (8). They also exhibit day-to-day and even year-to-year stability in the number of body movements (1). There are many approaches to the measurement of physical activity in the ambulant person carrying out his or her ordinary daily routine (7, 11, 15).

The present discussion will be restricted to use of the self-report diary and movement-activated electronic instruments, focusing on applications to ambulatory blood pressure monitoring (ABPM). The systems presented will illustrate general problems associated with the acquisition and management of 24 hour records of physical activity and have applications well beyond blood pressure monitoring.

An efficient system for ambulatory activity monitoring permits convenient data acquisition, automated data downloading and scoring, and low-cost management of large volumes of data that have been collected from many subjects over extended periods of time. When activity monitoring produces massive quantities of data, as is often the case, there are distinct advantages to be gained by using monitoring systems that are computer-based. Two specific computer-based systems will be illustrated.

ACTIVITY DIARIES

Activity during blood pressure (BP) monitoring is often recorded by having the patient keep a behavioral diary on the day of monitoring. The patient is typically instructed to record all significant events immediately following each BP reading. The aim of the diary is to capture the "when, where, what, and how" of each BP reading; <u>when</u> was the reading taken; <u>where</u> was the person located at the time of the reading (e.g., work, home, car, other); <u>what</u> was the person doing at that time (e.g., subject chooses one of ten activities); <u>how</u> did the person feel (e.g., subject chooses one of three mood states); and <u>how</u> was the body positioned (sitting, standing, reclining)? When blood pressure is taken every 15 minutes during sixteen waking hours, the diary described above will generate 21 (number of diary variables) X 64 (number of waking readings) = 1,344 scores. When the diary information is to be used in research or in a computer-generated clinical report, the 1,344 scores must be entered into the computer manually from the keyboard.

The great volume of behavioral data in ABPM poses a major problem both for the patient and the technician or clinician. Patient acceptance of the diary is often far from ideal; and the quantity of information provided by the patient may vary from the obsessional detailed to none at all, even when the diary format is standardized. Chesney and Ironson (3) have reviewed the problems associated with the construction and use of activity diaries, including response bias and other psychometric problems.

The gathering and processing of activity information for ABPM are so time-consuming as to pose a formidable barrier to the wider use of ABPM. To lower this barrier, the method of logging behavior must be interesting enough to motivate the patient, and simple enough to avoid disrupting the normal flow of patient activities. The information obtained must be easily accessible to the investigator for clinical report writing and data analysis.

THE CAD SYSTEM

To deal with these problems, we developed a computer-assisted diary (CAD) (14). The CAD system enables the user to monitor the behavior conditions surrounding ambulatory blood pressure readings, to extract critical features of the data, and to readily access and use the information. The system was designed to meet the specific performance criteria that it (a) be clear and simple to use, (b) have good patient acceptance, (c) monitor activities that have been shown to be related to ambulatory blood pressure, (c) have a low user error rate, (d) provide automatic computer checks for errors, (e) be implemented on an IBM-compatible microcomputer, (f) download diary information to the computer automatically rather than manually, and (g) yield quantitative diary information that is usable both for research and for clinical evaluation. The result is the computer scorable diary card and the associated computer software described here and elsewhere (14).

We initially considered using a small, hand-held programmable microcomputer to log diary information. But we abandoned the idea, because the operation of these devices is too complex and the fear of computers of some people is too great to ensure reliable performance. Instead, we developed the mark sense diary card shown in Figure 1.

Following each BP reading, the subject marks boxes on the card to indicate the time of the reading, his location (work, home, car, other), his body position (sitting, standing, reclining), his activity (working, watching television, reading, talking, walking, eating, talking on the telephone, drinking a caffeinated beverage, smoking, drinking an alcoholic beverage, and other), the number of people he is having a face-to-face interaction with, and his emotion or mood (happy, angry, tense, rushed, tired, feeling goals are blocked, and other).

There are places on the card where the subject can write comments; as well as locations, activities, and moods other than those printed on the card. It takes approximately 30-45 seconds to mark the diary card each time blood pressure is read. The diary card is printed on both sides, with two records on each side, so that each card can accommodate diary information for four BP readings. When blood pressure is read every 15 minutes, the subject fills out one card per hour.

Prior to a BP recording, the subject receives detailed written instructions describing the use of the diary and the operation of the BP monitor. Upon returning to the clinic or laboratory following a 24 hour BP recording, the person rates the recording for the quality of sleep, problems with the BP recorder, problems with the diary cards, the extent to which monitoring interfered with the individual's customary routine, the level of stress on the day of monitoring relative to the usual level of stress, and the level of physical activity (body movement) on the day of monitoring relative to the usual levels of activity. This information is transferred to a "header" card. The header card and diary cards are placed into the hopper of a card reader, and the information is downloaded directly into a microcomputer for automatic and rapid computer-assisted data scoring, data analysis, and clinical report writing. Data analysis and clinical report generation can be conducted within minutes.

Any practical activity diary is powerfully constrained by the need for economy of time in logging activities. Consequently, items printed on the diary card were carefully chosen for their fertility as "root" categories from which additional activity and mood information could be derived. Besides activities and moods listed earlier, the CAD computer program combines diary card information to score the diary log for additional activities (driving a car, household chores, desk work, attending a meeting, relaxing, sleeping) and mood states (stress, frustration). In all, each diary record for a single BP reading is scored for 36 variables -- 4 locations, 3 body positions, 17 activities, 9 moods, 1 social behavior, 1 behavioral efficiency estimate, and 1 comments score). The total number of diary scores for a typical 24 hour BP recording is about 2300.

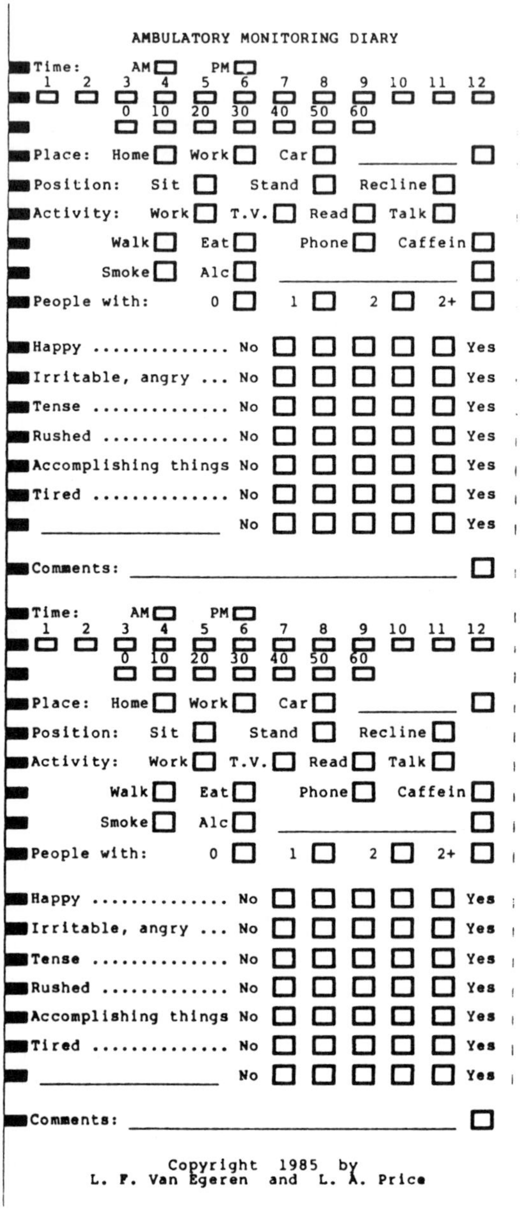

AMBULATORY MONITORING DIARY

Time: AM ☐ PM ☐
1 ☐ 2 ☐ 3 ☐ 4 ☐ 5 ☐ 6 ☐ 7 ☐ 8 ☐ 9 ☐ 10 ☐ 11 ☐ 12 ☐
0 ☐ 10 ☐ 20 ☐ 30 ☐ 40 ☐ 50 ☐ 60 ☐

Place: Home ☐ Work ☐ Car ☐ ________ ☐

Position: Sit ☐ Stand ☐ Recline ☐

Activity: Work ☐ T.V. ☐ Read ☐ Talk ☐
Walk ☐ Eat ☐ Phone ☐ Caffein ☐
Smoke ☐ Alc ☐ ________ ☐

People with: 0 ☐ 1 ☐ 2 ☐ 2+ ☐

Happy .... No ☐ ☐ ☐ ☐ ☐ Yes
Irritable, angry ... No ☐ ☐ ☐ ☐ ☐ Yes
Tense .... No ☐ ☐ ☐ ☐ ☐ Yes
Rushed .... No ☐ ☐ ☐ ☐ ☐ Yes
Accomplishing things No ☐ ☐ ☐ ☐ ☐ Yes
Tired .... No ☐ ☐ ☐ ☐ ☐ Yes
________ No ☐ ☐ ☐ ☐ ☐ Yes

Comments: ________ ☐

Time: AM ☐ PM ☐
1 ☐ 2 ☐ 3 ☐ 4 ☐ 5 ☐ 6 ☐ 7 ☐ 8 ☐ 9 ☐ 10 ☐ 11 ☐ 12 ☐
0 ☐ 10 ☐ 20 ☐ 30 ☐ 40 ☐ 50 ☐ 60 ☐

Place: Home ☐ Work ☐ Car ☐ ________ ☐

Position: Sit ☐ Stand ☐ Recline ☐

Activity: Work ☐ T.V. ☐ Read ☐ Talk ☐
Walk ☐ Eat ☐ Phone ☐ Caffein ☐
Smoke ☐ Alc ☐ ________ ☐

People with: 0 ☐ 1 ☐ 2 ☐ 2+ ☐

Happy .... No ☐ ☐ ☐ ☐ ☐ Yes
Irritable, angry ... No ☐ ☐ ☐ ☐ ☐ Yes
Tense .... No ☐ ☐ ☐ ☐ ☐ Yes
Rushed .... No ☐ ☐ ☐ ☐ ☐ Yes
Accomplishing things No ☐ ☐ ☐ ☐ ☐ Yes
Tired .... No ☐ ☐ ☐ ☐ ☐ Yes
________ No ☐ ☐ ☐ ☐ ☐ Yes

Comments: ________ ☐

Copyright 1985 by
L. F. Van Egeren and L. A. Price

FIG. 1. Mark-sense diary card.

The CAD system interfaces with manufacture supplied computer software for the Spacelabs, ICR BP monitors. When the Spacelab's BP report program is executed, CAD automatically inserts activity and mood labels into the report; obviating the need to enter them manually from the keyboard. CAD also creates a supplementary BP report, which can be printed at the end of Spacelabs' standard report. The supplementary report includes (a) a table containing the average systolic BP, diastolic BP, and heart rate for each of ten activities and five moods, (b) a table listing the five highest systolic pressures and five highest diastolic pressures during the BP recording, and (c) a summary description of the behavioral conditions under which the patient's blood pressure was monitored.

CLINICAL APPLICATIONS

An application of the CAD system is illustrated in Table 1 which presents an excerpt of the clinical report of the 24 hour BP recording of a man with mild hypertension who has a sedentary office job. The BP report was created by the Spacelabs' computer program. The activity and mood labels in the "Diary Activity" column were inserted automatically by the CAD computer

Table 1. SAMPLE OF PATIENT'S BLOOD PRESSURES AND ACTIVITIES

Time	Systolic	Diastolic	Mean	Heart Rate	Diary Activity
13:14	137	82	105	77	On phone, angry
13:29	162	97	108	78	Desk work, angry
13:45	142	78	116	72	On phone, tense
13:59	140	80	110	63	On phone
14:14	145	87	117	68	Desk work, rushed
14:29	155	91	106	80	Desk work, rushed
14:44	160	95	102	67	Rushed
14:59	150	83	110	74	Talking
15:14	160	83	106	80	Desk work
15:32	155	76	113	77	On phone, tense
15:44	166	92	115	73	On phone
15:59	176	88	118	77	Walking, tense
16:15	161	96	111	69	Desk work, rushed
16:29	161	100	107	94	Rushed, tense
16:44	122	81	85	81	Leave work, driving
16:59	206	92	111	80	Driving , rushed
17:14	145	76	98	73	At home, TV, talking
17:29	140	76	102	65	TV
17:44	130	83	98	68	TV
18:00	142	86	101	71	Eating, tense
18:14	152	90	108	75	Eating, TV
18:29	142	72	95	77	TV

program. The activity and mood information indicate what the person was doing and how he reported feeling at the time each blood pressure was read. For example, information inserted by CAD indicates that when the person's systolic pressure peaked at 206 mmHg at 4:59 P.M. he was driving home from work and feeling rushed. When his diastolic pressure reached 97 mmHg at 1:29 P.M., he was at his desk at work and feeling angry.

The CAD computer program created the summary information for this patient which appears in Table 2. The table relates blood pressure and heart rate to major categories of activity and mood. The table gives a synoptic view of the relationship between behavior and blood pressure for the particular person. It becomes clear, for example, that the person's blood pressure was higher at work than at home in the evening. Systolic pressure dropped slightly during sleep but was still considerably elevated (134 mmHg). Systolic and diastolic pressures were noticeably higher when the man was angry, tense or rushed, compared to feeling happy or relaxed.

TABLE 2. AVERAGE BLOOD PRESSURE DURING ACTIVITIES AND MOODS

	Systolic	Diastolic	Heart Rate	Readings
Activity:				
At work	151	86	76	32
At home	144	78	69	24
Sleeping	134	70	57	13
Walking	162	94	78	4
Talking	150	84	74	21
Driving	164	86	80	2
On telephone	147	82	73	6
Watching TV	144	76	68	19
Desk work	150	85	76	19
Meeting	NA	NA	NA	0
Mood:				
Happy	142	74	66	13
Angry	149	89	77	2
Tense	152	86	79	16
Rushed	151	86	76	27
Relaxed	139	69	62	7

NA = Not available; blood pressure not read during activity or mood.

Using header card information, the CAD program constructed and printed the following summary of information about the conditions under which the patient's blood pressure was monitored: "On the day of the blood pressure scan the patient's stress level was slightly above average and activity level was average. The patient experienced mild problems with the blood pressure monitor and no problems with the diary. The patient's normal routine was slightly disrupted by wearing the monitor and the patient slept poorly."

A recent empirical test of the accuracy and validity of the CAD system (14) indicated that the system met our most important performance criteria.

Subjects made relatively few errors in marking diary cards. The low error rate (less than 1%) and frequent written comments suggested that subjects were both willing and able to use the diary correctly.

The validity of the system was evaluated by determining whether activity categories were related to blood pressure in a way which was consistent with results of others using manual scoring of activity logs. The relation of mean systolic pressure to the activities of 32 normotensive working adults (16 males) with white collar, sedentary jobs who received 24 hour ambulatory BP monitoring on a work day was as follows: cigarette smoking (136 mmHg), driving a car (131 mmHg), walking (130 mmHg), drinking an alcoholic beverage (127 mmHg), drinking a caffeinated beverage (126 mmHg), household chores (126 mmHg), talking on telephone (125 mmHg), talking in general (124 mmHg), working in general (123 mmHg), eating (122 mmHg), watching television (121 mmHg), desk work (121 mmHg), reading (118 mmHg), attending a meeting (117 mmHg), relaxing (105 mmHg), and sleeping (104 mmHg). These results were in general agreement with expectations.

Existing diaries for ABPM lack adequate standardization (3). In the absence of standard-ization, making inferences about the effects of behavior on blood pressure will remain hazardous. Two people may differ in 24 hour blood pressure because of a difference in behavioral activity, or because blood pressure was maintained differently at comparable levels of activity. Currently, we cannot satisfactorily distinguish between these two important cases.

The use of computer-automated standardized activity diaries for ambulatory monitoring can potentially introduce the following benefits: a) better quantification of behavioral information; b) greater accessibility of this information for diagnostic and research purposes; c) greater comparability of data gathered at different centers; d) the possibility of developing activity-standardized blood pressure norms for use with patients; and e) significant reductions in clinician and technician time. For these reasons, the use of a computerized activity diary for ambulatory blood pressure monitoring, as well as for other kinds of clinical monitoring, merits further investigation and trial applications.

ELECTRONIC MOTION SENSORS

The strength of the activity diary is its specificity. It provides detailed information on each activity reported. The diary, however, has several major disadvantages. It disrupts the patient's routine, lacks objectivity, requires good patient cooperation, and, unless the system is computerized, places heavy time demands on the technician whenever the activity data must be coded and prepared for analysis or for clinical report generation. An electronic motion detector can often be an attractive alternative to, or supplement for, the activity diary. This is especially so because of new design technology, which has significantly expanded the capability, and removed some of the more serious limitations, of older instruments.

To be practical for tracking human activity levels during a normal daily routine a motion sensor must meet certain criteria. It must be able to: a) accurately measure body motility (linear displacement and angular rotation of body); b) distinguish between common everyday activities, most of which have low energy costs; c) distinguish between individuals and populations; and d) maintain high reliability and low sensitivity to noise in a wide range of work and home environments.

Many movement-activated recorders are the size of a large wristwatch. They can be attached to the arm, the ankle, or the waist. They monitor and quantify motility by converting mechanical motion into an electrical signal. There are many ways of making this conversion, which are not equally satisfactory (11). Reliability and validity studies of automated activity monitors usually involve examination of monitor values during the application of test movements or during physical activities that have been directly observed under naturalistic conditions (12).

PCD INSTRUMENT

Early actimeter designs were modified self-winding wristwatches that accumulated counts of movements. Technology has advanced considerably since then. An activity monitor of advanced design, manufactured by Precision Control Design (PCD), is shown in Figure 2. Technical aspects of its development have been described by Redmond and Hegge (11). The device is sensitive to small movements and can record the duration of movement (presumed to have some relation to the amplitude of movement) as well as the frequency of movement can accumulate data over operator-selectable periods from 2 seconds to 5 minutes, and can record continuously for up to 9 days (when data are stored in cumulative units of 1 minute).

The PCD actigraph is a self-contained microcomputer housed in a 2.5 X 3.5 X .75 inch lightweight aluminum case. The unit interfaces with an IBM-compatible microcomputer for operator selection of patient identification, start time, length of accumulation period, and for downloading of data. A piezoelectric flexible element translates body movement into an electrical signal. The instrument can be adjusted to detect g forces down to .01 g, which may be too sensitive to distinguish hand tremors from background noise. At a threshold setting of .05 g for translation movements (linear displacements), the sensor responds to rotational movements of 20 degrees. The sensor can record movement frequencies in the .25-5 Hz range (with maximum effort, a person can voluntarily shake his wrist as fast as about 4 HZ). Controlled tests in our laboratory indicated that the PCD monitor responds to movements occurring on two spatial axes. By proper orientation of the actigraph on the body, the restriction to two axes of movement need not be problematic. With normal human activity, there is considerable overlap, or redundancy, in the cumulative values when movements are recorded on three separate axes (11).

Illustrative Application

Six 24 hour activity recordings made by the PCD monitor are shown in Figure 3. Actigraphs A and B are wrist and waist recordings of movement durations in a 41 year old woman with a sedentary job. Each spike is a 1-min cumulative total. Figure 3C is a movement duration wrist actigraph of a 14 year old girl. The three lower graphs show the movement frequencies of a 54 year old man (wrist and waist, 3D and 3E) and a 14 year old boy

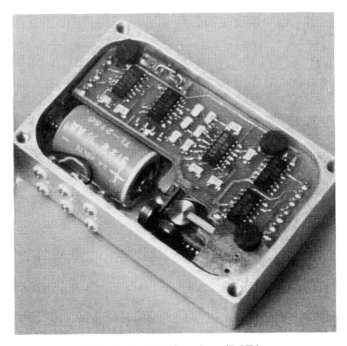

FIG. 2. Activity monitor (PCD).

with an elevated risk for coronary heart disease (wrist, 3F). Subjects wore the wrist monitor, but not the waist monitor, to bed.

They also wore a blood pressure monitor during the 24 hour period of observation. In agreement with expectations, the actigraphs show that there is greater minute-to-minute change in movement amplitude (duration) than in movement frequency, and greater wrist motility than waist motility. The waist actigraph in Fig. 3B shows a 30 minute burst of motion from 12:10 PM to 12:40 PM during vigorous walking exercise. The wrist actigraph in Fig. 3F shows extremely restless sleep beginning at 11:30 PM in the high-risk boy. Studies comparing sleep actigraphs with traditional sleep EEG recordings show close agreement between measures of sleep onset, sleep duration, and arousals during sleep (9). In general, the less the body movement during sleep the better the quality of sleep. Activity recordings offer an opportunity for low-cost monitoring of sleep behavior while the patient sleeps at home. These recordings may be useful for diagnostic evaluation of sleep disorders such as sleep apnea (1).

The "notch" near the middle of the wrist actigraph in Fig. 3D occurred when the 54 year old man, napped from 5:50 PM to 6:30 PM. Low activity while reading before and after the nap is evident in the longer period of relative immobility, from 5:30 PM to 7:10, PM, in the man's waist actigraph (Fig. 3E). During the reading the man's wrist was active but his waist was inactive, as one would expect. A burst of high amplitude activity, from 6:15 PM to 8:40 PM, appears in actigraph 3C, while the 14 year old girl vigorously ran and biked.

08:00   **08:00**

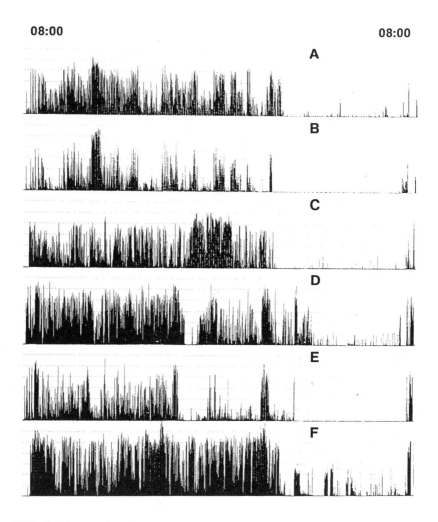

FIG. 3. Twenty-four hour actigraphs of wrist movement durations (A,C), waist movement durations (B), wrist movement frequencies (D, F), and waist movement frequencies (E). Recordings started at 8 AM. Each spike is the cumulative movement for one minute.

As the motor system makes a major demand on circulation, one might expect that simultaneous recordings of motility and blood pressure would show close correspondence. The mean one-hour values for 24 hour ambulatory recordings of 47 adults monitored on a work day shown in Figure 4 confirm this expectation. The typical diurnal rhythm in ambulatory blood pressure (13) is paralleled closely by a diurnal rhythm in ambulatory physical activity.

Electronic motion sensors have several important advantages. They do not interfere with the patient's activity, require little time from the

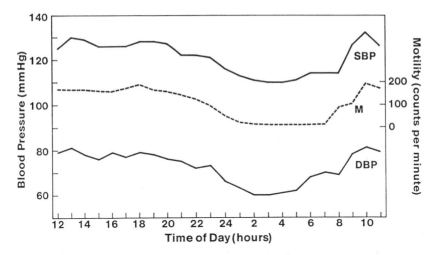

FIG. 4. Twenty-four hour systolic blood pressure (SBP), diastolic blood pressure (DBP), and motility (M). Mean of 47 subjects.

investigator or clinician and little effort by the patient, and provide a quantitative estimate of physical activity. Advanced designs can record both the frequency and the intensity of movement (11, 17). By means of commercially available instruments it is now possible to obtain 24 hour records of unimpeded motion by monitoring human activity continuously. Through continued advances in sensor technology many clinical applications of ambulatory activity monitoring that were once impractical or impossible are now becoming feasible.

ACKNOWLEDGEMENTS

The research reported was supported in part by grants RO1 HL38458 and HL34389 from the National Heart, Lung and Blood Institute. Portions of the material in this chapter have been published in Van Egeren and Madarasmi (1988) (cf. references).

REFERENCES

1. Aubert-Tulkens, G., Culee, C., Harmant-Van Rijckevorsel, K. and Rodenstein, D. (1987): Ambulatory Evaluation of Sleep Disturbance and Therapeutic Effects in Sleep Apnea Syndrome by Wrist Activity Monitoring. *American Rev. Resp. Dis.*, 136:851-856.

2. Barkley, R. (1977): The Effects of Methylphenidate on Various Types of Activity Level and Attention in Hyperkinetic Children. *J. Abn. Child Psychol.*, (4):351-369.

3. Chesney, M. and Ironson, G.: Diaries in ambulatory monitoring. In: *Handbook of Research Methods in Cardiovascular Behavioral Methods*, edited by N. Schneiderman, P. Kaufman and S.M. Weiss. Plenum, New York.

4. Crowley, T. and Hydinger-Macdonald, M. (1979): Bedtime Flurazepam and the Human Circadian Rhythm of Spontaneous Motility. *Psychopharm.,* 62:157-161.

5. Fentem, P., Fitton, D. and Hampton, J. (1976): Long-term recording of activity patterns. *Postgrad. Med. J.,* 52 (Suppl.7):163-166.

6. Kupfer, D., Weiss, B., Foster, F., Detre, T., Delgado, J. and McPartland, R. (1976): Psychomotor Activity in Affective States. *Arch. Gen. Psychia.,* 30:765-768.

7. LaPorte, R., Montoye, H. and Caspersen, C. (1985): Assessment of Physical Activity in Epidmiologic Research: *Problems and Prospects. Public Health Reports,* 100 (2):131-146.

8. Montoye, H., Washburn, R., Servais, S., Ertl, A., Webster, J. and Nagle, F. (1983): Estimation of energy expenditure by a portable accelerometer. *Med. Sci. and Sports Exer.,* 15:403-407.

9. Mullaney, D., Kripke, D., Messin, S. (1980): Wrist-Actigraphic Estimation of Sleep Time. *Sleep,* 3 (1):83-92.

10. Porrino, L., Rapoport, J., Behar, D., Sceery, W., Ismond, D. and Bunney, W. (1983): A Naturalistic Assessment of the Motor Activity of Hyperactive Boys. *Arch. Gen. Psychia.,* 40:681-687.

11. Redmond, D. and Hegge, F. (1985): Observations on the design and specification of a wrist-worn human activity monitoring system. *Behav. Res. Meth. Inst. Comput.,* 17 (6):659-669.

12. Renfrew, J., Moore, A., Grady, C., Robertson-Tchabo, E., Cutler, N. and Rapoport, S. (1984): A method for measuring arm movements in man under ambulatory conditions. *Ergonomics,* 27 (6):651-661.

13. Sundberg, S. (1989): Noninvasive, automatic 24-h ambulatory blood pressure monitoring in normotensive subjects. *Eur. J. Appl. Physiol.,* 56:381-383.

14. Van Egeren, L. and Madarasmi, S. (1988): A Computer-assisted Diary (CAD) for Ambulatory Blood Pressure Monitoring. *Amer. J. Hyperten.,* 1:179S-185S.

15. Webster, J., Messin, S., Mullaney and Kripke, D. (1981): Transducer design and placement for activity recording. *Med. Biol. Eng. Comput.,* 20:741-744.

16. Wehr, T., Sack, D., Rosenthal, N., Duncan, W. and Gillin, J. (1983): Circadian rhythm disturbances in manic-depressive illness. *Federation Proceedings,* 42(11):2809-2814.

17. Wong, T., Webster, J., Montoye, H. and Washburn, R. (1981): Portable accelerometer devices for measuring human energy expenditure. *IEEE Trans. Biomed. Eng. BME.,* 28:467-471.

Medical Monitoring in the Home and Work Environment,
edited by Laughton E. Miles and Roger J. Broughton.
Raven Press, New York © 1990.

CONTINUOUS BODY TEMPERATURE MONITORING AT VARYING LEVELS OF PHYSICAL EXERTION IN CROSS-COUNTRY BICYCLISTS

Jonathan H. Mermin[1] and *Charles A. Czeisler

Neuroendocrinology Laboratory, Division of Endocrinology
*Department of Medicine, Harvard Medical School
Brigham and Women's Hospital
221 Longwood Avenue, Boston, Massachusetts 02115

INTRODUCTION

The increasing use of ambulatory body temperature monitoring in human subjects for the diagnosis of disorders of the circadian sleep-wake cycle necessitates a clearer understanding of the factors which affect daily variations in the thermoregulatory system. Observed body temperature reflects both the output of the endogenous circadian oscillator as well as responses evoked from various stimuli such as activity, sleep, and postural changes (5). Numerous studies have examined the acute effects of exercise on human thermoregulation including the influence of such variables as ambient temperature, humidity, degree of hydration, posture, and type and intensity of exercise on body temperature (2,3,4,9,12,17,20,21). None of these studies, however, has employed continuous body temperature monitoring. Typically, body temperature has been monitored for less than 2 hours, with data collected for less than 45 minutes after the cessation of exercise. Furthermore, even these short-term studies have failed to account for the endogenous circadian variation of body temperature, despite the demonstration that the absolute height of the temperature rise due to exercise at different times of the day follows the circadian pattern of body temperature at rest (7,11,18).

These issues may account for the equivocal results which have been reported regarding whether or not body temperature remains above or below baseline in the period following exercise (3,4,10,22,23). Therefore, in our investigation of the thermoregulatory response to exercise in cross-country bicyclists, we monitored rectal temperature and the rest-activity cycle continuously.

---

[1] Present address: Stanford University School of
Medicine, Stanford, California 94305

METHODS

Subjects

Two 18-year-old men were recruited from a group of undergraduates planning a bicycling trip across the United States. Both subjects had consistent sleep-wake schedules as derived through histories, with no transmeridian travel in the preceding 4 months and no previous exposure to shift work. Subjects had no evidence of medical, psychiatric, or sleep disorders as determined by clinical history, physical examination, chest radiograph, electrocardiogram, clinical biochemical screening tests, and a psychological questionnaire (Minnesota Multiphasic Personality Inventory). Informed consent was obtained from both subjects.

Physiologic Recording

Ambulatory data collection involved measurements of rectal temperature, non-dominant wrist activity, meal times, sleep-wake times, and the beginning and ending of bicycling events. Data was collected through a small, portable, battery-operated computer (Vitalog). Information from the Vitalogs were transferred to a floppy disk through an Apple II-C computer every 2-3 days.

The Vitalog was worn at the waist, held in place by a belt. Rectal temperature was measured using a disposable plastic thermistor (Yellow Springs Instrument Co.) inserted 10 cm into the rectum. Wrist activity data was collected on the non-dominant arm using a wrist band containing 6 mercury switches sensitive to movement. Meal times, sleep-wake times, and bicycling events were recorded by the Vitalog using a numerical code. All sensors were worn 24-hours a day except for swimming and showering, or defecating in the case of the temperature thermistor.

Experimental Conditions

For both subjects body temperature, non-dominant wrist activity, and sleep-wake times were continuously monitored for 11 weeks. The first period of the protocol consisted of measuring for two weeks all the above mentioned functions during the subjects' normal daily life as college students (home monitoring). Each subject came to the laboratory five times during this two week period to have data from the Vitalog transferred to a floppy disk via an Apple computer.

The second section of the protocol involved a two day period inside the laboratory during which each subject partook in normal activities while confining himself to one room. During this time the subjects remained on the sleep-wake schedule that they had been following during home monitoring.

Upon waking the morning after laboratory monitoring, the subjects began a "constant routine," a 40-hour period of enforced supine wakefulness in constant indoor light, with their daily nutritional intake equally distributed into hourly liquid aliquots. This regimen is designed to expose the endogenous component of the circadian rhythm of core body temperature by minimizing the masking effects of sleep-wake and light-dark transitions and exogenous environmental and behavioral stimuli (1,6,14,16).

The subjects then returned to a period of home monitoring for several days following the constant routine until they began a 58-day period of bicycling approximately 90 miles per day (exercise monitoring). In total, each subject traveled 4,500 miles during this period, from the east to the west coast of the United States. Sleep schedules were generally regular, with the subjects waking an hour later the morning after crossing each time zone. Sleeping conditions consisted of a sleeping bag placed on a carpeted floor or wrestling mat, or occasionally a bed. Physical conditions during cycling varied greatly in ambient temperature (15-38 degrees C), altitude, and humidity.

Upon returning by plane to the laboratory both subjects participated in another session of laboratory monitoring during which they maintained the sleep-wake schedules they had been following during the period of exercise monitoring. Upon the completion of this two-day period, they participated in another constant routine.

Data Analysis

To examine average daily variations in body temperature, average waveforms were educed for home monitoring and exercise monitoring for each subject using mid-sleep time as reference. Days during exercise monitoring in which the subjects did not bicycle, and days during home monitoring in which they bicycled during a training run, were eliminated from analysis. Information from the wrist activity sensor was used along with event markers entered into the Vitalog to determine the subjects' sleep-wake times.

To examine the acute effects of exercise and subsequent rest on body temperature we measured the magnitude of temperature changes immediately following the beginning and end of exercise. An exercise event was defined as a period of bicycling for at least 20 minutes which was preceded by a rest of at least 20 minutes. If a bicycling event was interrupted by a rest of less than 5 minutes then it was considered a single exercise period. A rest event was defined as a period of rest of at least 20 minutes immediately following a period of exercise. Exercise and rest events within 90 minutes of sleep times were eliminated from analysis. The change in body temperature due to ending an exercise event was determined by measuring the difference in temperature between the event code marking the cessation of cycling and the next event code marking the initiation of an exercise event. The change in body temperature due to initiating an exercise event was determined by measuring the change in temperature between the event code marking the initiation of an exercise event to the peak of the subsequent temperature rise.

In order to investigate the morphology of the body temperature curve for a more extended period (2 hours) after the initiation and cessation of periods of strenuous exercise, we further examined a subset of exercise events which were preceded by at least 90 minutes of rest and recovery periods consisting of at least 120 minutes. Using the times of the onset of bicycling events as reference points, we averaged the temperature data immediately preceding and following these points across all events. This resulted in a composite average waveform of the response of body temperature to the initiation of cycling. We analyzed the temperature data for rest periods using the same technique. To control for time-of-day effects, we compared these data to baseline temperature data collected at the same times of day during randomly assigned days of home monitoring. This constituted our baseline data.

RESULTS AND DISCUSSION

As shown in Figure 1, the average educed waveform of the body temperature cycle during exercise monitoring days was remarkably similar to that recorded under baseline home monitoring conditions, notwithstanding the fact that the subjects were bicycling 90 miles per day during exercise monitoring. Both the amplitude and the morphology of the body temperature cycle were essentially the same under both conditions.

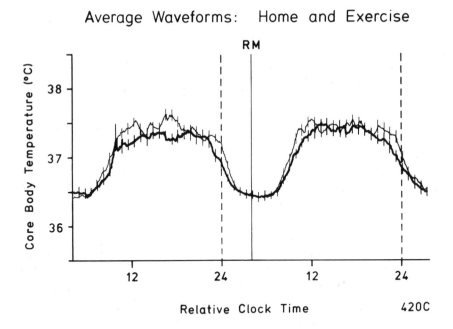

FIG. 1. Average educed waveforms (+S.E.M.) for home monitoring (bold line) and exercise monitoring (light line) are shown superimposed on the same axes. Both waveforms are similar in amplitude and morphology even during waking hours, when activity is most varied.

In fact, we found that the subjects' average daytime temperature curves were very similar under all four conditions of study: exercise monitoring, home monitoring, laboratory monitoring, and even the constant routine, when the subjects were relatively inactive in bed during the daytime. During the night, the subjects' average temperature curves were also essentially the same under all conditions except for the constant routine, when core body temperature was approximately 0.25 degrees C higher than it was during baseline home monitoring.

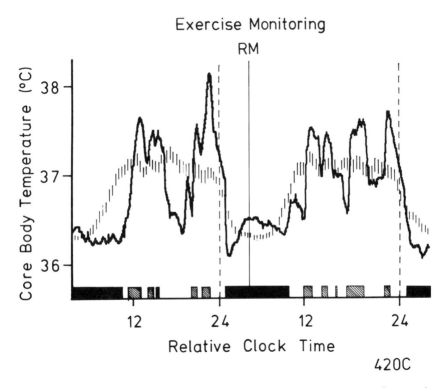

FIG. 2. Core body temperature for two individual days of exercise monitoring (bold line) is superimposed on the average educed waveform (+S.E.M.) of exercise monitoring for subject 420C (vertical hatch marks). Solid bars on the abscissa denote sleep episodes, and the hatched bars represent episodes of exercise. Significant increases in body temperature are seen during episodes of exercise with subsequent decreases in temperature below the average during periods of rest. These temperature fluctuations may result in the similar average waveforms seen in Fig. 1, since the timing of exercise and rest events differ for each day of exercise monitoring.

The unexpected similarity between the average daytime body temperature curves during exercise and home monitoring appear to be in contrast to data from numerous past studies which show body temperature increasing during periods of exercise (3,4,8,10,13,22,23). Examination of unaveraged temperature data from single days of recording during exercise monitoring revealed that individual bouts of exercise induced an acute rise in body temperature in our subjects as well (Figure 2). However, these exercise-induced temperature increases were followed by decreases in body temperature below baseline at the termination of exercise events. This is in contrast to unaveraged temperature data from single days of home monitoring, which closely adheres to the average waveform, as seen in Figure 3.

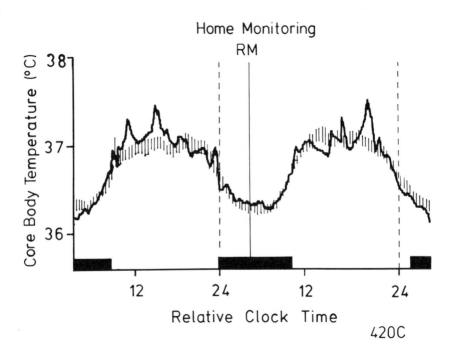

FIG. 3. Core body temperature for two individual days of home monitoring (bold line) is superimposed on the average educed waveform (+S.E.M.) of home monitoring for subject 420C (vertical hatch lines). Solid bars on the abscissa denote times of sleep. The example period of home monitoring closely adheres to the average waveform.

In order to quantify the acute effects of exercise and subsequent rest on body temperature, we measured the magnitude of temperature changes during these periods. The average temperature rise associated with exercise periods was 0.63 degrees C for subject 422C and 0.66 degrees C for subject 420C. The average temperature fall subsequent to cessation of exercise was 0.63 degrees C for subject 422C and 0.63 degrees C for subject

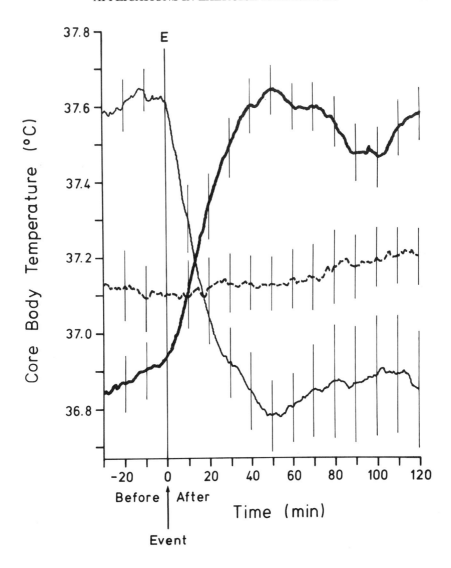

FIG. 4. Body temperature data (+S.E.M.) following the initiation of an exercise event (bold line), the cessation of exercise (light line), and under baseline conditions at the same times of day (dashed line). The vertical line marked E designates the onset of these events. The temperature increases associated with exercise onset and the decreases after the cessation of exercise (and onset of rest) are of approximately the same absolute value but in opposite directions.

420C. The similarity of these values might initially appear to indicate that the exercise-induced increase in temperature was simply superimposed upon the baseline temperature curve. However, careful examination of the unaveraged data in Figure 2 reveal that during exercise, the temperature rose above baseline, only to fall below baseline during intervening periods of rest. Due to recovery from a preceding bout of exercise, the body temperature was often depressed prior to the start of exercise bouts.

In order to investigate the generality of this finding, we averaged temperature data immediately following the initiation or cessation of an exercise event and compared it with paired data from the same subject during baseline home monitoring conditions, matched for the time of day (Figure 4).

Analysis of the data in this manner reveals that although there was indeed an increased average body temperature above baseline following the start of exercise, there was also a decrease in body temperature below baseline following the cessation of exercise. In fact, the baseline data lies nearly midway between the temperature values during periods of exercise and periods of rest. Since the exercise and rest periods occurred at varying times each day, the evoked responses to these events had little net effect on the average waveform of the body temperature cycle during the daytime (Figure 1) despite the considerable variations in the subjects' physical activity and environment.

In addition, we found that the level did not change during the night in association with varying levels of activity performed during the prior day. The constant routine, however, was associated with a marked increase in nighttime temperature. It thus appears that modification of the subjects environment and behavioral state during the night can have a much more powerful effect on nocturnal temperature than daytime activity.

It has been reported (13,15) that marathon runners have a tendency to become markedly hypothermic in the recovery period after a race. Data from our study suggest that this phenomenon may be more common than previously suspected and occurs to some extent after less severe exercise. One might speculate that the elevated body temperature during exercise induces an anti-pyrogenic response which depresses the hypothalamic set point. Upon the cessation of exercise, this response may result in an overcompensatory drop in body temperature.

The similar average temperature waveforms which we recorded under diverse field conditions suggest that average body temperature rhythms do not vary significantly with changes in physical activity. Although exercise acutely raises body temperature, a proportional decrease in temperature occurs during rest periods following strenuous exercise. The mechanisms underlying this phenomenon invite further investigation.

ACKNOWLEDGEMENTS

This research was supported, in part, by a grant from the United States Olympic Committee. The authors wish to thank N. Salafsky, S. Sullivan, A. Ward, J. Ronda and W. Freitag for their assistance.

REFERENCES

1. Aschoff, J. (1960): *Cold Spring Harbor Symp. Quant. Biol.*, 25:11.

2. Blomstrand, E., Kaijser, L., Martinsson, A., Bergh, U. and Ekblom, B. (1986): *Acta Physiol. Scand.*, 127:477-484.

3. Chappuis, P., Pittet, P. and Jequier, E. (1976): *J. Appl. Physiol.*, 40(3):384-392.

4. Christensen, S.E., Jorgensen, O.L., Moller, N. and Orskov, H. (1984): *Acta Endocrinol.*, 107:295-301.

5. Czeisler, C.A. (1978): *Thesis*, Stanford University.

6. Czeisler, C.A., Brown, E.N., Ronda, J.M., Kronauer, R.E., Richardson, G.S. and Freitag, W.O. (1985): *Sleep Res.*, 14:295.

7. Davies, C.T.M. and Sargeant, A.J. (1975): *British J. Ind. Med.*, 32:110-114.

8. De Meirleir, K., Arentz, T., Hollmann, W. and Vanhaelst, L. (1985): *British Med. J.*, 290:739-740.

9. Deutsch, D.T. and Knowlton, R.G. (1980): *Arch. Phys. Med. Rehabil.*, 61:298-303.

10. Downey, J.A. and Darling, R.C. (1962): *Appl. Physiol.*, 17(2):323-325.

11. Faria, I.E. and Drummond, B.J. (1982): *Ergonomics* 25(5):381-386.

12. Greenleaf, J.E., Castle, B.L. and Card, D.H. (1974): *Acta Physiol. Pol.*, 25(5):397-409.

13. Maron, M.B., Wagner, J.A. and Horvath, S.M. (1977): *Appl. Physiol.*, 42(6):909-914.

14. Mills, J.N., Minors, D.S. and Waterhouse, J.M. (1978): *J. Physiol.*, 285:455.

15. Minors, D.S. and Waterhouse, J.M. (1985): *Chronobiol. Int.*, 1:205.

16. Nadel, E.R. (1984): *Clinics in Chest Med.* 5(1):13-20.

17. Nadel, E.R., Holmer, I., Bergh, U., Astrand, P.O. and Stolwijk, J.A.J. (1973): *Life Sci.*, 13(7):983-989.

18. Reilly, T. and Brooks, G.A. (1982): *Ergonomics*, 25(11):1093-1107.

19. Reilly, T. and Brooks, G.A. (1986): *Int. J. Sports Med.*, 7:358-362.

20. Saltin, B. and Hermansen, L. (1966): *J. Appl. Physiol.*, 21(6):1757-1762.

21. Sawka, M.N., Pemental, N.A. and Pandolf, K.B. (1984): *Eur. J. Appl. Physiol.*, 52:230-234.

22. Simpson, K.H., Green, J.H. and Ellis, F.R. (1986): *J. Clin. Pharmac.*, 22:579-586.

23. Tanaka, M., Bolle, M.A., Brisson, G.R. and Dion, M. (1979): *Eur. J. Appl. Physiol.*, 42:263-270.

Medical Monitoring in the Home and Work Environment,
edited by Laughton E. Miles and Roger J. Broughton.
Raven Press, New York © 1990.

AMBULATORY MONITORING IN THE AVIATION ENVIRONMENT

Linda J. Connell and R. Curtis Graeber

NASA Ames Research Center
Aerospace Human Factors Research Division
Mail Stop: 239-21
Moffett Field, California 94035

INTRODUCTION

The immediate and long-term physiological effects of time zone travel are critical considerations in aviation. People whose lifetime careers involve repeated flights across continents at ever increasing speeds and distances find themsleves exposed to numerous variables that may affect well-being, performance, quality of life, and possibly longevity. Many of the issues surrounding the impact of these changes on the biopsychological milieu have been documented in laboratory research (13), but rarely in the actual field situation of transport aviation. With the advent of recent technological advances in microprocessor instrumentation, it has become feasible to propose real-time, continuous physiological measurement of flight crewmembers during performance of their duties on the flight deck (5).

Research is presently in progress to document changes in circadian rhythms, sleep, and alertness among a variety of flight crews (3,4). Within this broad investigative study, a core set of data gathering procedures has been implemented, of which ambulatory monitoring has been a major part. Continuous ambulatory monitoring has not only been feasible and suitable for physiological data collection, but it is both a reality and a success within commercial and military air transport operations. This chapter will illustrate the application and acceptability of ambulatory physiological monitoring in a wide variety of settings within the home and work environments of the pilot.

ENVIRONMENTS IN COMMERCIAL AND MILITARY AVIATION

Due to the versatility and portablility of ambulatory monitors, data collection methods have been readily adaptable to the changing situations of field research within the commercial and military aviation systems. Whether flying 90 passengers from Pittsburgh to Boston or transporting cargo to Incirlik AFB, Turkey, the lack of interference in the operation of normal duties has been a crucial variable in the success and validity of physiological monitoring. Crewmembers, company managers, and regulatory authorities had to be assured that the research monitoring would not hamper a pilot's performance, especially if an in-flight emergency should arise. In addition to being unobtrusive, another requirement of any ambulatory instrumentation is freedom of movement to allow the volunteer to pursue his or her normal activities while at home or in the work environment. It is important that the monitoring unit adapts to the individual and that the person does not substantially modify his or her behavior in order to adapt to the device. It has also been necessary that the ambulatory monitoring equipment meet the requirements of aviation operations conducted within a wide variety of environments, from the tropical heat of Bombay to the arctic weather of Andoya, Norway. The equipments's tolerance of such extremes has led to the successful collection of data during the performance of flying duties in aircraft ranging from commercial jets (DC-9, B727, B737, and B747) to military transports (USAF-MAC: C-5, C-9, C-130, and C-141) and P-3 patrol aircraft to four types of helicopters operating in the North Sea. The collective database contains continuous physiological and behavioral information on approximately 400 flight crewmembers, and represents the largest database of its kind in aeromedical research.

PHYSIOLOGICAL-BEHAVIORAL MONITORING

The current protocol uses the Vitalog PMS-8 monitoring system (Redwood City, CA) to record the following three physiological parameters every two minutes: heart rate, non-dominant wrist activity, and body temperature. At the same time, volunteer flight crewmembers record information in a dailylog regarding sleep timing, exercise, duty schedules, meal timing, meal content, caffeine intake, health symptoms, and self-assessments of sleep quality, mood, and fatigue. Additional information is collected in a background questionnaire on demographics, aviation experience, and usual at-home sleep, exercise, and meal behavior. Included in this questionnaire are scales for morningness-eveningness and personality assessments (1,7,12).

Collection of physiological and daily log data begins with 2-3 days baseline recording at home prior to the scheduled flight duty and continues throughout the trip. A trained cockpit observer accompanies the crewmembers for the entire flight duty period (commonly 3-4 days for domestic patterns, and 7-10 days for international patterns), thus providing flight deck observations by phase of flight from all flight segments. Using a combined format (structured and open-ended), the observer records time-linked observations of operational events related to flight countermeasures or adaptive strategies used by these experienced aviators to ameliorate fatigue or circadian disruption. Finally, to assess recovery, physiological monitoring and daily log data collection continues for up to four days post-trip.

APPLICATION OF VITALOG MONITOR

Every type of physiological monitor has unique characteristics for application and maintainance. The Vitalog PMS-8 system is an 8K, solid-state unit consisting of a portable recorder (12 oz., 6.0 x 3.4 x 1.3 in.) powered by rechargeable nickel-cadmium batteries with color-coded sensor cables and worn in a pouch on a belt. The amount and type of data collected is selected through the available software options. Sampling interval, value tables, parameter selection, and many other unique characteristics of data collection can be programmed into the recorder via an interface with a personal computer system.

Choosing an appropriate sampling rate involves a trade-off between frequency of data points required and memory storage available in the recorder. In the present protocol, a two minute sampling rate on three parameters saturates the memory storage capability in approximately 10 days. However, due to the unique characteristics of the rechargeable battery, the battery life is the limiting variable affecting the length of the data recordings. The data, therefore, must be read-out into a computer for disk storage every 4-6 days. After re-initialization of the PMS-8, data collection resumes.

The three parameters monitored in the present study were selected to provide information on circadian rhythms, sleep, and operational impact. The circadian rhythmicity in continuous core body temperature is assessed via a small, flexible rectal themistor. The themistor (Yellow-Springs, Series 400) has been specially tailored in our laboratory as a result of suggestions from subjects and researchers wearing the device. To ensure correct and consistent placement just within the rectal sphincter, a small, plastic bead about 7mm in diameter is secured 10cm from the thermistor tip. Three coats of white silicon are subsequently applied to the sensor for a smooth, continuous surface and aesthetic appearance.

Heart rate values (r-wave) are collected with three color-coded electrode leads applied to the chest. After attachment of button-type ECG electrode pads (Syncor Inc.) to the clips, the self-adhesive pads are placed on the chest. The red lead is placed on the outer, lateral aspect of the right side of the chest at approximately nipple level. The white lead is similarly placed on the left side. This basic configuration allows for right to left telemetry across the chest. The green lead serves as the gound lead and is placed on the left over the bottom rib. The instrumentation stores the average heart rate (beat/min) over the specifed sampling period as the mid-point value of the binning table established by the resarcher.

Non-dominant wrist activity is measured with a small, watch-size device on a wrist strap. There are many devices available to record activity, including accelerometers (6). In the present project, a device that has an array of three mercury tilt switches aligned in three planes sends a movement signal from any plane to the PMS-8 monitor which stores the total number of movements within the sampling period. As with heart rate, a binning table installed via the software programming is utilized, and the mid-point value of the specific bin is recorded as the data point. Consistent placement on the wrist is encouraged for data integrity, and, because the activity sensors cannot be cross-calibrated, the same wrist sensor is worn by the participant throughout the study. All activity data must be either standardized statistically for comparison, or a within-subjects design must be utilized. An example of the typical data obtained from these physiological recordings and daily log is presented in Figure 1.

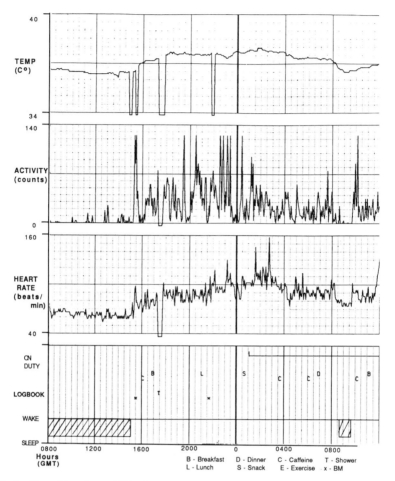

FIG. 1. Graphic plot of Vitalog PMS-8 physiological data time-linked with the daily log information.

CONCURRENT SUBJECTIVE REPORT

To reinforce data continuity as well as to gather valuable information on subjective responses, some form of a diary or daily log is necessary to allow the reliable assessment of ambulatory physiological responses. A pocket-size paper format that provides the opportunity and encourages a person to record information about the time and type of their daily activities, such as sleep, awakenings, exercise, personal care and work. Other variables that may have physiological impact, such as meals, medication, caffeine, and general symptoms may also be recorded.

Aside from providing direct information about the issue being investigated, the subjective record is invaluable when attempting to assess absent or artifactual data. Distinguishing artifactual from reliable functioning of the instrumentation is a continuous requirement for valid data collection.

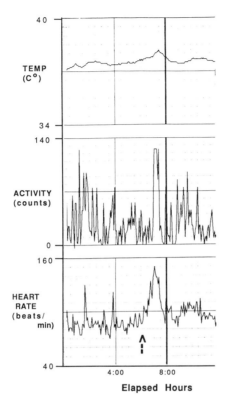

FIG. 2. Example of the physiological response of a pilot to aerial refueling in a C-141 military aircraft. Arrow indicates beginning of air-to-air hook-up; each small grid square equals 30 minutes.

If, for instance, the heart rate channel appears erroneous, there may be a question of a poor signal due to possible equipment malfunction. Logbook information reporting that the volunteer was exercising at the time may reveal that sweating was most likely interfering with good conduction and that there was no equipment failure. Entries in a logbook that indicate times of showers or bowel movements can explain missing data (i.e., leads off). Additionally, it is important to provide an open-ended comment section not restricted by an inflexible format allowing the volunteer the opportunity to report other helpful information.

In addition to the importance of data integrity and continuity, time-coordinated logging of significant events allows direct comparison to the physiological record for addressing specific research issues. For example, in the aviation environment, the physiologic impact of operational events is of interest. It is important to note that a heart rate response of 150 beats/min during a duty flight period was related to an aerial refueling manuever (Figure 2). Another significant time-coordinated event of interest is the physiological response to exercise. It is important to identify core body temperature rises and heart rate increases that are linked to exercise (Figure 3) as opposed to those linked to circadian fluctuations. Sleep

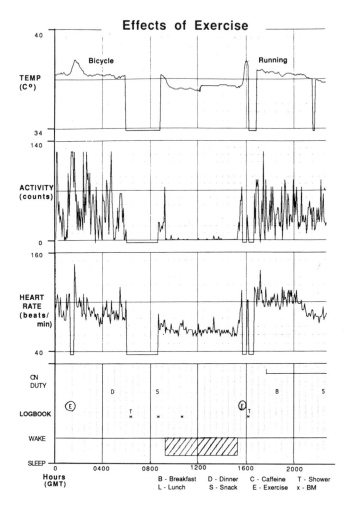

FIG. 3. Typical physiological responses in heart rate, activity, and body temperature during exercise (onset indicated by circled E in logbook record).

quality and quantity are of major interest, therefore reliable logbook information about when a person goes to bed, to sleep, and awakens is crucial when no direct measurements are available (i.e., EEG). Confirming physiological changes (e.g., decreases in heart rate, temperature, and activity) as sleep related events assists in analyzing how numerous awakenings or displaced circadian cycles affect sleep duration and quality. In addition, the masking effects of activity and sleep are major methodological considerations which must be addressed for the accurate quantification and description of circadian rhythms (2). Diligent and reliable records on the rest/activity cycles enable the researcher to meet this requirement.

DATA PROCESSING

Consideration for the immense volume of data that is generated by continuous recording of physiological parameters cannot be de-emphasized. One of the major benefits of the abundant data obtained from ambulatory monitoring can become a major stumbling block, if procedures and capabilities are not developed to cope with immense data strings. For instance, a four-day recording of one parameter sampled every two minutes will yield approximately 70,000 data points. Imagine the database required for 400 records approximately 10 days in length on three parameters. In the present study, an interactive database (Relational Interactive Management, Boeing Co.) on a VAX 750 mainframe computer has been programed to store and allow manipulations of this volume of data.

The actual processing of the raw data involves several steps. In the interest of illustration, one method of handling large quantities of ambulatory data will be discussed. This process has evolved after considerable problem solving and has been tailored to the experiences of the present project. Therefore, it may not apply to other types of ambulatory monitoring in detail; but it may be helpful in terms of the general approach.

In order to maintain accurate inventories and to track equipment use, it is necessary to devise utilization logs to be completed by the field researchers. Such inventories are particularly helpful in keeping data collection costs, in terms of time and money, at a minimum. The experience of losing 4-6 days of data due to poor equipment handling can be disappointing to the researcher, but it becomes even more difficult to explain the loss to the volunteer who experienced the inconvenience, for example, of wearing a rectal temperature sensor during that time. Of course, a utilization log should contain entries concerning the time-coordination of initialization, readout, and hook-up, but it should also report the use history of all recorders, cables, and wires. This enables the efficient tracking of any inoperable equipment during trouble shooting and facilitates prompt removal from the useable inventory. Battery voltages are tracked and recorded at initialization, readout, and before and after charging, thus providing an extensive charge-discharge history on each battery. Consequently, changes in the expected, unique characteristics of nickel-cadmium batteries can be detected early to prevent data loss from poor battery functioning. Of course, during data collection the field observer should always have a spare, initialized PMS-8 recorder plus accessories available for exchange in the event of any data disruption from equipment failure.

After readout of the PMS-8 monitor via an interface cable to an Apple IIe, the raw data is stored on a floppy disk and reviewed through a plotting program. Any irregularities in data collection are noted on the utilization log. Back-up diskettes are created at this time. The back-up diskettes are kept at the field site while the originals are transported to the laboratory. Back-ups are maintained at all times in case of the possibility of inadvertent computer or disk failure.

The raw diskette data, after reformatting from binary to ASCII, is transferred to the mainframe computer. The files are linked from readout of one record to restart of another for that crewmember's data collection period. The data are then automatically edited by conservative criteria (see Table 1) to eliminate obvious artifacts, such as inaccurate temperature changes associated with thermistor slippage or unintentional heart rate/activity data generated when the wires are removed from the subject but still connected to the device. The data are replotted and finally hand edited for only the most obvious errors. The completed data string is then entered into the interactive database (RIM, Boeing Co.) along with entries from the daily log, observer log, and background questionnaire. This database is fully interactive allowing flexibility for comparisons between objective and subjective variables. For example, mid-cruise heart rate on the third day of flight for all pilots in a Boeing 747 can be compared to

TABLE 1. Computer Editing Criterion - Physiologic Data

Set to default/null values, if:		
Temperature	$<34.5^{o}$ or $>40.0^{o}$	change 0.25^{o} in 2 min.
Activity	>250	heart rate = 0 and temp = 0
Heart Rate	<40 or >170	

the same time period for co-pilots. Another example of interactive flexibility could be determining the mean heart rate and activity level during sleep after time zone shifts of 8 or more hours for all flight crewmembers. In summary, this type of database allows manageable, but thorough exploration of research and operational issues.

SUBJECT ACCEPTANCE AND COMPLIANCE

Time and effort is well spent in assuring acceptance of physiological monitoring equipment and reliable adherence to the recommended protocol. This is especially important when the person is ambulatory and not always under direct researcher supervision. The quality of the resultant data can only benefit from increasing the level of motivation and understanding towards the rationale of the research. In order to accomplish this goal, a major effort was undertaken to coordinate and establish good communication and acceptance between the aviation and research communities. Following presentations of the proposed research to airline management and pilot groups, contact was initiated by distribution of a pamphlet and letter. These items were prepared to educate the flight crewmembers and prepare them for the initial research contact. After selection of target flight sequences, crewmembers assigned to these flights were contacted by telephone and given a full disclosure of the research protocol. An effort was made in this first conversation to educate the person on the history of the research, the scientific rationale for the data collection measures being utilized, and the relevance to their everyday life and career.

The physiological monitoring equipment, although addressed in general terms in the introductory pamphlet and letter, was discussed fully. The size, weight, and method of wearing the Vitalog PMS-8 were presented. Whenever possible, references were made to tangible items with which the volunteer would most likely be familiar (i.e., the Vitalog PMS-8 is similar in size to a standard portable cassette player used outdoors). The body temperature measurement was the portion of the protocol most often resisted, due to the unusual rectal placement. Therefore, when describing the temperature measurement, the wire was referred to as a "sensor", not as a "probe". The size of the thermistor was described as the "size of a shoelace" in order to arrest the common tendency to visualize something much larger and more threatening. The importance of obtaining circadian rhythm information and the rationale for core body temperature was stressed.

The daily maintenance of the equipment and the impact on daily living was discussed with numerous suggestions and options offered for personal care and methods of wearing the recorder in order to decrease the intrusion. Specific suggestions for wearing the device during exercise and sleeping were mentioned. It was especially important that there were clear instructions concerning acceptable times to remove the equipment and when it was especially important to be hooked-up. Reasonable limits and expectations toward this type of continual data collection can help to increase compliance. The emphasis was on adapting the system to the specific, individual situation and not vice versa. The rejection rate with this type of recruitment was as low as 15% among a group of U.S. commercial air carriers.

At the time of hook-up, one of three methods was used to maintain continuity. Whenever possible, the preferable method was a one-to-one demonstration. If this was not feasible, a videotape was included with the equipment demonstrating the hook-up and requirements of the daily log. The least preferable method, written instructions, was only utilized when the person did not have access to a videotape recorder. A follow-up telephone call (by the researchers) was made (to all volunteers) the day after hook-up. The volunteer crewmember had access to one of the researchers 24 hours a day for any question, concerns, or problems.

Equal in importance to a thorough introduction to ambulatory monitoring is feedback. At the time of the first readout with the field observer, the data is plotted and the crewmember is able to compare his or her own logbook entries to the actual physiologic record. Basic explanations are provided by the field observer regarding circadian rhythms, sleep, and the impact of typical operational events. This has a positive effect on continued compliance and increased accuracy of record keeping. Additionally, after the data processing, a continuous plot of the completed record is always mailed to the volunteer along with a letter of appreciation.

CURRENT AND FUTURE TECHNOLOGIES

In addition to the main protocol described above for ambulatory monitoring with the Vitalog system, other portable technologies have been utilized in the on-going research in the aviation environment. In an attempt to quantify objective sleep parameters in flight crewmembers, portable EEG recorders (Oxford Medilog) were successfully utilized on several crewmembers flying multiple flights between Tokyo and London. Research with these EEG monitors is continuing and will address other issues of waking/alertness states of flight crewmembers flying extended international routes. Since prolonged exposure to altitude might be expected to reduce circulating oxygen and therefore increase sleepiness, these recordings will be supplemented by measurements of arterial oxygen saturation obtained from the finger using non-invasive pulse-oximetry spectrometry. Thus, multiple ambulatory technologies may be utilized to provide a more comprehensive understanding of biomedical phenomena in real-world environments.

The development of portable physiological measurement devices is rapidly expanding. Other current technologies covering a wide range of variables are available for application to a variety of home and work environments. For instance, sleep EEG measurements are presently being transmitted over telephone lines from home to the laboratory (11). Heart rate functioning of ventricular efficiency can be monitored with the use of an ambulatory vest for more accurate measures of ischemic sequelae (10). Ambulatory blood pressure monitoring has been found to have greater reproducibility and predictability than clinic measurements (9). Additionally, methods are being developed to assess levels of cerebral oxygen sufficiency from non-invasive transillumination spectrometry (8). Some of these recent innovations are being evaluated for their applicability to aerospace medicine. Recent trends in commercial aviation may increase the demand for such "in-flight" measurement capability. For instance, the predicted pilot shortage has increased attention to the medical fitness of pilots, especially those beyond 50 years of age. Ambulatory monitoring could be the most valid, reproducible method available to address these workplace issues. The potential contribution of ambulatory monitoring technology to the understanding of human performance in aviation is significant, especially considering the safety aspects of this high risk environment. These portable devices are now capable of unobtrusively sampling physiological events that were illusive in the not-so-distant past. The resulting increase in real-time, on-site monitoring will undoubtedly improve our understanding about how variables such as lifestyle, job demands, and environmental factors affect worker well-being and health.

REFERENCES

1. Eysenck, H.J. and Eysenck, S.B. (1968): *Eysenck Personality Inventory. Educational and Industrial Testing*, San Diego, CA.

2. Gander, P.H., Connell, L.J. and Graeber, R.C. (1986): Masking of the Circadian Rhythms of Heart Rate and Core Temperature by the Rest-Activity Cycle in Man. *J. Biol. Rhythms*, 1 (2): 119-135.

3. Gander, P.H. and Graeber, R.C. (1987): Sleep in Pilots Flying Short-Haul Commercial Schedules. *Ergonomics*, 30 (9):1365-1377.

4. Graeber, R.C. (1982): Alterations in Performance Following Rapid Transmeridian Flight. In: *Rhythmic Aspects of Behavior*, edited by F.M. Brown and R.C. Graeber, pp. 173-212. Erlbaum, New Jersey.

5. Graeber, R.C., Foushee, H.C., Gander, P.H. and Noga, G.W. (1985): Circadian Rhythmicity and Fatigue in Flight Operations. *Journal of the UOEH*, 7 (Suppl.):122-130.

6. Groves, D. (1988): Beyond the Pedometer: New Tools for Monitoring Activity. *Physician and Sportsmed.*, 16 (6):160-166.

7. Horne, J.A. and Ostberg, O. (1976): A Self-Assessment Questionnaire to Determine Morningness-Eveningness in Human Circadian Rhythms. *Int. J. Chronobiol.*, 4:97-110.

8. Jobsis-VanderVliet, F.F., Piantadosi, C.A., Sylvia, A.L., Lucas, S.K. and Keizer, H.H. (1988): Near-Infrared Monitoring of Cerebral Oxygen Sufficiency. I. Spectra of Cytochrome C Oxidase. *Neurol. Res.*, 10 (1):7-17.

9. Pickering, T.G. (1987): Strategies for the Evaluation and Treatment of Hypertension and Some Implications of Blood Pressure Variability. *Circulation*, 76 (1-2):I77-82.

10. Rozanski, A. and Berman, D.S. (1987): Silent Myocardial Ischemia. I. Pathophysiology, Frequency of Occurrence, and Approaches Toward Detection. *Am. Heart. J.*, 114 (3):615-626.

11. Sewitch, D.E. and Kupfer, D.J. (1985): A Comparison of the Telediagnostic and Medilog Systems for Recording Normal Sleep in the Home Environment. *Psychophysiology*, 22 (6):718-726.

12. Spence, J.T. and Helmreich, R.L. (1983): Achievement- Related Motives and Behavior. In: *Achievement and Achievement Motives: Psychological and Sociological Approaches*, edited by J.T. Spence. W.H. Freeman & Co., New York.

13. Wever, R. (1979): *The Circadian System of Man*. Springer-Verlag, New York.

Medical Monitoring in the Home and Work Environment,
edited by Laughton E. Miles and Roger J. Broughton.
Raven Press, New York © 1990.

CIRCADIAN EFFECTS OF VARYING ENVIRONMENTAL LIGHT

Daniel F. Kripke and Lois Watanabe Gregg

Department of Psychiatry
University of California
San Diego, Calfornia 92161

INTRODUCTION

Earth's 24-hour cycle of daylight and darkness is known to synchronize the circadian rhythms of many plants and animals. Although social cues were believed most important in synchronizing human circadian rhythms (9), recent data show that light is also an extremely powerful synchronizer and phase-setter of the human circadian system (10,11). Unlike familiar laboratory species, however, for major effects, the human circadian system requires several hours of exposure to illumination of the order of 2000-4000 lux or more (11). Such illumination intensities are rarely achieved by customary artificial indoor lighting, though at moderate latitudes, outdoor illumination is 2000 lux in prevailing weather conditions from soon after sunrise until shortly before sunset. Most primates are diurnal and spend all of the day in daylight. From the modest human circadian sensitivity to light, it would seem that our circadian systems are also adapted to exposure to outdoor light much of the daylight hours.

With the invention of artificial light, modern man has loosed his dependence on daylight. The majority of Americans today spend most of their waking hours in artificial lighting. Total light exposure, the timing of light exposures and the intensity of light exposures have thus changed markedly from the natural conditions to which our prehistoric ancestors were adapted. Many scientific models preserve the romantic notion that the contemporary population is exposed to something resembling the natural photoperiod. This is hardly correct.

To describe the actual patterns of contemporary illumination exposures, our group has developed an ambulatory monitoring system to continuously monitor a subject's illumination exposure. The system is based on a photometric transducer connected to the Vitalog PMS-8 monitoring computer (4,6). To obtain the almost 180 degrees circular field of sensitivity which is probably characteristic of the suprachiasmatic nucleus neurons which respond to light synchronization, we adapted our transducers to a wide angle of sensitivity. Because a variety of data suggests that the circadian system may have peak sensitivity to green light (with a sensitivity spectrum similar to rhodopson), we filtered our inputs to match maximal sensitivity to the green portion of the spectrum. Preliminary experiments have suggested that illumination at the wrist correlates ($r = 0.89$) with illumination at the forehead striking the eyes, and there is no systematic bias (5). Therefore, for convenience, we have mounted our transducers on wrist bands. To simultaneously record wrist activity, we have incorporated acceleration transducers into the wrist-mounted sensors.

With this technology, Okudaira et al. (6) showed that subjects in our urban environment were exposed to daylight illumination for only brief and scattered episodes during the 24 hours. Savides, et al. (7) then studied a group consisting mainly of medical students and medical researchers. Even in sunny San Diego in the summer, the average subject only experienced illumination exceeding 2000 lux for about 1.5 hours per 24 hours. Moreover, remarkable inter-individual variability was found in the timing as well as in the durations of bright light exposures.

The current study examined the day-to-day variability in illumination for a single individual over a much longer period of time. Though no single individual is likely to be typical of a population, intensive study of an individual allows us the first information on the intra-individual variance in illumination. Also, this study quadrupled the total round-the-clock illumination measurements which had up to that time been collected.

METHODS

To minimize factors related to poor outdoor weather and work schedules, a medical student agreed to be studied in the equable environment of Oahu, Hawaii, housed just four miles from Waikiki beach. Having given informed consent, and having been assigned to collect and analyze the data as an independent study project, the volunteer was free to pursue a flexible schedule. From June 23 to August 25, 1985, a healthy 23 year-old, right-handed female student wore a special data recording system which consisted of the Vitalog PMS-8 computer monitor connected to a wrist actigraph and light transducer.

The light transducer was a photoresistor (CL9P911 photo-conductive resistor), a fixed resistor, and a battery network connected to the Vitalog analog-to-digital converter (4). The spectral sensitivity of the system was adjusted by affixing a 15 x 15 mm green Kodak Wrattan Gelatin Filter (#38) so that the transducer peak sensitivity was at about 520 nm. A Kodak neutral density attenuator film (Density 1.0, #173 4532) placed directly atop the green filter allowed the range of sensitivity of the system to be adjusted to approximately 1 to 50,000 lux, covering the range from dim twilight to direct sunlight. The neutral density film also broadened the transducer's circular receptive angle to about 180 degrees (5). The wide receptive angle minimized directional aspects of measurement. A calibration curve was obtained by illuminating both the Vitalog light transducer and a photometer (UDT Model 40X with cosine-corrected photometric filter) with varying controlled white light intensities and referencing the transducer output to the photometer lux measurements. The light transducer was sampled once at the end of every minute and the value recorded.

The wrist actigraph transducer consisted of a small weight soldered off-center onto a spring-like wire connected to a peizoceramic element which was excited whenever the transducer was moved in any direction. The activity transducer was sampled several times a second. The average activity amplitude recorded represented the most active 2 second interval during each minute. Both the light and activity transducers were mounted on the dominant right wrist, oriented like a wristwatch dial.

The subject wore this recording system 24 hours a day for 62 days while continuing habitual daily activities during her summer at home in Hawaii, removing the system only while showering or swimming. When not wearing the system, the transducer was placed in lighting as similar to the subject's environment as was possible, e.g. on the beach when the subject was swimming. Every 24 to 48 hours, data were transferred from the Vitalog system to an Apple II+ computer for storage and analyses. In addition, daily sleep and activity diaries were diligently kept. Of the 62 recorded days, 23 days worth of data were excluded from analysis due to equipment and human failures.

To roughly identify illumination exposures with powerful affects on the circadian system, an arbitrary threshold of 2000 lux was selected. For each 24-hour period, from midnight to midnight, the number of minutes of 2000 lux illumination were totalled. For the same 24-hour period, the median time of bright illumination for that day was calculated. This was achieved by totalling the number of minutes of 2000 lux, and finding the midpoint time (half the bright illumination before and half after this midpoint). The means and standard deviations were then calculated over the 39 day period for (a) the total number of minutes in each day of 2000 lux and (b) the median time of illumination with 2000 lux.

From the sleep diary data and activity recordings, sleep latency, sleep onset, and sleep duration were estimated. The wrist actigraph output has been shown to provide a good estimator of sleep. The time of sleep onset was determined by adding four minutes to the time of the last movement as recorded by the wrist actigraph. Sleep latency was calculated by subtracting the time of "lights out" (as determined by a clear drop in the Vitalog illumination value) from the time of sleep onset. Sleep duration was the time from sleep onset to the time of awakening, as indicated by activity.

RESULTS

Figure 1 is a condensed plot of the valid 39 days of data with each spike representing an average of 10 minutes with 2000 lux. This illustrates the large variability of timing and duration of bright light exposure (2000 lux). The day-to-day variability can best be appreciated in Figures 2 and 3. Figure 2 illustrates the number and percent of days that the subject experienced various durations of 2000 lux. For example, in 8 out of 39 days (20.5% of days), the subject received a total of less than 30 minutes of 2000 lux, while in 2 out of 39 days (5% of days), she experienced more than 6 hours of bright light exposure. The mean number of minutes of 2000 lux for a 24-hour period was 131 minutes +/- SD 99 minutes. Figure 3 illustrates the distribution of median times at 2000 lux. For example, on 10 of the 39 days (or 26% of days) half the minutes of 2000 lux were before and half were after median times between 10:30 and 11:30 am. Though 67% (26/39) of the days had a median time of bright light exposure between 10:30 am and 2:30 pm, great variability was observed, with 5% (2/39) of

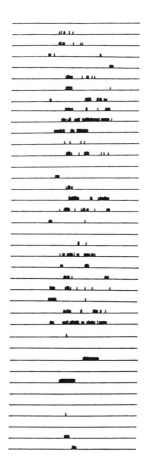

FIG. 1. Each horizontal line represents one 24-hour illumination recording from midnight to midnight. The vertical bars each represent 10 minutes when the mean illumination exceeded 2000 lux.

days with median times between 7:30 and 8:30 am and 8% (3/39) of days with median times between 5:30 and 6:30 pm. The mean and standard deviation of median time of exposure of 2000 lux was 12:30 pm +/- 147 minutes. To explore possible effects of light exposure variations upon sleep each night, correlations were computed among variables: (a) sleep duration, (b) sleep latency, (c) sleep onset time, (d) wake-up time,

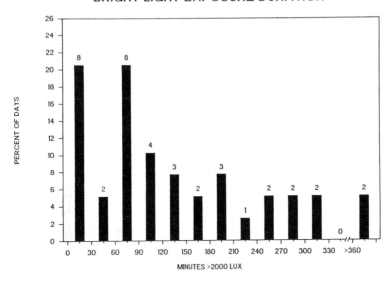

BRIGHT LIGHT EXPOSURE DURATION

FIG. 2. The distribution of daily durations of exposure to illumination exceeding 2000 lux.

(e) the previous day's number of minutes 2000 lux, (f) previous day's median time of 2000 lux. Data for 39 days were included in all analyses except the variables of sleep duration, sleep latency, and sleep onset. Sleep duration and sleep onset could only be determined on 37 of the 39 days because of ambiguities in the time of sleep onset on two of the days. Sleep latency was determined on only 18 of the 39 days because on 21 days, the time of "lights out" was either ambiguous from the Vitalog values or was inconsistent with the time recorded in the sleep diary. The Pearson product-moment correlation coefficients were determined (Table 1). Several were found to be significant. Sleep onset, sleep duration, and wake-up time were related as might be expected, with a later onset leading to a later wake-up, and sleep duration related both to earlier sleep onset and later wake-up. A later median time of bright light exposure was not associated with significant changes in sleep latency or sleep onset; nevertheless, a later median time of bright light exposure was associated with later wake-up times and consequently longer sleep durations.

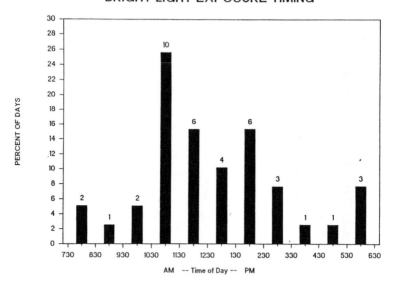

BRIGHT LIGHT EXPOSURE TIMING

FIG. 3. The distribution of daily timing of exposures to illumination exceeding 2000 lux. Each bar represents the number of days where the median time for illumination >2000 lux fell in a particular hour of the day.

DISCUSSION

Though Hawaii is famous for the availability of sunshine and equable weather, and a flexible schedule permitted their enjoyment, it is striking that the subject experienced an average of only 131 minutes of outdoor light a day.

Wever et al. (11) suggested that light does not strongly synchronize human circadian rhythms until exposures of 4000 lux are maintained for 3 to 8 hours, a finding supported by Czeisler et al. (2) Though our volunteer did not restrain herself from enjoying the outdoors, she spent more than 3 hours in 2000 lux on only 30% of the days. On 21% of the days, she received less than 30 minutes of bright light. Savides et al. (7) found that 5 researchers, whose schedules may be more representative of working Americans, averaged only 26 minutes of 2000 lux. This evidence suggests that the bright light exposures experienced in contemporary society are often insufficient for maximal synchronization of circadian rhythms.

The timing of bright light exposures are crucial in synchronizing human

Table 1: Associations of variables: analysed by Pearson product- moment correlation.

	Minutes >2000 lux (N=37)	Median time >2000 lux (N=37)	Sleep Latency (N=18)	Sleep Onset (N=37)	Sleep Duration (N=37)	Wake-Up Time (N=37)
-Mean	131	12:30	7.5 min.	00:22	428 min.	07:30
+ SD	99	147 min.	4.4 min.	63 min.	78 min.	69 min
Minutes >2000 lux		0.10	0.21	-0.15	0.09	0.04
Median time >2000 lux			0.10	-0.07	0.39**	0.38*
Sleep latency				0.04	0.19	0.32
Sleep onset					-0.53+	0.30
Sleep duration						0.64+

(* $p<0.05$, ** $p<0.025$, + $p<0.001$)

circadian rhythms. Our intra-individual results show that the main daily exposure to illumination 2000 lux can be experienced in almost any portion of the daylight hours. On the majority of days, the median times of 2000 lux occurred between 10:30 am and 2:30 pm, but median times occurred as early as 7:30 am and as late as 6:25 pm, a range of almost eleven hours. Given light's phase-setting effects on the human circadian system, this variability in duration and timing of exposures could produce frequent aberrations of circadian rhythm phase. It would be predicted that such aberrations could affect both sleep and mood.

Our data showed no significant correlations of: (a) minutes 2000 lux with median time of lux 2000, sleep latency, sleep onset, or sleep duration; (b) median time of lux 2000 with sleep latency or sleep onset. However, our data do suggest that there was a relationship between median time per day experiencing illumination 2000 lux and sleep duration, which resulted from the significant correlation between the median bright illumination time of each day and the wake-up time the following morning. In other words, the later in the day the volunteer was exposed to bright light, the longer she slept that night; the earlier she experienced bright light, the earlier she awoke the next morning. These results suggest that variations in each day's illumination experience resets the phase of the underlying circadian oscillator sufficiently to influence the time of awakening, as predicted by several circadian models (3,8,12). It is interesting to note that there was a significant negative correlation between sleep onset and sleep duration (r=-0.534, p.001) as suggested by the models of Czeisler et al. (3) and Zulley et al (12).

Another possible mechanism must be considered. There is evidence to suggest that a rebound effect occurs after evening light suppression of melatonin secretion causing higher mid-sleep melatonin production (1). Later, illumination exposures causing greater rebound might explain the correlation between time of bright light exposure and sleep duration to the extent that increased late-night melatonin might prolong sleep duration.

This study illustrates the extreme variability in light exposures experienced by one individual in a locale with minimal weather changes in a limited portion of the year. It is likely that people in other parts of the world experience even greater ranges of light exposures. Such intra-individual variations in light exposure could account for frequent variations in mood and sleep experienced by insomniacs and persons with affective instability. Future research should aim to more precisely identify the role of illumination experience in these disorders with a view toward treatment with planned illuminations. Our data suggest that the timing of bright light affects sleep duration. Further investigations should explore how the timing of bright light exposure affects the occurrence of insomnia, low mood, melatonin excretion, and chronobiologic disorders.

ACKNOWLEDGEMENTS

Supported by: NIMH RSDA MH00117, MH38822, AG02711, HL 07491, and the Veterans Administration.

REFERENCES

1. Beck-Friis, J. Borg, G. and Wetterberg, L. (1985): Rebound Increase of Nocturnal Serum Melatonin Levels Following Evening Suppression by Bright Light Exposure in Healthy Men: Relation to Cortisol Levels and Morning Exposure. In: *The Medical and Biological Effects of Light,* edited by R.S. Wurtman, M.J. Baum and J.T. Potts, Jr., pp. 371-375. The New York Academy of Sciences, New York.

2. Czeisler, C.A. and Allan, J.S. (1987): Acute Circadian Phase Reversal in Man via Bright light Exposure: Application to Jet Lag. *Sleep Research,* 16:605.

3. Czeisler, C.A., Weitzman, E.D., Moore-Ede, M.C., Zimmerman, J.C. and Knauer, R.S. (1980): Human Sleep: Its Duration and Organization Depend on its Circadian Phase. *Science,* 210:1264-1267.

4. Kripke, D.F., Webster, J.B., Mullaney, D.J., Messin, S. and Fleck, P. (1981): Measuring Sleep by Wrist Actigraphy. In: *ʃArmy Final Technical Report #4,* AD#A124200, pp. 1-45.

5. Kripke, D.F., Mullaney, D.J., Savides, T.J. and Gillin, J.C. (In press): Phototherapy for Nonseasonal Major Depressive Disorders. In: *Seasonal Affective Disorders and Phototheraphy,* edited by N. Rosenthal and M. Blehar. The Guilford Press, New York.

6. Okudaira, N., Kripke, D.F. and Webster, J.B. (1983): Naturalistic Studies of Human Light Exposure. *Am. J. Physiol.,* 245:R613-R615.

7. Savides, T.J., Messin, S., Senger, C. and Kripke, D.F. (1986): Natural Light Exposure of Young Adults. *Physiol. Behav.,* 38:571-574.

8. Strogatz, S.H., Kronauer, R.E. and Czeisler, C.A. (1986): Circadian Regulation Dominates Homeostatic Control of Sleep Length and Prior Wake Length in Humans. *Sleep,* 9(2):353-364.

9. Wever, R.A. (1979): The Circadian System of Man: Results of Experiments under Temporal Isolation. Springer-Verlag, New York.

10. Wever, R.A. (1985): Use of Light to Treat Jet Lag: Differential Effects of Normal and Bright Artificial Light on Human Circadian Rhythms. In: *The Medical and Biological Effects Of Light,* edited by R.J. Wurtman, M.J. Baum and J.T. Potts, Jr., pp. 282-306. The New York Academy of Sciences, New York.

11. Wever, R.A., Polasek, J. and Wildgruber, C.M. (1983): Bright Light Affects Human Circadian Rhythms. *Pflugers Arch.,* 396:85-87.

12. Zulley, J. and Campbell, S. (1985): The Coupling of Sleep-Wake Patterns with Rhythm of Body Temperature. In: *Proceedings of the Seventh European Congress on Sleep Research, Sleep `84,* edited by W.P. Koella, E. Ruther and H. Schulz, pp. 81-85. Gustav Fischer Verlag, New York.

Medical Monitoring in the Home and Work Environment,
edited by Laughton E. Miles and Roger J. Broughton.
Raven Press, New York © 1990.

AUTOMATED BLOOD PRESSURE MONITORING IN THE DIAGNOSTIC AND THERAPEUTIC ASSESSMENT OF HYPERTENSION

Michael A. Weber, Deanna G. Cheung and Joel M. Neutel

Hypertension Center
Veterans Administration Medical Center
University of California, Irvine
Long Beach, California 90822

INTRODUCTION

Establishing the diagnosis of hypertension and assessing its response to treatment can be facilitated by automated whole-day blood pressure monitoring with non-invasive portable devices. It has been shown that a meaningful proportion of patients with office-diagnosed hypertension exhibit apparently normal whole-day blood pressure values when tested with the monitoring procedure. This technique appears to be indicated in patients with milder forms of office hypertension in whom there are no physical changes, personal or family history, or other clinical findings to support a diagnosis of hypertension requiring treatment. Whole-day measurements may sometimes be of value in assessing the individual patient who does not appear to be responding adequately to treatment. There is a growing use of automated monitoring in clinical trials of antihypertensive drug efficacy. Placebo responses are eliminated or minimized by this technique; and statistical analysis of efficacy can be made with fewer patients than would be required if conventional measurements were used. It is also possible to assess the duration of treatment effects and to make recommendations on the frequency of administration of antihypertensive medications. Automated measurements may be especially useful for monitoring the effects of treatment during the early morning hours, when the blood pressure often rises sharply.

The measurement of blood pressure in the office has become a routine part of the physical examination. Data obtained by this technique have been used to define the prognosis and natural history of hypertension and are used in most research studies that evaluate the pathophysiology of human hypertension or assess its response to differing forms of therapy. Moreover, practicing clinicians use the conventionally-measured blood pressure in order to make clinical diagnoses of hypertension and to make decisions concerning its treatment. But, as discussed below, the sphygmomanometer-measured blood pressure is inconsistent; and, despite its usefulness in establishing prognostic information in large populations, it can be a misleading measurement in the individual patient.

Lightweight, automated, portable monitoring equipment has made it convenient and safe for blood pressure to be measured on a 24-hour basis in ambulatory subjects. Studies with this technique have started to establish its role in clinical hypertension and to document its relationship to cardiovascular changes. The whole-day blood pressure measured in the ambulatory patient correlates more closely than conventional readings with echocardiographically-measured indices of cardiac left ventricular muscle mass (4,3). In turn, this echocardiographic index has been shown to have strong prognostic implications for cardiovascular disease (1). Other investigators have used a point score system based on clinical evaluations of target organ involvement in normotensive and hypertensive patients, and have shown that the whole-day blood pressure value is predictive of cardiovascular status (16). The same investigators have shown that blood pressure variability during the day, a measurement that can be derived from the whole-day monitoring procedure, also correlates strongly with the status of the cardiovascular system. Blood pressure monitoring technology has not yet been available for a sufficient time for us to have accumulated clear data concerning its role in predicting long-term cardiovascular prognosis; but preliminary studies with semi-automated equipment have suggested that this method is superior to the conventionally-measured blood pressure in forecasting major events (11).

It appears that the major uses for whole-day ambulatory blood pressure monitoring are for the diagnosis of hypertension and for evaluating response to treatment, especially the efficacy and duration of action of investigational antihypertensive drugs.

DIAGNOSTIC CONSIDERATIONS

There is evidence that conventional methods for assessing blood pressure may lead to erroneous diagnoses of hypertension in some patients. Even in carefully performed clinical trials, in which patients have been diagnosed only after several conventional readings have been shown to be clearly in the hypertensive range, there have been marked placebo responses that have brought into question the accuracy of the original diagnosis in many study participants (14). It has also been shown that in up to 30% of hypertensive patients the blood pressure remains within the normal range following discontinuation of therapy (6), again suggesting that the original diagnosis may have been erroneous.

It is usually recommended that physicians delay a diagnosis of hypertension until high blood pressure readings have been confirmed during several office visits, preferably over a period of a few weeks. Although this careful approach may help identify some individuals whose initial blood pressure values might have been falsely high, there is growing evidence that conventionally obtained blood pressure readings sometimes provide values that are not representative of the true blood pressure status. Recently we have described patients whose whole-day blood pressure monitoring values were normal despite consistently hypertensive readings during multiple visits to the office, including a 4 to 6-week period of placebo administration (22). Using intra-arterial methods of monitoring, other investigators have observed that the mere approach of a physician to the patient for the purpose of measuring blood pressure can raise the readings by approximately 27/14 mm Hg (13). Interestingly, this response is not attenuated over time, even after several contacts with the physician.

A recent large-scale comparison of hypertensive and normotensive patients has verified that over 20% of patients diagnosed as having hypertension by standard clinical means appear normal when evaluated for the full 24-hour period (17). These authors also found that the high office readings were sustained during multiple visits, and concluded that this phenomenon was not one of simple anxiety but instead reflected a conditioned response to the medical environment. Thus, they have argued that the doctor-patient relationship might have a unique impact on blood pressure, and that these hypertensive reactions are not necessarily indicative of responses to other stresses or stimuli during routine daily activities. Finally, an experience in our own clinic has verified these findings: as shown in Figure 1, when we compared groups of age and sex-matched normotensive and hypertensive patients (diagnosed clinically by multiple visit criteria), we found a considerable overlap between the two groups in their whole-day systolic and diastolic blood pressure values (5).

INDICATIONS FOR THE PROCEDURE

It is clearly not necessary to perform whole-day automated blood pressure monitoring in all patients in whom a diagnosis of hypertension is being considered. A decision to diagnose hypertension and to initiate treatment is readily supported in patients whose conventionally-measured high blood pressure readings are associated with clinical or laboratory evidence for target organ involvement. Additionally, the presence of other cardiovascular risk factors also seems to justify a more ready acceptance of the diagnosis of hypertension. And the presence of a strong family history of hypertension, or possibly of premature cardiovascular disease, facilitates the diagnosis and early treatment of hypertension. Thus, the ideal candidate for diagnostic blood pressure monitoring is the patient whose blood pressures are found consistently in the mild to moderate hypertension range and in whom there is no supportive clinical or historical information favoring the diagnosis of hypertension or its need for treatment.

As yet there is no clear agreement on how to make diagnostic interpretations of whole-day blood pressure monitoring data in individual patients. One of the most simple methods for analyzing data is to average all values obtained during the 24-hour period. This value appears to be a powerful and reproducible reflection of the whole-day blood pressure, provided that the averages are based on readings obtained at consistent intervals throughout the entire 24-hour period. It is then possible to interpret the whole-day blood pressure value by using diagnostic criteria derived previously from epidemiologic studies with conventionally-measured blood pressures. Based on 100 subjects, we have found that there is a reasonably consistent relationship between office measured blood pressures and whole-day blood pressure values both in normotensive volunteers and in patients with mild to moderate essential hypertension (see Figure 2). Overall, the whole-day blood pressure averages are 10/5 mm Hg lower than the office values (19), presumably because whole-day

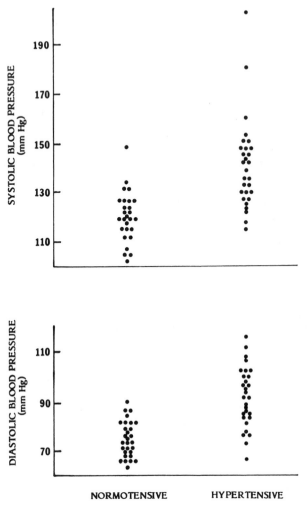

FIG. 1. Whole-day averages for systolic and diastolic blood pressures in 29 pairs of age-matched hypertensive (by conventional office criteria) and normotensive men. With permission from (5).

averages include the lower readings that occur typically at night. Thus, the diagnostic blood pressure criteria of 140/90 mm Hg recommended by the Joint National Committee on the Detection, Evaluation, and Treatment of High Blood Pressure (9) would correspond to whole-day averages of 130/85 mm Hg. Other investigators, using separate statistical methods for choosing 24-hour diagnostic criteria, have proposed similar diagnostic values (17,10).

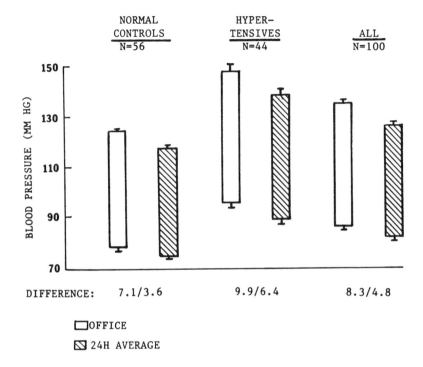

FIG. 2. Conventional office blood pressure measurements and whole-day blood pressure averages in normotensive volunteers and patients with mild to moderate hypertension (diagnosed by conventional office criteria). Differences refer to the average of the differences between the office and the whole-day values. Adapted from (19).

Of course, other approaches to diagnosis are possible, including such criteria as the incidence of readings throughout the day that fall above a given arbitrary level, or the use of chronobiologic concepts such as the hyperbaric index that take into account the actual time duration of increased blood pressure values (7). It is also possible to visually scan the 24-hour data and determine on an empirical basis, by clinical experience and judgement, whether there appears to be consistent evidence for hypertension or whether high blood pressure readings can be explained by stimuli or events that have occurred during the day.

VALUE OF THE TEST

Despite the growing experience with automated ambulatory blood pressure monitoring, this technique has not yet been universally accepted for the diagnosis of hypertension. It has been suggested, for example, that this technique be regarded as investigational rather than clinical until, among other things, "normative" data for blood pressures measured with this method are established (8). Unfortunately, this type of information, especially if it is to be linked to large population studies of cardiovascular prognosis, would be logistically difficult and expensive to obtain. It could also be argued that long-term studies of the natural history of untreated hypertension might be unethical. This type of information, however, may not be necessary for there are already abundant epidemiologic and actuarial data linking casual or conventional blood pressures with cardiovascular outcome. The chief attribute of the whole-day monitoring procedure is to determine whether or not a particular individual patient has a sustained increase in blood pressure. Once that question is answered, then prognostic and therapeutic assumptions can be extrapolated from the established epidemiological experiences.

Some observers have also expressed concern at the potential financial cost of performing large numbers of blood pressure monitoring procedures. But, as discussed above, this technique should only be recommended in those patients in whom the diagnosis of hypertension cannot be reasonably established by more standard clinical means. It should also be noted that antihypertensive therapy usually is a lifelong commitment, and incurs the expenses of physician visits, clinical tests, medications, and the cost of the patient's time lost from work. Thus, even if only a minority of patients studied with the monitoring technique are found not to be in need of therapy, this approach would still appear to be cost effective.

One important question, however, remains unanswered: Are patients whose conventional blood pressures appear high, but whose 24-hour monitoring values fall within the normal range, truly normal? It could be argued that their higher casual readings, even if they occur only in the physician's office, make them different from individuals whose blood pressure are always normal. In a previous study using standard blood pressure measurements, we subdivided patients into those whose hypertension was sustained during serial clinic visits and those whose blood pressures fell into a borderline or normal range. Measurements by echocardiography of left ventricular wall thicknesses and muscle mass were virtually identical in the two groups, and were significantly higher in each of them than in normal controls (20). Thus, it is possible that patients with non-sustained hypertension, including those with high office blood pressures but normal 24-hour values, might in some instances have cardiovascular target organ changes that are suggestive of true hypertensive disease. Clearly, this issue demands further study.

EVALUATION OF TREATMENT

Automated blood pressure monitoring is useful for assessing progress in patients receiving antihypertensive treatment. It can be used for studying the effectiveness of therapy of individual patients in clinical practice and also for measuring the efficacy and duration of action of antihypertensive agents being studied in clinical trials. The main purpose of blood pressure monitoring in routine clinical practice is to evaluate patients in whom antihypertensive treatment, as assessed by conventional means, does not appear to be successful. In most of these patients there will not be a previous monitoring period as a basis for comparison, and the interpretation of the findings must be somewhat empirical. A recent report described patients whose blood pressure control measured in the conventional clinical setting was relatively unsatisfactory, and who were then examined by a monitoring procedure (18). In some of these patients, the apparently poor response to treatment was confirmed by the longer-term blood pressure values; but in others, it was evident that the treatment blood pressure measurements were far lower than those observed in the clinic and that alterations in their therapeutic regimens would not appear necessary.

Whole-day ambulatory blood pressure monitoring has been used successfully to evaluate new antihypertensive agents (23,24,15). A strength of this technique is that there appears to be no placebo response, and that determinations of efficacy can be made with fewer patients than would be required, if conventional measurements were used (2). It is possible to compare blood pressure values obtained throughout the day during baseline and treatment monitoring periods. Comparisons can be based on the blood pressures for the day as a whole or on selected shorter periods. Typically the day is divided into 12 two-hour periods, and it is possible to utilize statistical testing of differences between corresponding periods during the pre-treatment and treatment monitoring procedures. Determining duration of antihypertensive efficacy is a particular strength of this technique, especially as data can be obtained during sleep and the important early morning hours around the time of arousal.

The value of this technique was shown in a recent study in which the effects of an antihypertensive agent given twice daily were compared with its effects when given just once daily (21). We found that the once-daily administration was at least as effective as the twice-daily regimen for the first 20 hours of the monitoring period; it was only near the end of the whole-day observation, during the early morning hours that cannot readily be studied by conventional clinical methods, that we found a relative loss of efficacy during the once-daily regimen. An interesting approach to drug evaluation was recently reported with the converting enzyme inhibitor, captopril (24). Whole-day non-invasive monitoring in a group of 31 hypertensive patients receiving this drug, given just once daily, indicated a moderate antihypertensive response. But if patients with relatively poor responses to this treatment (n=10) were removed from analysis, the monitoring data then revealed that the once-daily administration of captopril in the remaining 21 patients provided meaningful antihypertensive efficacy throughout the entire 24-hour period. Thus, in this experience, the automated monitoring technique was used not so much to determine efficacy as to measure the duration of effect in patients already shown to have antihypertensive responses to this form of therapy.

We have used whole-day blood pressure monitoring in yet another fashion to evaluate the antihypertensive effects of the calcium channel blocking agent, diltiazem (22). In a group of 15 patients, all of whom had been shown to have hypertensive blood pressure values by repeated conventional measurements prior to the start of the study, we found that twice-daily administration of diltiazem produced a moderate antihypertensive response that was sustained throughout the full 24-hour period. However, we noted that the baseline blood pressure monitoring procedure performed immediately prior to the initiation of therapy indicated that 6 of the 15 patients failed to meet the criteria for the diagnosis of hypertension (as discussed earlier). If we now analyzed the blood pressure effects of diltiazem in this "non-confirmed" hypertensive subgroup, we found that there was no significant change in blood pressure with treatment. On the other hand, the monitoring data in the remaining nine hypertensive patients indicated that diltiazem produced antihypertensive effects throughout the 24-hour period that were clearly more powerful than those observed for the original full treatment group. By using the diagnostic properties of whole-day monitoring in addition to its ability to determine efficacy and duration of action of antihypertensive treatment, it was possible to quantify treatment effects in those patients for whom treatment appeared to be most justified.

SUMMARY

Our growing experience with automated non-invasive whole-day ambulatory blood pressure monitoring has revealed that this technique is valuable in the diagnosis of hypertension and in assessing its response to therapy. Further research in the realm of diagnosis is still required to more closely associate data obtained with the monitoring procedure with the underlying status of the cardiovascular system. It is also important to further study those patients whose hypertension is not confirmed by the monitoring technique. Are these patients truly normal, or do they exhibit some stigmata of target organ change? The experiences with ambulatory monitoring in assessing efficacy of antihypertensive treatment have been encouraging, and innovative uses of this method are allowing an improved understanding of the properties of new and established antihypertensive agents. By better defining the hypertensive process, this technology may help establish new criteria for characterizing optimal approaches to treatment.

REFERENCES

1. Casale, P.N., Milner, M. and Devereux, R.B. (1985): Value of Echocardiographic Left Ventricular Mass in Predicting Cardiovascular Morbid Events in Hypertensive men. *Circulation*, 72:130.

2. Conway, J., Johnston, J., Coats, A., Somers, V. and Sleight, P. (1988): The Use of Ambulatory Blood Pressure Monitoring to Improve the Accuracy and Reduce the Numbers of Subjects in Clinical Trials of Antihypertensive Agents. *J. Hypertension*, 6:111-116.

3. Devereux, R.B., Pickering, T.G., Harshfield, G.A., et al. (1983): Left Ventricular Hypertrophy in Patients with Hypertension: Importance of Blood Pressure Response to Regularly Recurring Stress. *Circulation*, 68:470-476.

4. Drayer, J.I.M., Weber, M.A. and DeYoung, J.L. (1983): BP as a Determinant of Cardiac Left Ventricular Muscle Mass. *Arch. Intern. Med.,* 143:90-92.

5. Drayer, J.I.M., Weber, M.A. and Nakamura, D.K. (1985): Automated Ambulatory Blood Pressure Monitoring: A Study in Age-Matched Normotensive and Hypertensive Man. *Am. Heart J.,* 109:1334-1338.

6. Gould, B.A., Mann, S., Davies, A.B., Altman, A.G. and Raftery, E.B. (1981): Can Placebo Therapy Influence Arterial Blood Pressure? *Clin. Sci.,* 61:478S-482S.

7. Halberg, F., Drayer, J.I.M., Cornelissen, G. and Weber, M.A. (1984): Cardiovascular Reference Data Base for Recognizing Circadian Mesor- and Amplitude-Hypertension in Apparently Healthy Men. *Chronobiologia,* 11:275-341.

8. Hunt, J.C., Frohlich, E.D., Moser, M.,Roccella, E.J. and Keighley, E.A. (1985): Devices Used for Self-Measurement of Blood Pressure. *Arch. Intern-Med.,* 145:2231-2234.

9. Joint National Committee on Detection, Evaluation, and Treatment of High Blood Pressure. (1984): The 1984 Report of the Joint National Committee on Detection, Evaluation, and Treatment of High Blood Pressure. *Arch. Intern-Med.,* 144:1045-1057.

10. Krakoff, L. R., Eison, H., Phillips, R.H., Leiman, S.J. and Lev, S. (1988): Effect of Ambulatory Blood Pressure Monitoring on the Diagnosis and Cost of Treatment for Mild Hypertension. *Am. Heart J.,* 116:1152-1154.

11. Linsell, C.R., Lightman, S.L., Mullen, P.E., Brown, M.J. and Causon, R.C. (1985): Circadian Rhythms of Epinephrine and Norepinephrine in Man. *J. Clin. Endocrinol. Metab.,* 60:1210-1215.

12. Mancia, G., Parati, G., Pomidossi, G., Colombo, A., Cuspidi, C., Lattuada, S., Antivalle, M., Rindi, M., Libretti, A., Gianfranco, B. and Zanchetti, A. (1987): Evaluation of the Antihypertensive Effect of Once-a-Day Captopril by 24-Hour Ambulatory Blood Pressure Monitoring. *J. Hypertension,* 5, 5:S591-S593.

13. Mancia, G., Parati, G., Pomidossi, G., Grassi, G., Casadei, R. and Zanchetti, A. (1987): Alerting Reaction and Rise in Blood Pressure During Measurement by Physician and Nurse. *Hypertension,* 9:209-215.

14. Meyers, A. and Dewar, H.A. (1975): Circumstances Attending 100 Sudden Deaths from Coronary Artery Disease with Coroners' Necrosis. *Br. Heart J.,* 37:1133-1143.

15. Nissinen, A., Koistinen, A., Tuomilehto, J., Sundberg, S. and Gordin, A. (1986): Sustained Release Verapamil in Hypertension--Results from a Noninvasive Ambulatory Blood Pressure Monitoring and a Clinical Study. *Eur. J. Clin. Pharmacol.*, 31:255-260.

16. Parati, G., Pomidossi, G., Albini, F., Malaspina, D. and Mancia, G. (1987): Relationship of 24-Hour Blood Pressure Mean and Variability to Severity of Target Organ Damage in Hypertension. *J. Hypertension,* 5:93-98.

17. Pickering, T.G., James, G.D., Boddie, C., Harshfield, G.A., Blank, S. and Laragh, J.H. (1988): How Common is White Coat Hypertension? *JAMA.,* 259:225-228.

18. Porchet, M., Bussien, J.P., Waeber, B., Nussberger, J. and Brunner, H.R. (1986): Unpredictability of Blood Pressures Recorded Outside the Clinic in the Treated Hypertensive Patient. *J. Cardiovasc. Pharmacol.,* 9:332-335.

19. Weber, M.A. and Drayer, J.I.M. (1986): Role of Blood Pressure Monitoring in the Diagnosis of Hypertension. *J. Hypertension,* 4, 5:S325-S327.

20. Weber, M.A., Drayer, J.I.M. and Baird, W.M. (1986): Echocardiographic Evaluation of Left Ventricular Hypertrophy. *J. Cardiovasc. Pharmacol.,* 8, 3:s61-s69.

21. Weber, M.A., Tonkon, M.J. and Klein, R.C. (1987): Blood Pressure Monitoring for Assessing the Duration of Action of Antihypertensive Treatment. *J. Clin. Pharmacol.,* 27:751-755.

22. Weber, M.A., Cheung, D.G., Graettinger, W.F. and Lipson, J.L. (1988): Characterization of Antihypertensive Therapy by Whole-Day BP Monitoring. *JAMA.,* 259:3281-3285.

23. White, W.B., Smith, V.E., McCabe, E.J. and Meeran, M.K. (1985): Effects of Chronic Nitrendipine on Casual (Office) and 24-Hour Ambulatory Blood Pressure. *Clin. Pharmacol. Ther.,* 38:60-64.

24. Zachariah, P.K., Sheps, S., Schirger, A., Spiekman, R.E., O'Brien, P.C. and Simpson, K.K. (1986): Verapamil and 24-Hour Ambulatory Blood Pressure Monitoring in Essential Hypertension. *Am. J. Cardiol.,* 57:74D-79D.

Medical Monitoring in the Home and Work Environment,
edited by Laughton E. Miles and Roger J. Broughton.
Raven Press, New York © 1990.

AMBULATORY ECG MONITORING TO DETECT MYOCARDIAL ISCHEMIA

Saul B. Freedman

Hallstrom Institute of Cardiology
University of Sydney and Royal Prince Alfred Hospital
Missenden Road, Camperdownts
NSW, 2050 Australia

INTRODUCTION

Ambulatory ECG monitoring first became possible with the development of battery operated tape recorders. The first of these recorders was designed by Dr. Holter in 1961 (21) and resulted in the name "Holter monitoring" applied to this technique. Initial instruments were heavy and cumbersome. But there have been huge technological advances since, so that current devices are small, light and intelligent. The initial clinical application of Holter monitoring was to detect cardiac arrhythmias; and while periodic attempts were made to look at myocardial ischemia (34), this was impeded by technological limitations of the early devices (20).

Recent interest in silent ischemia has spurred the technological improvements which have made it possible to reliably detect ischemia in the ECG of ambulatory patients. This review will focus on the technical requirements of ambulatory ischemia monitors, because of the fundamental importance of these considerations for producing ECG signals adequate for evaluation. In addition, the application of this technique in the diagnosis and management of patients with coronary disease, will be compared with standard diagnostic techniques.

ECG CHANGES IN ISCHEMIA

Ischemia causes a change from aerobic to anaerobic metabolism in the myocardium, which results in the accumulation of lactic acid, reduced pH and high energy phosphate stores, and local accumulation of extracellular potassium. The resultant alteration in resting membrane potential, and changes in amplitude and duration of the cardiac action potential, produce characteristic changes in the electrocardiogram, notably in the ST segment (23). When ischemia is subendocardial, as is usual during exercise testing and ambulatory monitoring, there is depression of the ST segment, while subepicardial or transmural ischemia seen in patients with vasospastic angina or myocardial infarction, causes ST segment elevation. Peaking or psuedo-normalization of T waves also occurs with ischemia, but is less specific, and is not universally accepted as denoting ischemia unless occurring reversibly at the time of symptoms. Changes in the QRS complex, such as alteration in R and S wave amplitude are not usually accepted as reliable indicators of ischemia.

The usual ST criteria for diagnosis of ischemia are borrowed from exercise stress testing: > 1 mm (0.1 mV) planar or downsloping ST depression at the J point, or > 1mm ST elevation (12). A slowly up-sloping ST depression is usually accepted, if the ST is still depressed > 2 mm at 80 ms after the J point. All the same interpretation problems of exercise testing (i.e., false positive and false negative tests, uninterpretable ECG's as with left bundle branch block, or drug or hypertrophy induced depolarization changes) apply equally to ambulatory electrocardiography. Additionally, as body position can vary enormously through the day, spurious ST deviation associated with postural changes must be distinguished from ischemic ST shifts (6,15). Failure to consider these changes is a shortcoming of many of the manual and automated commercial systems.

FREQUENCY AND PHASE REQUIREMENTS

The importance of adequate low frequency response for accurate reproduction of the ECG was noted by Berson and Pipberger in 1959 (3), and is readily apparent in the characteristic distortion seen when high pass filters are set at 0.15 Hz in ECG monitors. As a result, the American Heart Association has recommended that ECG recorders have a linear frequency response between 0.05 and 100 Hz for accurate reproduction of the wave form (28). The apparent frequency dependence of ST segment display results from the use of analog amplifiers and filters in ECG recorders. In general, these amplifiers have a phase response approximately 1 decade worse than their frequency response and it is this relationship which has made the AHA low frequency response criterion clinically useful.

In a number of recent studies it has been shown that phase and not frequency is important for accurate ST segment representation (4,25,36). Firstly, digital filters with linear frequency response to 0.05 Hz but with phase distortion at that frequency, produced quite severe distortion of the ECG waveform. Secondly, digital filtering of low frequencies up to 2 Hz without phase shift, produced no distortion of the waveform. This might be predicted from the Fourier theory, which states there are no frequencies in the waveform below the fundamental (equal to the heart rate, i.e. 1 Hz at 60/min)(17). Frequency information below this is responsible for baseline wander, and is undesirable as it makes ambulatory ECG interpretation difficult.

Most new ECG recorders use digital technology and digital filtering with linear phase filters to remove frequencies below 0.5 Hz without phase distortion, and these produce high quality, accurate, ECG waveforms. Manufacturers still quote conformation to the AHA frequency response standards, although clearly this is not so, and it is likely that the American Heart Association will reexamine its criteria in the light of these findings.

TAPE RECORDERS

Most ambulatory monitors are low speed tape recorders, typically running at 3 3/4 inches/min, and using either cassette or reel to reel high-fidelity logging magnetic tape. The recorders are usually AM, with a limited frequency response, often quoted only for the front-end. While this frequency performance may conform to the AHA criteria, manufacturers seldom indicate the frequency response of the overall system, including play-back and hard copy. In my experience, and as found by Bragg-Ramschel et al. (4), frequency and phase problems largely result from tape replay and can be substantial. For some of the available AM systems, overall frequency and phase response are inadequate for accurate reproduction of the ST segment.

A very simple test of a monitors' performance is to record a range of ECG's with and without resting ST changes simultaneously using a high quality standard recorder and the Holter recorder, and compare the output of both. Monitors with the poorest frequency and phase performance perform worst (4). The performance of AM recorders can be improved by paying special attention to the playback heads and amplifiers, and by high speed playback, as used in a number of commercial systems. Other suggestions have been to play the tape backwards to reverse the phase shift, but this also reverses the ECG making interpretation difficult. A novel approach in one commercial system uses a high-pass filter during the initial recording to produce a known degree of phase distortion and remove baseline wander, with subsequent digital phase rectification by computer (Marquette).

An alternative solution to the problems of AM recorders is to use FM recorders which are linear in phase and frequency to DC. Monitors such as the Oxford FM recorder are able to accurately reproduce ST segments, but are less reliable and produce wow and flutter contributing to baseline wobble which again makes ECG interpretation difficult (4).

PLAYBACK

Most of the ambulatory ECG systems in the past used a form of audio-visual superimposition to allow the operator to rapidly scan a 24 hour tape, typically at 60 times real-time, with ECG complexes superimposed on the screen by an R wave trigger. An audio signal can be added and this method is usually quite adequate for detecting ectopic beats and unusual rhythms. Its use is less appropriate for detection of ST segment change, as baseline wander may make it very difficult to visualize ST segment shifts, and short episodes of ischemia can easily be missed. The technique is also liable to error from observer fatigue (35).

Another technique produces a complete disclosure of the 24 hour ECG so that every complex is shown but is relatively compressed and miniaturized. This can be displayed on a TV screen or on hard copy, and again is very useful for the detection of arrhythmias, but small shifts in the ST segment can be very difficult to see in this format (15).

A more reliable technique utilizes compressed analog signals, replaying the tape at rapid speed (e.g., 60 x real-time) with output to a recorder with good high frequency response (e.g., photographic recorder or Mingograph),

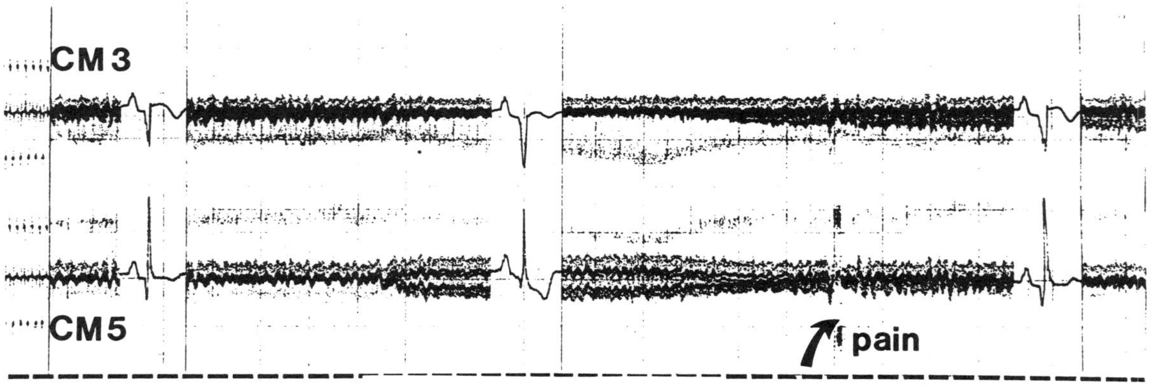

FIG 1. Example of a compressed analog printout (1min=2cm) of a Holter ECG in leads CM3 and CM5. Calibration signals (0.1mV) are shown on the left. The compressed trace initially shows a thick baseline (isoelectic ST segment) as shown in the expanded CM5 complex on the left, with gradual separation of the thick baseline (ST depression) as seen in the middle. There is also a gradual change in R&S wave amplitude followed by a gradual resolution of ST depression. Pain (arrowed), indicated by the patient event signal on the tape, occurred very late in the episode. In the following 10 mins, there was an almost identical ischemic episode, which was completely silent (episode not shown in Fig.).

running at slow speed. The ECG baseline shows up as a thick line, while ST segment elevation or depression, is detected by separation of the baseline. An example of this is shown in Figure 1.

Many commercial systems will also produce trend graphs of the ST level measured at a user defined interval after the detected R wave. Episodes of ST elevation or depression seen in the trend graph can later be verified by tape playback at real-time, as for episodes detected by the compressed analog technique (15). More recently, computer programmes which measure multiple parameters including the ST segment level have been devised; and these can produce ST segment trends and show the relationship of changes to alterations in R and S wave amplitude, ST segment area, heart rate, etc., making the interpretation of the ECG more certain. This technique appears to have the highest accuracy, when compared with AV superimposition, ST trend, and full disclosure systems, as reviewed by Gallino et al. (15). However, each new technique must be validated independently for accuracy in detection of ischemia. To do this ideally, an annotated ischemia ECG data base should be established, similar to currently available arrhythmia data bases.

REAL-TIME ANALYSIS

The most significant recent improvement in technology has been the development of microprocessors which digitize and analyse the ECG in real-time, storing the measured standard parameters for subsequent display with examples of detected ECG abnormalities. Such systems have no moving parts and eliminate the problems of frequency and phase distortion introduced by tape recorders. Initially these devices were limited by the size of memory available to record samples of the ECG, and early models could store only four brief periods of ECG (22). The current availability of miniature chips with huge RAM memory enables the storage of all parameters and all ECG complexes in one or two leads, over a 24 to 48 hour period.

One of the first such devices (QMED Monitor One) was specifically designed for the detection of ischemia in real-time, and has the capacity to notify the wearer of the occurrence of an ischemic episode. This system was verified in our laboratory during exercise stress testing and showed fairly good sensitivity and specificity as well as predictive accuracy for ischemia, provided the physician could verify ischemic ECG samples (22). The main problem was with specificity, because movement artefact produced spurious detection of ST change; and with only four ECG strips available for verification, false positives were possible. Current models of this and other monitors have overcome the problem with extended memories to allow appropriate verification. The trend for manufacturers is to record all complexes to also permit a full disclosure, if required.

ELECTRODES

An often overlooked but extremely important consideration in ambulatory recording is the type and placement of electrodes. Mostly, these have been Ag/AgCl electrodes, which can give excellent quality recordings for extended periods, provided the following pitfalls are avoided:

1. High (>5 K.Ohm) skin resistance, caused by inadequate abrasion of the horny layer of the epidermis.

2. Dislodgement of the adhesive portion of the electrode because of inadequate degreasing and cleansing of the underlying skin, or inadequate adhesive tape anchoring of leads and electrodes.

3. Severe muscle tremor and body movement artefact caused by placing electrodes over muscle or loose skin folds rather than over bony points.

One commercially available system (QMED) has chosen capacitance electrodes as are used for long term ECG monitoring in astronauts. These electrodes do not require the same degree of skin preparation, although it is important that points 2 and 3 noted above are followed.

CHOICE OF LEAD SYSTEM

Because most ambulatory ECG monitors have the capacity to record only 1 or 2 leads, these should be chosen to give the maximum sensitivity for detection of ischemia. On the basis of the stress test literature, these two leads should include either CM5 or CS5 (reference electrode over the centre of the manubrium sternae or the right subclavicular fossa, with the positive electrode in the V5 position). These are bipolar leads and have been shown to have a high sensitivity for ischemia (12,29). Most holter manufacturers also recommend the use of an inferior lead. Attention is rarely given to electrode positioning: and I would recommend either a modified lead II (negative electrode in the right subclavicular fossa and positive electrode over the left lower antero-lateral rib-cage) or a modified lead III (negative electrode in the left subclavicular fossa and positive electrode on the left lower antero-lateral rib cage). Another 2-lead system recommended by Tzivoni and Stern (37) is CM3 and and CM5, with a reported sensitivity approaching that of the 12-lead ECG for detecting ischemia during exercise. If a V2 lead is required, the negative electrode can be placed either in the left or the right subclavicular fossa or on the back between the scapulae.

If a previous positive 12-lead exercise ECG is available, then the leads showing the maximal ST segment change during ischemia should be chosen for ambulatory monitoring; and this should increase the sensitivity for ischemia detection.

One commercially available system (COMPAS) uses 3 electrodes (V2, V5 and lower anterolateral rib cage) to construct a modified central terminal of Wilson with each of the leads acting as a unipolar lead. Unfortunately the ECG produced in this way has little semblance to a standard ECG, distorts ST segments, and should probably not be used.

USES OF AMBULATORY ISCHEMIA MONITORING

1. Diagnosis of Coronary Artery Disease

The major purpose of ambulatory ST monitoring in the early literature was diagnostic. Reports indicated adequate sensitivity for the diagnosis of coronary disease (35). But it is likely that the exercise ECG is more sensitive, as the degree of exertion produced on the treadmill is usually greater than occurs in everyday life and is more likely to provoke ischemia. This has been borne out by a number of recent studies which indicate that episodes of ischemia on ambulatory recording usually occur in patients with a low exercise tolerance, especially if there is an early positive exercise ECG (7).

When used as a diagnostic tool, ambulatory monitoring has the same problems of diagnostic accuracy as the exercise stress test, because there is a variable but substantial incidence of positive ST segment responses in normal subjects (1,8,30). These false positives must be taken into consideration, if ambulatory electrocardiography is to be used as a screening test for coronary disease. This is because the predictive accuracy of a positive test may be relatively low, especially if screening is performed in groups with a low expected prevalence of coronary disease (10). This author would therefore not recommend ambulatory ST segment monitoring as a screening tool for the diagnosis of coronary artery disease.

2. Detection of Ischemia

In the last five years, the widespread acceptance that ischemia is often silent, has re-awakened interest in continuous ECG recordings to detect it. Most studies indicate that chest pain is a late and inconstant accompaniment of myocardial ischemia, with patients unaware of up to 90% of ischemic episodes (5). It has therefore become important to attempt to determine the total ischemic burden in each patient: i.e. the total daily duration of both painful and painless ischemic episodes. Ambulatory ECG recordings are particularly suited to this purpose, and this is probably the main indication for ambulatory ST monitoring.

Occasionally, ischemia is purely silent, as in some patients with diabetes and in others who have a high pain threshold (11,16), although usually patients experience both painful and silent ischemia. Silent episodes occur commonly at times of mental stress, as shown by radionuclide studies (9,31) which also demonstrate that the ECG lacks sensitivity in comparison to changes in myocardial perfusion or function. Silent ischemia seems to respond to therapy in much the same way as painful ischemia (27), so when a patient has been rendered painfree by therapy, painless episodes are often (but certainly not invariably), also either diminished or absent.

We compared the incidence of ischemic episodes on ambulatory recording with the predischarge exercise test in patients with unstable angina or small infarction at hospital discharge. Exercise was more sensitive than ambulatory recordings for detecting ischemia, although this may be due in part to the choice of the single ECG lead on the ambulatory recorder (14). In those patients with a positive exercise ECG, a significant proportion had numerous episodes of silent ischemia during the ambulatory recording which was not anticipated from the history. Silent ischemia was more common in patients with a low exercise tolerance, especially where the test was positive at low work levels. Obviously this type of information might influence therapy, although patients with a positive exercise ECG at low work levels would be considered for revascularization regardless of the occurrence of silent ischemia.

A novel approach to therapy has used ambulatory ECG monitoring with a real-time device to signal the occurrence of ischemia to the wearer, who is instructed to take nitroglycerin even if asymptomatic at the time (2). This approach resulted in a much smaller total ischemic time for each patient, and could prove useful in overall management.

3. Prognostic Significance of Silent Ischemia

A number of reports have suggested that silent ischemia detected by continuous ECG recording has an adverse prognostic significance. This has been shown in patients with unstable angina for both short and long term outcome (18,19,24,26) as reviewed recently (13,32). In our experience, the incidence of silent ischemia detected in this way is low in unselected patients with unstable angina, which limits its usefulness (39). We found that recurrence of rest pain was a more valuable predictor of adverse outcome.

Silent ischemia detected by ambulatory recording may also denote an adverse prognosis in patients with stable effort angina (33,38). Research on this aspect is only preliminary, and the results have not been compared with other readily available clinical predictors of prognosis such as exercise testing or radionuclide ventriculography. My own suspicion is that ischemia detected in this way would not add greatly to other prognostic information, but further research in this area is certainly warranted.

REFERENCES

1. Armstrong, W.F., Jordan, J.W., Morris, S.W. and McHenry, P.L. (1982): Prevalence and Magnitude of ST Segment and T Wave Abnormalities in Normal Men During Continuous Ambulatory Electrocardio-graphy. *Am. J. Cardiol.,* 49:1638-42.

2. Barry, J., Campbell, S., Nabel, E.G., Mead, K. and Selwyn, A.P. (1987): Ambulatory Monitoring of the Digitized Electrocardiogram for Detection and Early Warning of Transient Myocardial Ischemia in Angina Pectoris. *Am J Cardiol.,* 60:483-88.

3. Berson, A.S. and Pipberger, H.V. (1966): The Low Frequency Response of Electrocardiographs, a Frequent Source of Recording Errors. *Am. Heart J.,* 71:779-789.

4. Bragg-Ramschel, D.A, Anderson, C.M. and Winkle, R.A. (1982): Frequency Response Characteristics of Ambulatory ECG Monitoring Systems and Their Implications for ST Segment Analysis. *Am. Heart J.,* 103:20-31.

5. Chierchia, S., Lazzari, M., Freedman, S.B., Brunelli, C, Maseri A. Impairment of Myocardial Perfusion and Function During Painless Myocardial Ischaemia. *J. Am. Coll. Cardiol.*, 1:924-30.

6. Colquhoun, D., Richards, D., Bailey, I., Fletcher, P., Kelly, D. and Harris, P. (1984): Nocturnal ST Segment Monitoring of Healthy Males at Rest in Bed (Abstr). *Aust. N.Z. J. Med.*, 14: Supp 2:576.

7. Crea, F., Kaski, J.C., Fragasso, G., Hackett, D., Stanbridge, R., Taylor, K.M. and Maseri, A. (1987): Usefulness of Holter Monitoring to Improve the Sensitivity of Exercise Testing in Determining the Degree of Myocardial Revascularization After Coronary Artery Bypass Grafting for Stable Angina Pectoris. *Am. J. Cardiol.*, 60:40-3.

8. Deanfield, J.E., Ribiero, P., Oakley, K., Krikler, S. and Selwyn, A.P. (1984): Analysis of ST Segment Changes in Normal Subjects Implications for Ambulatory Monitoring in Angina Pectoris. *Am. J. Cardiol.*, 54:1321-25.

9. Deanfield, J.E., Shea, M., Ribeiro, P., de Landsheere, C.M., Wilson, R.A., Horlock, P. and Selwyn, A.P. (1984): Transient ST Segment Depression as a Marker of Myocardial Ischemia During Daily Life. *Am. J. Cardiol.*, 54:1195-200.

10. Diasmond, G.A. and Forrester, J.S. (1979): Analysis of Probability as an Aid in the Clinical Diagnosis of Coronary Artery Disease. *N. Engl. J. Med.*, 300:1350-8.

11. Droste, C. and Roskamm, H. (1983): Experimental Pain Measurement in Patients With Asymptomatic Myocardial Ischemia. *J. Am. Coll. Cardiol.*, 1: 940-5.

12. Ellestad, M.H. (1986): Stress Testing. *Principles and Practice.* Third edition. FA Davis, Philadelphia.

13. Epstein, S.E., Quyyumi, A.A. and Bonow, R.O. (1988): Myocardial Ischemia - Silent or Symptomatic. *N. Engl. J. Med.*, 318:1038.

14. Freedman, S.B., Wilcox, I., Doyle, S.J., McCredie, R., Harris, P.J. and Kelly, D.T. (1988): Silent Ischemia on Ambulatory Recordings After Unstable Angina or Small MI: Relationship to Results of Stress Testing (Abstr). *Circulation*, 78: Suppl II-469.

15. Gallino, A., Chierchia, S., Smith, G., Croom, M., Morgan, M., Marchesi, C. and Maseri, A. (1984): Computer System for Analysis of ST Segment Changes on 24 Hour Holter Monitor Tapes: Comparison with Other Available Systems. *J. Am. Col. Cardiol.*, 4:245-52.

16. Glazier, J.J., Chierchia, S., Brown, M.J. and Maseri, A. (1986): Importance of Generalized Defective Perception of Painful Stimuli

as a Cause of Silent Myocardial Ischemia in Chronic Stable Angina Pectoris. 58:667-672.

17. Golden, D.P., Wolthius, R.A. and Hoffler, G.W. (1973): A Spectral Analysis of the Normal Resting Electrocardiogram. *IEEE Trans. Biomed. Eng.*, 20:366-372.

18. Gottlieb, S.O., Weisfeldt, M.L., Ougang, P., Mellits, E.D. and Gerstenblith, G. (1986): Silent Ischemia as a Marker for Early Unfavourable Outcomes in Patients with Unstable Angina. *N. Engl. J. Med.* 314:1214-1219.

19. Gottlieb, S.O., Weisfeldt, M.L., Ouyang, P., Mellits, E.D. and Gerstenblith, G. (1987): Silent Ischemia Predicts Infarction and Death During 2 Year Follow Up of Unstable Angina. *J. Am. Coll. Cardiol.*, 10:756-60.

20. Hinkle, L.E., Meyer, J., Stevens, M. and Carver, S.T. (1967): Tape Recordings of the ECG of Active Men. Limitations and Advantages of the Holter - Avionics Instruments. *Circulation,* 36: 752-765.

21. Holter, N.J. (1961): New Method for Heart Studies: Continuous Electrocardiography of Active Subjects Over Long Periods is Now Practical. *Science,* 113:1214.

22. Jamal, S.M., Mitra-Duncan, L., Kelly, D.T. and Freedman, S.B. (1987): Validation of a Real-Time Electrocardiographic Monitor for the Detection of Myocardial Ischemia Secondary to Coronary Artery Disease. *Am. J. Cardiol.*, 60:525-7.

23. Janse, M.J. (1981): *Electrophysiological Changes in Acute Myocardial Ischaemia. What is Angina?*, edited by D.G. Julian, K.I. Lie, L. Wilhelmsen and A.B. Hassle. pp. 160-70. Molndahl, Sweden.

24. Johnson, S.M., Mauritson, D.R., Winniford, M.D. et al. (1982): Continuous Electrocardiographic Monitoring in Patients with Unstable Angina Pectoris: Identification of High-Risk Subgroup with Severe Coronary Disease, Variant Angina, and/or Impaired Early Prognosis. *Am. Heart J.,* 103:4-12.

25. Lambert, C.R., Imperi, G.A. and Pepine, C.J. (1986): Low Frequency Requirements for Recording Ischemic ST Segment Abnormalities in Coronary Artery Disease. *Am. J. Cardiol.,* 58:225-229.

26. Nademanee, K., Intarachot, V., Singh, P.N., Josephson, M.A. and Singh B.N. (1986): Characteristics and Clinical Significance of Silent Myocardial Ischemia in Unstable Angina. *Am. J. Cardiol.,* 58:2613-3313.

27. Pepine, C.J., Hill, J.A., Imperi, G.A. and Norvell, N. (1988): Beta-Arenergic Blockers in Silent Myocardial Ischemia. *Am. J. Cardiol.,* 61: 18B-21B.

28. Pipberger, H.V., Arzbacher, R.C., Berson, A.S., et al. (1975): Recommendations for Standardization of Leads and of Specifications for Instruments in Electrocardiography and Vectorcardiography: Report to the Committee on Electrocardiography, American Heart Association. *Circulation,* 52:11-31.

29. Quyyumi, A.A., Crake, T., Mockus, L.J., Wright, C.A., Frickards, A.F. and Fox, K.M. (1986): Value of the Bipolar Lead CM 5 in Electrocardiography. *Br. Heart J.,* 56:372-

30. Quyyumi, A.A., Wright, C. and Fox, K. (1983): Ambulatory Electrocardiographic ST Segment Changes in Healthy Volunteers. *Br. Heart J.,* 50: 460-64.

31. Rozanski, A., Vairey, C.N., Krantz, D.S., Friedman, J., Resser, K.J., Morell, M., Hilton-Chalfen, S., Hestin, L., Bietendorf, J. and Berman, D.S. (1988): Mental Stress and the Induction of Silent Myocardial Ischemia in Patients with Coronary Artery Disease. *N. Engl. Med.,* 318:1005-12.

32. Selwyn, A.P. and Ganz, P. (1988): Myocardial Ischemia in Coronary Disease (Editorial). *N. Engl. J. Med.,* 318:1058-60.

33. Shook, T.L., Glasser, S.P., Crawford, M.H., Bhatia, S.J.S., and Stone, P.H. (1987): Discordance Between Ambulatory Electrocardiography and Exercise Testing for Assessment of the Severity of Ischemia (Abstr). *Circulation,* 76: Suppl IV-362.

34. Stern, S., Tzivoni, D. (1973): Dynamic Changes in the ST Segment During Sleep in Ischemic Heart Disease. *Am. J. Cardiol.,* 32:17-20.

35. Stern, S., Tzivoni, D. and Stern, Z. (1975): Diagnostic Accuracy of Ambulatory ECG Monitoring in Ischemic Heart Disease. *Circulation,* 52:1045-49.

36. Taylor, D. and Vincent, R. (1985): Artefactual ST Segment Abnormalities Due to Electrocardiograph Design. *Br. Heart J.,* 54:121-128.

37. Tzivoni, D., Benhorim, J., Gavish, A. and Stern, S. (1985): Holter Changes During Treadmill Exercise Testing in Assessing Myocardial Ischemic Changes. *Am. J. Cardiol.,* 55:1-5.

38. Vaghaiwalla, M.F., Nademanee, K., Intarachot, V., Josephson, M.A., Robertson, H., Harwood, B. and Singh, N. (1987): Prognostic Significance of Silent Myocardial Ischemia in Chronic Stable Angina

Based on Correlation with Coronary Angiography (Abstr). *Circulation,* 76: Suppl IV-78.

39. Wilcox, I., Harris, P.J., McCredie, J.R., Doyle, S.J., Tweedy, S., Kelly, D.T. and Freedman, S.B. (1988): Silent Ischemia: An Insensitive Prognostic Indicator in Unselected Patients with Unstable Angina (Abstr). *Circulation,* 78: Suppl II-24.

Medical Monitoring in the Home and Work Environment,
edited by Laughton E. Miles and Roger J. Broughton.
Raven Press, New York © 1990.

TRANSFERRING EEG POLYSOMNOGRAPHY TO THE HOME ENVIRONMENT

Jack R. Smith

Electrical Engineering Department
University of Florida
Gainesville, Florida 32611

INTRODUCTION

Instrumentation is now available for monitoring sleep in the home. The data collected can vary from a simplified description of the night's sleep to a complete acquisition and/or analysis of the EEG/EOG data which can be played back on a polygraph located in the sleep lab. Just as EEG analysis had to await the electronic amplifier, home recording requires portable EEG amplifiers capable of accurately recording EEG signals in a home environment containing large amounts of ambient noise. These amplifiers are now available, and home recordings are now possible. The user can chose between obtaining a summary of the data with automated analysis or collecting and transmitting to the laboratory the same polysomnography data obtained had the patient slept in the laboratory.

The following discussion first describes the instrumentation requirements for collecting and analyzing polysomnography data. Reduced instrumentation requirements will usually reduce the system cost and at the same time reduce the quality of the data collected. The reduced data quality may still be adequate for the intended study. The tradeoffs between system requirements and data are discussed. Various methods for collecting and/or analyzing the data are then described; and finally, additional descriptors of the EEG/EOG data that can be obtained from an automated analysis are described.

INSTRUMENTATION REQUIREMENTS

The type and cost of the home monitoring instrumentation is somewhat dependent on the information sought. The amount of information to be obtained is both a clinical and a research problem. Instrumentation is needed for both data acquisition and analysis. Instrumentation is available for acquiring the polysomnography data in the home and then reproducing it in the laboratory. Laboratory polygraph recordings provide a standard of comparison for determining instrumentation requirements. Certain studies require less information, and the instrumentation requirements are reduced accordingly. Sleep studies normally include four EEG/EOG/EMG/data channels recorded with low frequency time constants of .1 to .3 seconds. The polygraph is capable of accurately reproducing signals up to approximately 100 Hz. There may be information in higher frequency components of the EEG; but if so, the higher frequency activities are not yet of interest to polysomnographers. A good quality polygraph can resolve signals as small as one or two microvolts in peak amplitude and has sufficient dynamic range to linearly display signals of approximately 500 microvolts peak-to-peak amplitude. Respiration signals, NPT signals and heart rate are much slower than EEG signals, and they can be recorded with amplifier channels with less than 1/10 the bandwidth of EEG channels. The following section illustrates the practical significance of this reduced bandwidth on data storage and display.

Digital Specifications

Although the signals to be analyzed are analog signals it is often the case that they are converted to digital signals for storage and/or analysis. Whereas analog signals can be described in terms of bandwidth and dynamic range, the equivalent specifications for digital signals are sampling rate and number of bits per sample. One byte (8 bits) can represent 256 different values, so if the values are equally spaced one byte can represent a signal which varies + 128 microvolts with samples spaced one microvolt apart (one microvolt resolution), and it can represent a signal which varies between + 256 microvolts with samples spaced two microvolts apart. One byte of data is sufficient to accurately represent EEG data provided care is taken to ensure that the accuracy of the data representation is not diminished during signal processing. Shannon's sampling theorem states that no information is lost if the sampling rate is twice the bandwidth of the signal; it is important to note that the term bandwidth as used by Shannon refers to the frequency spectrum occupied by all signals and not to the conventional -3db bandwidth, which is usually much smaller. A rule of thumb is that an analog signal should be sampled at a rate which is five to ten times the analog signal's -3db bandwidth. Studies in our laboratory indicate that a sampling rate of 1000 Hz is needed to completely describe the information of an EEG signal obtained with polygraph amplifiers, but that a sampling rate of approximately 250 Hz per channel is adequate for the EEG. Adequate is here defined as enabling the system to detect waveforms with about the same accuracy as the EEGer. The resolution depends on the waveforms of interest. Smith (9) found that a much slower sampling rate is sufficient to describe delta activity, but to distinguish, for example, between spindle and beta activity, a much faster sampling rate is required. It is possible to reduce the sampling rate somewhat by interpolating between samples. In our laboratory we sample each EEG signal 500 times per second and store the data at 250 samples per second. The advantage of sampling at a faster rate than that at which the data is stored (oversampling) is that it is much easier to minimize any phase distortion introduced by the prefilters (anti-aliasing filters).

Figure 1 contains an epoch of data with a spindle noted in the EEG channel. Figure 2 contains the EEG channel (with an expanded time scale) and illustrates the effect of a reduced sampling frequency on the waveform

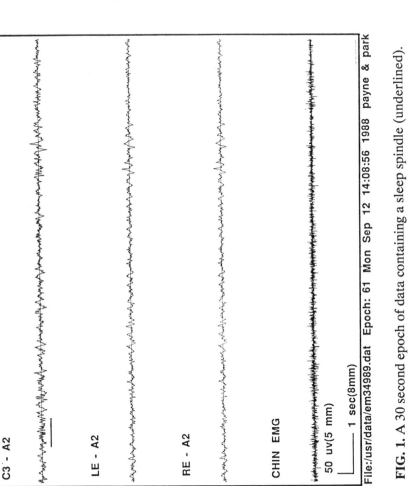

FIG. 1. A 30 second epoch of data containing a sleep spindle (underlined).

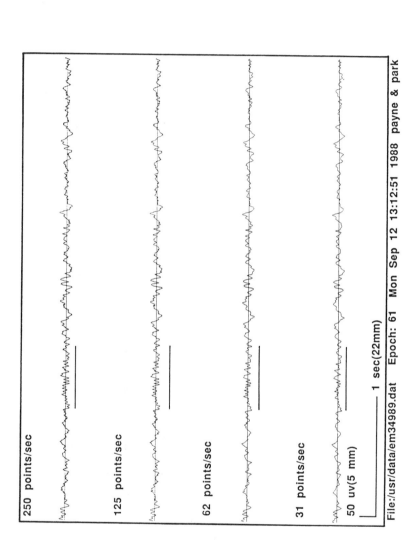

FIG. 2. The EEG of Figure 1. (expanded time scale) shown at various sampling rates.

appearance. Each tracing is presented with the data sampled at a different rate. Linear interpolation is used to fill in the points between samples. Figure 2A displays the data with a sampling rate of 250 samples per second, 2B at a sampling rate of 125 samples per second, 2C at 62.5 samples per second and 2D at 31.25 samples per second. The figure illustrates the degradation in the quality of the displayed data as the sampling rate is decreased. The degradation is greater for faster components. The sampling rate and bandwidth necessary to represent a signal has additional implications, such as in the use of electronic monitors for displaying polysomnography signals. A high quality monitor has approximately 1200 pixels in each row; a PC monitor has many fewer pixels. Each horizontal pixel can represent one sample (ignoring the # of pixels in each column-- the number of pixels per column determines the amplitude resolution) thus twelve hundred samples can be represented in one row. If 30 seconds of data are displayed on the screen, the equivalent sampling rate is 1200/30 or 40 samples per second. This is adequate resolution for displaying slowly varying data such as respiration signals, delta activity, and rapid eye movements, but it is not adequate to distinguish between the faster activities such as sleep spindles and beta activity. If 10 seconds of data are displayed the equivalent sampling rate is 120 samples per second. The implication is that a computer monitor can display data with about the same resolution as a polygraph, but not when thirty seconds of data are displayed on the screen.

To summarize: Each EEG channel requires an analog bandwidth of 100Hz; a heart rate channel requires approximately the same bandwidth. Lower frequency signals such as respiration can be recorded with channel bandwidths of 10Hz or less. Very slowly varying signals such as oxygen saturation and NPT require an even lower bandwidth. To digitally store one channel of EEG data requires approximately 250 samples per second or 900,000 (900K) bytes per hour (each sample is 8 bits (1 byte) long). An eight hour recording of four channels will require almost 30 million bytes (Mb) of storage. Each low frequency channel, such as heart rate, NPT and respiration will require fewer than 90K bytes per hour. An eight hour recording consisting of four EEG channels and four low frequency channels will occupy approximately 32 megabytes of data. The digitization of an eight hour recording consisting of seven EEG channels and eight low frequency channels of data will require 55.6 megabytes of storage. A very short time ago it was not possible to economically store this amount of data during monitoring in the home environment; but today there are several instrumentation options available for storing this information.

INSTRUMENTATION OPTIONS

The instrumentation to select for polysomnography in the home environment depends on the information required. Factors to be considered include: number of data channels--the fewer channels the lower the cost--although the cost for different data channels can differ. For example, it takes much less storage capacity to record a respiration channel than to monitor an EEG channel. The more channels the more information is obtained and the more redundancy is included in case of a failure in one of the channels; but the recording and analysis costs will increase as the number of data channels; increases. This is no different from what occurs in the laboratory. It is a clinical decision on the amount of information required (the clinician may not know how much information is being used). The point is that the information to be returned determines the system design and in some sense the cost, although there is not always a correlation between cost and performance.

The first decision to be made in selecting the instrumentation is whether or not to collect all of the raw data for subsequent analysis in the laboratory or to rely on automated analysis and transmit only the results of the analysis to the sleep laboratory. The advantages of the latter approach are the large data reduction, which allows for a much less expensive storage and transmission media; and it efficiently accomplishes the data reduction necessary for interpreting the data. The main disadvantages are that one must rely on the adequacy of the automated analysis and unexpected data may appear which the automated analysis has not been programmed to handle.

Complete Data Acquisition

Direct data transmission

EEG/EOG data can be sent directly to the sleep laboratory via a radio frequency link or over a telephone line. Both methods require a frequency multiplexor at the subject end and a demodulator at the receiving end of the data link. Such instrumentation is commercially available. Six to ten data channels can be frequency multiplexed onto one 2 kilohertz signal and transmitted over a standard telephone line. This provides a much cheaper data channel than r-f transmission (such as telemetry), although r-f transmission could be cheaper if data from several beds at the same site are to be transmitted to a remote location. The future for r-f transmission of signals does not appear as bright as that of the direct data transmission via fiber optic cables. Disadvantages of telephone transmission include tying up the telephone line for the duration of the recording.

Tape recording

This was the most frequently used method of data acquisition before the advent of relatively inexpensive digital data acquisition systems, and it is still widely used. A limitation of tape recording is that most tape-recorders are not able to record eight hours of data without changing the tape. The relatively long recording times require low speed recording, usually with fm. FM tape recorders provide the best quality recordings. Tape recording with polygraph quality output requires that each EEG channel have an analog bandwidth of approximately 100Hz. This is not the case with many of the small tape recorders used for ambulatory monitoring. Many of the very low speed recorders have a bandwidth of 30Hz. Whether or not this bandwidth provides sufficient information depends upon the information required from the study.

Computer storage

An alternative to a tape recorder today is a personal computer with an A/D converter and a large digital storage capacity. It has been demonstrated that an eight hour recording of seven EEG channels and 8 lower frequency channels can be digitized and stored in a 55.6 Mb file. The playback of this data would not be distinguishable from that recorded in the laboratory. The data can then be reconverted to an analog signal and played back in the laboratory onto a polygraph or viewed with a paperless EEG machine. The capability to store such large data files has recently become available to relatively lightweight (transportable) computers which can be used in the home.

Today's three practical storage media are Winchester disks, digital magnetic tapes and laser disks (write once read many times (WORM's)). The Winchester disk, although it is already present in most computers, is not an attractive alternative if one wants to keep a permanent record of the data. Once the Winchester drive is filled, as it soon will be if used to store raw polysomnography data, it can no longer accept additional data. If a permanent copy of the record is needed the data stored on the Winchester can be transferred to a digital tape or to a laser disk. Digital tape is the least expensive approach. Tape drives with sufficient capacity and speed to accept the polysomnography data are readily available. The disadvantage of magnetic tape is that to analyze the tape data, one must first enter it in the computer; this is a relatively slow process, requiring up to one hour to reenter a night's data.

A laser drive system is a much better, but more expensive, alternative if one wants to quickly access a record or a particular epoch of the record. This ability to go to quickly find a particular segment of data in the storage media is referred to as "random access." Laser drives with removal cartridges holding from 100 to more than 1000 megabytes of data are now available as are erasable optical cartridges. Thus a single cartridge can hold one or more night's of data. The laser disk media costs to store a night's data are rapidly decreasing and are now comparable to the costs of the polygraph recording paper, and much more convenient to store. The simultaneous acquisition and storage of all of the polysomnography data will require customized software regardless of which storage medium is selected. The computer used for the data acquisition and storage can also be used for an automated analysis of the data and for report generation. Computer storage also does not require the use of the telephone.

AUTOMATED ANALYSIS

Sleep analysis can be interpreted as a data reduction problem: at least the analysis of sleep contains a data reduction aspect. Sleep staging, for example, consists of reducing 30 seconds of data to one byte of data and an eight hour record to fewer than 1000 Mb. Since a thirty second epoch of four channels of EEG data contains approximately 30,000 bytes of data, the sleep staging of an epoch represents a data reduction by a factor of thirty thousand. A report which simply describes the number of epochs for each sleep stage is a further data reduction to less than five bytes of data. Data reduction is necessary, if sleep data are to be humanly manageable; yet the data reduction of sleep must not be so great that the important information is lost. Science requires paradigms for its rapid advancement (6). Sleep staging (SS) has been the driving paradigm behind the rapid growth of sleep as a research discipline by providing a quantitative and relatively objective method for describing a night's sleep data. Yet today SS provides an incomplete and inadequate description of the night's sleep. A subject reports that one night's sleep is much better than the next - yet sleep staging does not discriminate between them.

Does the clinician extract more information from the EEG than just the sleep stage? This is certainly the case. What information? This question cannot yet be answered completely. Sleep latencies and the number and duration of arousals are examples of additional information that is extracted from the sleep stage information. Other descriptors of the night's sleep EEG can be obtained either in the laboratory or on line in the home. Many of these descriptors are readily detectable by eye, but it is much too time consuming for most investigators to do. Sleep spindles, theta waves, delta activity, beta activity (an activity particularly difficult to detect visually), and rapid eye movements are examples of descriptors which can be used to more completely describe a night's sleep. The temporal distribution of one or more of these waveforms can also be used to more completely describe the data.

Another feature could be the amplitude and frequency content of individual waveforms. Delta activity is the one waveform that has been extensively studied (12). Some investigators, particularly Webb and Dreblow (15), have suggested that the only difference in the slow wave activity as a function of age is the amplitude. That is, Webb contends that if the amplitude criteria are reduced elderly subjects will have the same amount of stages 3 and 4 as do the younger subjects. This too can be monitored in the home environment. Individual waveform frequency components, such as the frequency components of the individual waves of which a spindle is composed, can also be monitored, although not as readily.

Several other physiological variables are also often monitored in order to better describe a night's sleep. The automated analysis of these signals, particularly respiration and NPT has received much less attention in the published literature, but the work done used instrumentation varying in size and complexity from small portable computers built for monitoring respiration signals (1) to relatively large laboratory computers (16). Today the same computer can be used for monitoring sleep EEG and respiration signals in the home.

Sleep Staging

Many different methods for automatic sleep staging have been published, and a few have been extensively evaluated with a broad range of subjects (10). Automated sleep staging can now be done in the home. The systems vary from small activity monitors to portable implementations of systems which could at one time only be implemented on large laboratory computers. The man/machine agreement of the automated systems depends on the subject population for which the system is evaluated. The agreement will not necessarily be the same for another subject population. EEG characteristics are age dependent. For example, sleep spindles increase in frequency with increasing age, and the frequency deviation within the individual spindles also increases with age (7). If the system is not designed to work with a subject population with a broad range of characteristics, extensive adjustments will be required for each recording (not only for each subject, but also for each night for the same subject); and the analysis can easily lose its objectivity.

Since the sleep stages are defined in terms of the waveforms that appear in the EEG, one approach to automatic sleep staging is based on the detection of the individual waveforms in the EEG. Smith et al. (13) obtained slightly better than 80% man/machine agreement when sleep staging records from subjects between 13 and 79 years of age. The agreement was much less for 5-year old subjects, as the human scorers used different scoring criteria, primarily because of the large amounts of delta activity present in most of the records. Hasan (2) obtained a similar agreement using a similar system.

The computer appears to be much better (more accurate, objective and consistent) at the detection of sleep EEG waveforms (alpha, beta, delta, sigma, theta and slow-waves) than is the human sleep scorer. Two independent laboratories, Johnson et al, (3) and Silverstein and Levy (8), using an automatic spindle detector of Smith et al, (11) obtained over 90% man/machine agreement for spindle detection. There has been no published study comparing the human detection of individual waveforms. The human appears to be better than an automated system at detecting rapid eye movements in REM sleep. This is partially due to the wide variability of individual waveforms and partially due to the contextual interpretation of REM activity. The published studies reporting the inter-laboratory human/human agreement (without an extensive training period) are not any better than the human/computer comparisons, but the best human agreement is obtained for REM sleep (5). This has been one of the stages of poorest performance for automated analysis. Neither human/human or computer/human agreement has been good for stage 1 sleep. This is in part due to the lack of objective criteria for stage 1 sleep. It does illustrate that with any record containing large amounts of stage 1 sleep the human/computer agreement will be less than with those records containing small amounts of stage one sleep. But in these cases human/human agreement will also be lower.

A HOME MONITOR

An expanded version of the sleep analyzer (SAC) first described by Smith and Karacan, (13) is now available in a portable version that can be used for home monitoring and data analysis. The system uses a portable amplifier system which obtains its power from the computer power supply. The system will accept an input signal from a portable oximeter. The computer monitors fifteen input signals, seven of which are each sampled at 500 Hz, one at 125Hz, three at 25 Hz (respiration signals) and the remaining four are each sampled at 5 Hz. The system automatically analyzes the EEG data by detecting the individual waveforms; the sleep stage is determined on-line. All fifteen input data channels can also be stored on an optical disk. The same computer can be used for additional automated analysis and can be used for reproducing the data in the laboratory on an electronic monitor or printing the original data on a printer or a polygraph.

REFERENCES

1. Ancoli-Israel, S., Kripke, D., Mason, W. and Messin, S. (1981): Comparisons of Home Sleep Recordings and Polysmonograms In Older Adults With Sleep Disorders. *Sleep,* 4:283-291.

2. Hasan, J. (1983): Differentiation of Normal and Disturbed Sleep by Automatic Analysis. *Acta. Physiol. Scandinavica.* Supplementum 526, 1-103.

3. Johnson, L.C., Hansan, K. and Bickford, R.G. (1976): Effect of Flurazepam on Sleep Spindles and K-Complexes. *Electroenceph. Clin. Neurophysiol.,* 40:67-72.

4. Keane, B., Smith, J.R. and Webb, W.B.,(1977): Temporal Distribution and Ontogenetic Development of EEG Activity During Sleep. *Psychophysiology,* 14:315-321.

5. Karacan, I. Orr, W.C., Roth, T., Kramer, M., Shurley, J.T., Thornby, J.F., Bingham, S.F. and Salis, P.J. (1978): Establishment and Implementation of Standardized Sleep Laboratory Data Collection and Scoring Procedures. *Psychophysiology,* 15:173-179.

6. Kuhn,T.S. (1962): *The Structure of Scientific Revolutions,* Chicago University Press.

7. Principe, J.C. and Smith, J.R. (1982): Sleep Spindle Characteristics as a Function of Age. *Sleep,* 5:73-84.

8. Silverstein, L.D. and Levy, C.M. (1976): The Stability of the Sigma Sleep Spindle. *Electroenceph. Clin. Neurophysiol.,* 40:666-670.

9. Smith, J.R., (1980): Automated EEG Analysis with Microcomputers. *Medical Instrumentation,* 14: 319-321.

10. Smith, J.R. (1986): Computer Analysis of Sleep Data. In: *Handbook of Electroencephalography and Clinical Neurophysiology, Vol. 2: Computer Analysis of the EEG and Other Neurophysiological Signals, Part B: Application in Clinical Neurophysiology* (edited by F.J. Lopes da Silva and W. Storm van Leuwen), Elsevier, Amsterdam.

11. Smith, J.R., Funke, W.F., Yeo, W.C. and Ambuehl, R.A. (1975): Detection of Human Sleep EEG Waveforms. *Electroenceph. Clin. Neurophysiology,* 38:435-437.

12. Smith, J.R., Karacan, I. and Yang, M. (1977): Otogeny of Delta Activity During Human Sleep. *Electroenceph. and Clin. Neurophysiology,* 43:229-237.

13. Smith, J.R., Karacan, I., and Yang, M. (1978): Automated Analysis of the Human Sleep EEG. *Waking and Sleeping*, 2:75-82.

14. Smith, J.R., Karacan, I. and Yang, M. (1979): Automated Measurement of Alpha, Beta, Sigma, and Theta Burst Characteristics. *Sleep,* 1:435-443.

15. Webb, W.B. and Dreblow, L.M. (1982): A Modified Method for Scoring Slow Wave Sleep of Older Subjects. *Sleep,* 5:195-199.

16. West,P. and Kryger,M.H. (1983): Continuous Monitoring of Respiratory Variables During Sleep. *Meth. Inform. Med.,* 22:198-203.

Medical Monitoring in the Home and Work Environment,
edited by Laughton E. Miles and Roger J. Broughton.
Raven Press, New York © 1990.

EVALUATION OF COMMERCIALLY AVAILABLE HOME RECORDING SYSTEMS FOR ALL-NIGHT SLEEP RECORDINGS: THE TELEDIAGNOSTIC AND OXFORD MEDILOG 9000 SYSTEMS

Deborah. E. Sewitch

Sleep Disorders Center, The Griffin Hospital, Derby Connecticut 06418;
and the Department of Psychiatry Yale University School of Medicine, New
Haven Connecticut 06519

INTRODUCTION

In the Spring of 1984 while at Western Psychiatric Institute and Clinic (WPIC), part of the University of Pittsburgh School of Medicine, I was asked to carry out a "feasibility" study for recording sleep in the home environment. The work was commissioned by a grant awarded to David J. Kupfer, M.D., from the John D. and Catherine T. MacArthur Foundation Research Network on the Psychobiology of Depression. This chapter is based on the final technical report (9) and the two subsequent journal articles (10,11) that followed.

The original Telediagnostic System described in this chapter has now been specifically redesigned for the clinical field of sleep disorders. It now transmits up to ten channels of electrophysiological data and is known as the TDS S-10 Telephonic Polysomnography System.

The only modification that I am aware of as having occurred with the Oxford Medilog 9000 System as it is described in this chapter is the fact that the HDX pre-amplifiers no longer need to be collodioned down to the individual's scalp along with the electrodes. There is also now a "Sleep Stager" that is available for use with the 9000 System.

Brief Comparative Literature Review

The Medilog System was first adapted for sleep monitoring by Wilkinson and Mullaney (12) using the older, 4-channel system. These researchers generated a single 24-hour recording on four normal subjects (3 males, one female). One brain and two eye channels were recorded. In an additional subject, a simultaneous record of sleep was written-out on a Grass polygraph. Again, only brain and eye movement data were recorded. The submental chin EMG was omitted from all of these test recordings. The 4-channel, Medilog system has also been used to screen eight, healthy elderly (85-94 years old) subjects with no sleep-wake complaints for sleep apnea and nocturnal myoclonus over a single night (13.5 hour period) (5). No EEG sleep was recorded.

The Telediagnostic System is an 8-channel (now 10-channel) telephone FM-multiplex data set. The Telediagnostic System was originally designed and developed by Parallel Data Systems, a medical electronics group in San Francisco now known as Telediagnostic Systems. The system was developed for regional, clinical electroencephalography, receiving-interpretation centers which serve a group of remote community hospitals to assist these hospitals in diagnostic testing (8). Coates, Rosekind and Thoresen (1,2,7) were the first researchers to adapt this system for home monitoring of EEG sleep. These authors presented a series of three publications on a study which adapted the Telediagnostic System to evaluate the long-term efficacy (one year) of behavioral self-management techniques in reducing sleep onset and maintenance insomnia in eight subjects (16-61 years old). All eight subjects were studied for three consecutive nights in the home environment using the Telediagnostic System and three consecutive nights in the laboratory environment. The home and lab sleep studies were separated by a one-week interval, and the order of home or laboratory sleep studies was counterbalanced across subjects. Mean values on standard sleep parameters were significantly correlated (Pearson product-moment correlations) between recording environments. The authors concluded that their "data does not argue for the superiority of sleep recordings in one location over another", (p.346,ref.2). There have been no further published applications of this system to sleep monitoring either in normals or sleep disorder patient subgroups. In addition, there have been no published reports on the utilization of either the Telediagnostic or Medilog Systems with psychiatric patient subgroups.

SPECIFIC AIMS

1.   To determine whether there are differences in standard electroencephalographic sleep parameters recorded in the home versus the laboratory environment.

2.   To determine whether electroencephalographic sleep measures recorded at home can reliably measure standard sleep parameters.

3.   To determine the feasibility of home environment monitoring of sleep, i.e., the advantages, pragmatic and economic, as well as disadvantages to carrying out such home sleep studies, with two types of systems (Medilog, and Telediagnostic).

SUBJECT SELECTION

A total of 19 healthy, normal subjects between the ages of 21 and 42 (mean age = 31.6; S.D. = 6.3 years) participated in the study as paid volunteers. There were 13 women and 6 men. A total of 5 of the 19 subjects elected to participate in both studies bringing the total number of subjects participating in both studies to 24 (13 subjects in the Telediagnostic study and 11 subjects in the Medilog study). The data from the home environment of 3 subjects who participated in the Telediagnostic study were technically unscorable giving a data loss rate of about 23% with the Telediagnostic System compared to the complete home environment data loss from only one subject (about 9%) with the Medilog System.

Both groups of subjects were comparable in terms of age and sex. All but 2 of the 13 women subjects were studied between days 2 and 10 of their menstrual cycle.

Screening Criteria

All subjects were administered the Schedule for Affective Disorders and Schizophrenia-Life (SADS-L) by the research nursing staff to rule out any Research Diagnostic Criteria (RDC) diagnosis and any family history (first-degree relatives) of depression or psychiatric illness prior to acceptance into either study. In addition, also subjects were given the Hamilton Rating Scale for Depression and all had scores of under 7 (first 17 items, one rater).

All subjects who participated in these two studies had no sleep-wake complaints and regular sleep-wake schedules which were further documented by a two-week sleep-wake log that each subject kept prior to beginning sleep studies. None of the subjects were on any prescribed medications and all denied any use of illicit drugs. None of the women subjects were on any pharmacological birth control regimens.

All subjects abstained from any alcohol throughout the two-week period of their sleep-wake logs and for the four nights of their monitored sleep studies. Subjects were also asked to restrict their caffeine intake to the morning and early afternoon only from the second week of their sleep-wake log until the end of their participation.

EVALUATION OF THE TELEDIAGNOSTIC SYSTEM

Apparatus

The Telediagnostic System is a portable, 16 pound unit which can transmit EEG data from any location, e.g., office, hospital, or patient home. The System was originally developed thirteen years ago and first presented to the American Medical Electroencephalo-graphic Association on May 15, 1971 (8). It uses a standard telephone line without any special telephone equipment to transmit electrophysiological data.

The T-7 Transmitter is battery operated. It has a built-in microphone speaker which provides two-way voice communication between transmitting facility and receiving facility. The TDS-AFR-J Receiver is fully compatible with any polygraph machine. It requires no frequency adjustments by receiving technician. It also has a built-in microphone and speaker to allow two-way communication between receiving and transmitting sites, and it has a built-in calibration circuit for verification that the system is operating properly. The T-7 Transmitter transmits a composite signal made up of all 8-channels (in the present study, all 4 channels) of data over the telephone line, while the TDS-AFR-J Receiver is basically a demodulation unit which demodulates the incoming signal into 8 (or 4) separate channels of data which are written out by the polygraph.

The front panel of the T-7 Transmitter has an electrode test function built into it. The appropriate 10/20 electrode system correspondence to applied electrode placement is dialed and the impedance between it and ground is read off of the meter's "Electrode" scale. The key element to remember is that this electrode impedance meter is hardwired to read the impedance between one selected electrode site and the ground electrode site. Thus, it is important that the impedance of the ground electrode by very low (2-3 K ohms) lest it artificially inflate the impedance meter reading with regard to the selected electrode site. The technical team was instructed to carry the standard laboratory, Grass impedance meter to check the impedance of individual electrode sites and in particular the ground (forehead) electrode site. All impedance readings off of the T-7 unit had to be below 7 K ohms.

Procedure

Subjects had their sleep studied in the home and laboratory environments in a counterbalanced order. This was accomplished by studying two subjects at a time, one in the home environment and one in the laboratory environment. Each subject was studied for four consecutive nights, two each in both the home and laboratory environments. After two nights in either environment, the two subjects being concurrently studied were read to switch environments.

Home Monitoring

The technical team phoned the subject several days prior to the nights of sleep studies in the home environment. Subjects were studied on their usual sleep schedule with bedtime remaining constant across both home and lab nights. Generally, the technical team arrived at the subject's home around 9 PM for an 11-11:30 PM bedtime with a freshly charged battery pack, the T-7, 8-channel telephonic EEG Transmitter, and a box of supplies for preparing the subject for his/her home sleep studies.

The technical team was instructed to attach the electrodes in an area where a window could be opened for adequate air ventilation since collodion and acetone are used in the scalp electrode applications. The subject and any family members who were observing were instructed not to smoke around these chemicals. A regular hair blow-dryer was used to dry the collodion. Subjects were given a small bottle of acetone (solvent to dissolve the collodion) and instructed on how to use it in the morning to remove their own electrodes.

Following "hookup", a test transmission of polygraphic data was initiated. The T-7 Transmitter was interfaced with a bedside telephone by means of a telephone adaptor. The technical team always carried a collection of telephone adaptors with different sized plastic snap-in male and female connector plugs. As was quickly learned, all modular type telephones do not have one standard connector plug size. The technical team also carried a 50-foot extension cord in case the subject's phone was outside of the bedroom.

At the conclusion of this transmission test, both sites disconnected from the phone line with the understanding that the laboratory would call the subject back at bedtime to initiate the night's sleep transmission. The technical team explained to the subject how to reconnect the transmitter.

The technical team made further arrangements with the subject for pick-up or dropoff of the transmitter unit. Some subjects elected to bring the T-7 Transmitter back to WPIC when they came into work following the second night of home sleep transmission. At that point, the technical team left and returned to the laboratory.

At the subject's bedtime, the laboratory phoned the subject for final transmission preparations. The laboratory specifically initiated the telephone call so that subjects would not be charged by the local phone company for eight hours of phone line usage. Subjects were also warned in advance of their home studies that their telephone lines would register as "busy" for the entire transmission period. Subjects were told to plug their mini electrode junction boxes into the Transmitter unit, plug the Transmitter into the phone line, switch the power to "on" and hang up the phone. From this point forward subjects were literally "talked" through the test transmission procedure. If the calibration and waking EEG signals received by the laboratory were embedded in electrical noise, both sites disconnected from the phone line and the telephone call was reinitiated from the laboratory.

With a successful signal transmission back to the laboratory, the subject was told "Good night" and further communication between the two sites was discontinued. Both sites turned the audio volume down on the respective Transmitter and Receiver units. During the night, subjects could disconnect from the Transmitter unit if necessary, without interfering in any way with continued transmission by simply unplugging from the unit just as a subject who wanted to go to the bathroom in the laboratory would simply unplug from the wall cabling to the polygraph. During the time the subject was unplugged, only electrical noise would be transmitted back to the laboratory until the subject plugged back into the Transmitter. As it happened, none of the subjects unplugged during the night.

Laboratory Monitoring

Subjects slept in bedrooms on the 13th floor of WPIC (the Sleep Center). They slept in complete privacy with no videotape monitoring and communicated with the technician in the control room via an intercom system. A Grass Model 78B, 24-channel polygraph was used for all sleep recordings.

Sleep recordings made utilizing either the home monitoring or laboratory monitoring systems consisted of the following three electrophysiological parameters: EEG, EOG, and submental chin EMG. The EEG was a monopolar, central scalp derivation (C4-Al + A2), while the EOG consisted of two monopolar eye derivations with the electrode placements just above the horizontal of the outer canthus (right electrooculogram) and just below the horizontal of the outer canthus (left electrooculogram). The submental chin EMG was bipolar. The EEG and EOGs were recorded using a low linear frequency filter of 0.3 Hz while, a low linear frequency filter of 10 Hz was used for the submental chin EMG. The high linear frequency filter was set at 30 Hz for the EEG and EOGs and 90 Hz for the EMG. Sleep recordings made in the laboratory or transmitted back to the laboratory were recorded on paper at a paper speed of 10mm/sec.

Results

Hand scored EEG was used to determine sleep continuity, sleep architecture, and two additional measures of REM sleep. All sleep was scored in 60-second epochs. Sleep continuity measures included sleep efficiency (the percentage of time spent asleep divided by the total recording time), sleep latency (the time from the beginning of the recording to the onset of stage 2 sleep), and sleep maintenance (sleep efficiency corrected for sleep latency). Sleep architecture measures included the distribution of total sleep time in the conventional stages of sleep; i.e. Stages 1, 2, delta, and REM. Delta sleep was regarded as the sum of Stages 3 and 4. The two additional REM sleep measures included REM sleep activity (an integrative measure of the frequency and intensity of rapid eye movements per minute of REM sleep) and REM sleep latency (the time from the beginning of Stage 2 sleep to the first REM sleep period, minus the awake time between sleep onset and the first REM period). The same modified Rechtschaffen and Kales (6) criteria were used to score all polygraph paper records generated by the home and the laboratory studies.

It should be mentioned that although the quality of the transmitted brain and eye movement signals was excellent and directly comparable to that produced by laboratory monitoring, the quality of the transmitted submental chin muscle signal was poor and essentially invalid during REM sleep. This turned out to be the case with the Medilog system as well.

The only marginally significant ($p = .054$) main effect occurred for sleep maintenance and the order of sleep recording. Sleep maintenance was significantly better in both environments when the subject was first sleep studied in the laboratory environment.

Since the intra-class correlation provides an estimate of the linear and/or nonlinear association between the independent and dependent variables when the independent variables are qualitative (3), i.e. environment and order of recording environments, the intraclass correlations were calculated for all nine of the sleep parameters tested. The intraclass correlations for five out of nine sleep variables were less than 0.50 suggesting that these sleep variables demonstrated a significant variability across subjects within the same treatment level. Thus, the measured sleep parameter differed from subject to subject independent of either environment or order of recording environment. Sleep latency, Stage 1%, Stage 2%, and delta% generated intraclass correlations in the range of 0.54 to 0.74 showing more homogeneity in these measures for different subjects within the same treatment level, i.e., a greater dependence or association with the two independent variables, environment and order of recording environment.

The conclusion drawn from Study 1 using the Telediagnostic System to transmit sleep data from the home versus the laboratory environments was that there were no significant differences in recording sleep parameters from the home versus the laboratory environments. Sleep maintenance or the continuity of the sleep state is significantly improved if the home transmission recordings are preceded by two nights of sleep monitoring in the laboratory suggesting an adaptation to sleep monitoring in general, independent of the actual recording environment.

EVALUATION OF THE MEDILOG SYSTEM

Apparatus

Oxford's Medilog 9000 Ambulatory Monitoring System has a long history of development (12 years) comparable to the Telediagnostic System. The Medilog recorder is small, battery-operated, and only 0.5 kg in weight. Its 4-channel predecessor was originally developed as a 24-hour EKG holter monitor recording both direct arterial pressure as well as the EKG in the form of a rhythm strip (4). In its present from, it is the 24-hour EEG analogue to the 24-hour EKG holter monitor. Its principal value is in its diagnostic value to clinical electroencephalography for intractable seizure activity . The cost of the Medilog 9000 Ambulatory Monitoring System was too prohibitive to purchase outright for the purpose of the present feasibility study. Therefore, a special arrangement with the Oxford Medilog, Inc. subsidiary in Clearwater, Florida, was made to rent the system.

Prior to rental of the Medilog System, I participated in a 1 1/2 day course on 9-channel basic ambulatory electroencephalography (the 9-channel recorder). When the Medilog System is purchased, a representative of the buyer is invited to take the course either on the 4-channel recorder and 4-channel Scanner (if purchased) or on the 9-channel (8-data channels) recorder and Scanner 9000 (if purchased). The course is very clear and comprehensive outlining everything that is needed in order to successfully use the System. Without the course, a great deal of time and effort would have been wasted, not to mention subject data loss and equipment failure due to improper handling. The Medilog System is a highly specialized system and therein lies its major disadvantage.

The Medilog 9000 recorder has the capability of recording 8-channels of electrophysiological data and a ninth channel for marking off events in time. The amplifiers and pre-amplifiers of the electrophysiological parameters being monitored are separated. The driver amplifiers are miniature electronic boards that are housed within a closed compartment in the recorder, while the HDX pre-amplifiers are miniature, black square tiles with a negative and positive pin sticking out of each side. These pre-amplifiers are attached by long, thing, black wire cables directly to the amplifier boards inside the recorder. Each pre-amp is color coded by channel according to the standard color coding for resistors. In the present study, only the first five channels were used so that the amplifier boards with their attached HDX pre-amps for channels 6-8 were removed. The electrodes that are used with the HDX pre-amps are specially designed shallow tin cup electrodes with a hole in the center. Each tin cup is attached to a 4 or 6 cm lead wire which plugs into one of the two pins on the HDX pre-amp.

There is no way to reference to linked or tied mastoids in this system so a modification in the running montage had to be made in order to use this system. Instead of running the standard laboratory montage, which could also be used with the Telediagnostic system, of C4-Al+A2, right EOG-Al+A2, left EOG-Al=A2, and left submental chin EMG-right submental chin EMG, the montage was altered to C4-Al, right EOG-Al, left EOG-A2, left submental chin EMG-right submental chin EMG, and C3-A2 (a back-up scalp derivation).

Although the 4 and 6 cm electrode lead lengths are perfectly adequate for the suggested bipolar, 8-channel montages that have been tested for maximal diagnostic value in clinical electroencephalography, these lengths are totally inadequate for standard sleep montages. The company, however, will custom make any lead length desired. Since in certain situations, it may be desirable to have the same scalp or mastoid derivation on two separate channels or tracings, the company also makes a bifuracated electrode enabling the technician to attach a single electrode placement to two separate HDX pre-amps and thereby two separate channels.

It is critical that one know ahead of time exactly what electrophysiological parameters are to be studied and where the sensors (electrodes) will be placed to study these parameters. Sample measurements were used to make potential electrode lead lengths for the desired sleep recording, running montage. This provided "average" lead lengths. For individual subject heads, there was sometimes too long a lead wire and, in the case of one male subject's head, too short a lead wire making the application more awkward.

Both the electrodes and the HDX pre-amps had to be completely glued down to the scalp with collodion and the individual's own the electrodes and HDX pre-amps. In the case of clinical electroencephalography where only scalp derivations are used, this works fairly well in practice. However, eight HDX pre-amps, sixteen electrodes, and a ground plug with two more electrodes, all collodioned to a person's scalp are difficult to hide much less to have glued to one's scalp. The solvent used to remove the collodion, acetone, is very toxic and large quantities are necessary to remove all of the collodion. In the case of a sleep recording in which eye movements and submental chin muscle activity were necessary, "hiding" these electrodes was impossible.

The Medilog 9000 recorder is battery operated and records data at the rate of 2 mm/second. The Scanner 9000 reads and displays the tape recorded data at 20, 40, and 60 times the recording speed, i.e., 40, or 80, or 120 mm/seconds. Sleep data can only be scored by the standard scoring criteria (6) at a recording speed of 10 or 15 mm/second. Therefore, the recorded tapes could not be scored by the standard criteria off of the Scanner 9000 display screen, since it did not permit adequate and detailed discrimination of all the waveforms essential to 20, 30, or 60 second, epoch-by-epoch, manual sleep staging. Consequently, the Scanner 9000 was used as an interface between tape recorded data (the audio cassette) and the 78B Grass polygraph. The data were read off of the cassette by the Scanner 9000 and then printed onto paper by the polygraph at a paper speed of 10 mm/second in order for it to be manually scored. Since there were at least eight hours of relevant data on each cassette, this meant that it took at least eight hours of additional technical time to produce a paper copy of the data at the correct paper speed for manual scoring.

The Medilog 9000 recorder requires four, double "A", 1.5 volt, alkaline batteries. These batteries must be replaced with brand new batteries following every 24-hours of use. Batteries must also be exactly 1.5 volts each. If the voltage drops by so much as a tenth of a volt, the recorder will stop several hours into the recording. Therefore, all batteries (about 100 were used in the present study) were kept in the refrigerator until used, the voltage of each battery was checked with a volt meter prior to use in the recorder, and all four batteries were discarded after one, 24-hour use.

Finally, the Medilog System requires that subjects/patients be wire-up in the laboratory. The only way to test out the system and particularly to test out whether anything is being recorded on cassette tape is to simultaneously record both on the cassette tape and to a write-out unit such as a polygraph or EEG machine. A monitor-writer coupling unit is included with the system to permit a simultaneous interface of both the recorder and the polygraph with any incoming signals from the amplifiers. This is the only test procedure for establishing whether the recorder is functioning properly prior to sending the subject out with it. Consequently, the subjects had to be wired and the system had to be tested in the laboratory prior to the recording of nocturnal sleep. One final statement should be made regarding the cassette tape. This is just a standard C-120 audio cassette tape. The company recommends their own, Maxell-UD, or TKD-LN-120, because all three have the same length "leader."

Procedure

As with the Telediagnostic System, subjects were sleep studied in the home and laboratory environments in a counterbalanced order. Each Subject was also studied for four consecutive nights, 2-each in both the home and laboratory environments.

Home Monitoring

Following the screening interview of a research nurse, the subject was again informed of his/her acceptance into the study, and an appointment was made to obtain informed consent. At this time the entire hook-up and testing procedure was explained in detail including the number of pre-amps and electrodes that would be glued to the scalp. The subject was asked to report to the laboratory at 6 PM on the nights of his/her Medilog studies for the hook-up and test procedure which would take about two hours. Subjects were told to wear a shirt or blouse that buttoned up the front or back, preferably, on those nights rather than one that had to be pulled up over the head. They were told not to wear a hat for those two days (static charge can short-circuit the pre-amps). They were also told that they would not be able to shower or swim (it was the beginning of summer) while wearing the Medilog. A bath could only be taken if there was a second person in the bathroom with the subject holding the recorder so that it could not fall into the bathtub. Subjects were also told that they could elect to wear the Medilog recorder for the entire 36-hour period or that it would be completely removed and reapplied after the first 18 hours. The subject was then given the names of the two technicians who would be at the laboratory to meet them at 6 PM.

The subject wire-up or hook-up procedure was done in stages. The placement of all scalp and facial electrodes and pre-amps and to be carefully "mapped-out" on the individual subject's head with the various electrode lengths available prior to any actual collodion application. The electrodes were all placed and collodioned or taped (face) down, first, leaving a small space where two input electrodes would join to the HDX pre-amp. Part of the awkwardness of the procedure stemmed from the fact that electrode wires had to be long and cross over a large area of scalp for the appropriate referencing montage, i.e., a bifurcated electrode was used at each mastoid site. This meant that the right mastoid had to join with the left central scalp electrode and the left outer canthus eye electrode, while, the left mastoid had to join with the right central scalp and the right eye electrodes.

The last step in this long and tedious procedure was to test the actual signals being recorded and produce a paper copy to document the quality of brain, eye, and submental chin muscle signals being recorded on tape. The subject was taken into the control room and interfaced with the polygraph via the Medilog monitor-writer coupling unit and the polygraph was turned on. A few basic tests were conducted. The subject was asked to sit quietly and close his/her eyes to provide a clear sample of relaxed wakefulness and an alpha rhythm. Then the subject was asked, with eyes still closed, to look to the right, back to center, left, and back to center. Several eye blinks were requested along with a cough and a clench of the jaw muscles. At this point the test was concluded and the polygraph turned off.

Subjects were asked not to chew any gum while wearing the Medilog and instructions about showers and swimming were repeated. The Medilog recorder includes a time event marker channel (9) and button. The subject was instructed to press the button once at bedtime and once when he/she awoke in the morning. Since there was no interest in any part of the tape recorded data except for the sleep period, marking these two events permitted the used of a "Scan for Event Marker" feature on the Scanner 9000 that could be used to isolate just the relevant sleep period portion of the data.

All eleven subjects complained about the length of the procedure. Four subjects elected to wear the Medilog Recorder for the entire period of their home sleep nights rather than go through the procedure a second time. These subjects were told that they could remove the facial electrodes by themselves the next morning and clip them into the hair so that they were less noticeable. They were also instructed on how to turn off the recorder the following morning but asked not to remove the cassette tape which would be removed that evening when they returned to the lab for regelling for all electrodes, placement of the facial electrodes, new batteries and a new cassette tape for the recorder. These subjects had to come into the laboratory for this procedure, since it also included a second interface with the polygraph for testing the pre-amps and for quality verification of the signals being recorded.

The three subjects who participated in both studies expressed a unanimous preference for the Telediagnostic System as did the entire technical staff. Eight of the eleven subject (73%) complained of excessive drying and scabbing of the skin and scalp areas where the electrodes had been applied. Tiny scabs formed at the electrode sites and then flaked away within 48-hours after the home nights. This pattern of dryness and scabbing did not occur following laboratory or Telediagnostic home nights where the standard Grass EC-2 electrode cream was always used. Although an occasional subject or patient might complain of sensitivity to the surgical tape used to secure the facial electrodes, such a problem is rare and usually attributed to highly sensitive skin. However, the electrode jelly that was specifically recommended for use with the Medilog System was not well tolerated at all by the normal subjects who participated in this study. In addition, all of the subjects complained of the large amounts of acetone required to remove all of the collodion in the hair.

Laboratory Monitoring

The laboratory recordings were carried-out as described in the report of the TeleDiagnostic Study.

Results

The Scanner 9000 was used only as a playback interface unit to the polygraph. When all of the tapes that could be played back and written-out on paper were completed, it was discovered, during the manual scoring of these records, that there was an inconsistent time discrepancy between what was calculated as time between "lights-out" and "lights-on" according to the subject's event markings and time between "lights-out" and "lights-on" according to the actual paper playback of the recorded data. The paper records demonstrated a totally idiosyncratic time loss from one playback to another. Time lost on the playback of tapes ranged from 6-39 minutes with a mean time loss of 16.69 minutes and a standard deviation of 11.03 minutes (median = 13 minutes0, and that excluded two extreme values of 4 and 56 minutes. There was no way of tracking where, why, or how this time was lost.

The quality of the brain and eye movement signals recorded and played back was excellent like that obtained with the Telediagnostic system and was definitely of laboratory quality. However, just as was the case with the Telediagnostic system, the submental chin muscle signal was of poor quality and at best, doubtful validity during REM sleep.

The identical nine, separate two-way, repeated measures ANOVA contrasts were carried out on the data from the Oxford Medilog 9000 study as had been carried out on the data from the Telediagnostic study. There were no significant main or interaction effects for any of the nine sleep parameters tested.

For the Medilog system, the intraclass correlations of only four sleep parameters, sleep efficiency, sleep latency, Stage 1%, and REM activity, were greater than 0.50 (0.55-0.81). It is interesting to note that only sleep latency and Stage 1% showed high intraclass correlations across both home monitoring systems. These two sleep parameters were the only sleep parameters to show enough stability across subjects and systems to reflect an environment or any other effect, if there had been one. The small intraclass correlations in many of the basic sleep parameters scored emphasize the significant individual variability and heterogeneity found even in the sleep of normal subjects.

COMPARISON OF THE TELEDIAGNOSTIC AND MEDILOG HOME MONITORING SYSTEMS

Statistical Comparison

Sleep latency and all three REM measures looked as though, they might be varying between systems. Therefore, four separate, split-plot repeated measures ANOVAs were performed with the monitoring system as the between subjects' factor and recording environment as the within subjects' factor. Only sleep latency showed a significant effect. This significant effect was not a main effect but rather an interaction effect ($F_{(1,18)} = 4.64$, $p < .05$) between monitoring system and recording environment. Using the Telediagnostic system, subjects took longer to fall asleep in the home environment as compared to the Medilog system. The reason for this was entirely unexpected and actually very funny. It turned out that the subjects in the Telediagnostic Study often invited friends, neighbors, and relatives to watch them being wired and prepared for "transmission of their sleep over the home telephone line." Pictures were taken for the "family album", etc.. By the time all of the "excitement" was over and it was time for sleep, many of these subjects had difficulty falling asleep!

Relative Advantages and Disadvantages

Comparisons: Each system has an application in basic and clinical sleep research and medicine. The most versatile, economically and manpower efficient system, and the system that does not require the subject/patient to come into the laboratory at all is the Telediagnostic system.

The Medilog system has evolved into a 24-hour EEG holter monitor analogue in clinical electro-encephalography to the 24-hour EKG holter monitor in cardiology. Its realistic application in sleep medicine or sleep research would be restricted to a diagnostic screening of sleep and wake distributions across the 24-hour day, i.e. to verify a sleep-wake schedule or regulation, disorder. It would be counterproductive in any project, research or diagnostic, that required a hardcopy of the sleep and waking periods across a 24-hour (or even an 8-hour sleep period) where standardized scoring into conventional stages by 20,30, or 60 second epochs was desired. Where the data simply need to be scanned on a screen for a "general impression" of sleep-wake regulation and/or possible abnormalities in other electrophysiological parameters (e.g., heart rate) across a 24-hour period, the Medilog system has a powerful potential. It would not be realistic to transmit electrophysiological data over a telephone line for 24-hour periods.

The Telediagnostic system is a relatively straight forward system to use and has a wide range of potential applications. Its two primary drawbacks are in terms of its total dependence on a "good" telephone line connection and the fact that it does not obviate the need for an all-night technician to monitor the transmission in the laboratory. The phone lines in a particular area where the system is to be used should be carefully checked before the study. Probably the most advantageous use of this system is within a medical center complex or university system linked by a single telephone network. In this case, the quality of the telephone connections is known and can be controlled.

REFERENCES

1. Coates, T.J., Rosekind, M.R. and Thoresen, C.E. (1978): *J. Behav. Ther. and Exp. Psychiat.*, 9:157-162.

2. Coates, T.J., Rosekind, M.R., Strossen, R.J., Thoresen, C.E. and Kirmil-Gray, K. (1979): *Psychophysiology*, 16-339-346.

3. Kirk, R.E. (1968): *Experimental Design: Procedures for the Behavioral Sciences.* pp 126-7. Brooks/Cole Pub. Co., Belmont, California.

4. Littler, W.A., Honour, A.J., Sleight, P. and Stott, F.D. (1972): *Brit. Med. J.*, 3:76-78.

5. Okudaira, N., Fukuda, H., Nishihara, K., Ohtani, K., Endo, S. and Torii, S. (1983): *J. Gerontol.*, 38:436-438.

6. Rechtschaffen, A. and Kales, A. (Eds.) (1968): *A Manual of Standardized Terminology, Techniques, and Scoring System for Sleep Stages of Human Subjects.* U.S. Department of Health, Education and Welfare, Public Health Service, Bethesda, MD.

7. Rosekind, M.R., Coates, T.J. and Thoresen, C.E. (1978): *J. Nerv. Ment. Dis.*, 166:438-441.

8. Schear, H.E., Rowe, W.J. and Pori, J.R. (1974): *Clin. EEG,* 5:24-30.

9. Sewitch, D.E., Kupfer, D.J. and Coble, P.A. (1984): Evaluation of Home Recording Methods for All-Night EEG Sleep Recordings. *Final Technical Report.* Commissioned by the John D. and Catherine T. MacArthur Foundation Research Network on the Psychobiology of Depression.

10. Sewitch, D.E. and Kupfer, D.J. (1985): *Sleep*, 8:288-293.

11. Sewitch, D.E. and Kupfer, D.J. (1985): *Psychophysiology*, 22:718-726.

12. Wilkinson, R.T. and Mullaney, D. (1976): *Postgrad. Med. J.*, 52(suppl. 7):92-96.

Medical Monitoring in the Home and Work Environment,
edited by Laughton E. Miles and Roger J. Broughton.
Raven Press, New York © 1990.

USE OF HOME MONITORING IN A SLEEP DISORDERS CLINIC

Khalil Kayed

Clinical Neurophysiology Section
Akershus Central Hospital, 1474
Nordbyhagen, Norway

INTRODUCTION

Standard polysomnography (PSG) is a complex technical procedure which is not limited to recording the sleep-wake cycle, but also provides information on several sleep-related physiological parameters. The latter may include simultaneous recording of respiration, cardiac, genitourinary, gastrointestinal and/or endocrine functions. PSG is a product of the sleep laboratory and is usually carried out in an institution committed to its effective application. Hospitals must be willing to provide the sleep laboratory with adequate recording equipment, facilities, personel, and budget. Technologists must be available to work at night. Likewise, a physician must be responsible for the overall direction of the laboratory. Certification standards have been developed by the American Sleep Disorders Association (ASDA) (formerly the Association of Sleep Disorders Centers [ASDC]).

Owing to fundamental differences between the American and the European medical systems, few specialized European laboratories have fulfilled the ASDA certification criteria. In Europe, most laboratories equipped for sleep recording have other daily neurophysiological responsibilities which limit their capacity to carry out additional night work; and medical technologists are not often available and willing to work at night. Moreover, in most of the European countries there are no well defined national plans on how and where sleep disorders should be diagnosed. There are also relatively few officially accredited clinical polysomnographers or other individuals suitably trained for directing such a sleep laboratory.

Consequently, there appears to be a great need for the development of ambulatory (or home) monitoring devices capable of unsupervised recording of sleep and associated physiological parameters. In the past few years, rapid advances in sensor technology, micro-electronics, data storage, and real-time data processing, have resulted in the development of some effective home physiological monitoring devices, some completely portable; and increasingly sophisticated systems will no doubt appear in the near future.

The aim of this chapter is to review our experience with the ambulatory monitoring systems that have been used routinely in our laboratory in the last 10 years. Our philosophy has always been that sleep can be recorded many ways and for many purposes. If one can obtain good quality data by practical and economic methods, why should one use more complex systems that are time consuming, expensive and frequently provide large amounts of unnecessary data?

THE RATIONALE OF AMBULATORY MONITORING IN HOME AND WORK ENVIRONMENT

Long term ambulatory monitoring originated in the field of cardiology where EKG recordings (Holter monitoring) used battery-operated, portable, single-channel tape recorders. Subsequently, multi-channel tape recorders were developed which could record sufficient information that long term ambulatory EEG recording became an established procedure in neurology, mainly for evaluation of patients with paroxysmal disturbances of cerebral function. Guidelines for the application of such devices in epilepsy were published by the American Electroencephalographic Society in 1985 (2).

Use of ambulatory devices in the field of sleep is still in its early phases of development, although some sleep disorders clinics now routinely carry out ambulatory sleep recordings. Several methods for evaluation of patients in home and work environment are now available for both clinical and research purposes. These devices record biological data by various techniques including analog tapes, solid-state monitors, telephone transmission systems, strip-chart recorders and local telemetric devices.

It is apparent that the main aim of long term monitoring is to make prolonged recording of sleep and its associated phenomena more practical than is possible using standard PSG. In a rapidly growing field in which new techniques are continuously introduced, these methods should be judged in terms of their relative strengths and weaknesses, and recommendations have to be made concerning the indications for their use. Like any diagnostic innovation, ambulatory recording should have some demonstrable advantage over other forms of evaluation, although it does not need to prove that it can and should completely replace other techniques.

Recent advances in integrated circuit technology have made it possible to develop portable systems that can easily be used by the patient for home monitoring. These systems can acquire long-term raw data which can be sent via radio-frequency or infra-red link to a receiver, transmitted via telephone line or stored in a portable computer placed at the subjects bedside. Together with data acquisition, sleep-wake staging and other analyses of physiological signals can be carried out. This means that it is now feasible to reproduce all the functions recorded in the sleep laboratory by standard polysomnographs. A newly introduced solid-state battery-driven portable EEG "The brain-Quick" (Micromed) has 24-channel insulated amplifiers, an EEG and polygraph tracing display on LCD monitor, and a hard disk incorporated in the unit for data storage. Similar devices can be used as satellite systems for PSG data acquisition while further data analysis can be carried out in a central sleep laboratory.

ADVANTAGES AND DISADVANTAGES OF AMBULATORY MONITORING

Among the advantages of ambulatory monitoring is the free mobility of the patient and the ability to record continuously the polycyclic sleep patterns across the sleep-wake cycle. Recent studies have shown that the first night effect encountered with in-lab studies does not exist (6,14). Ambulatory monitoring is cost effective as compared to standard PSG, and it has been found to be suitable for the evaluation of patients suffering for disorders of initiating and/or maintaining sleep (7). It has proven to be both feasible and suitable for physiological data collection in aerospace environment (8). Acceptance of the procedure by the patients has been shown to be high (13,9).

The disadvantages of ambulatory monitoring devices include the lack of guidelines and standards for their clinical application, technical specification, and safe use (especially when used by the elderly in their home environment). Some of the systems are still in their early phases of development and require further improvements both in hard and software. Most of the new ambulatory devices require further validation. Ambulatory systems should be built to tolerate occasional trauma and rough handling by subjects. They have to be user-friendly, including few and simple operative procedures. Some of the ambulatory equipment is not inexpensive, and some must be used with additional specialized and/or expensive equipment.

SLEEP RECORDING BY MOVEMENT SENSORS

The study of body movements during sleep has long been used as a measurement for the sleep-wake cycle and biological rhythms. Total body movement has been recorded using "a movement artifact cable" placed under the mattress (3) or by using static charge sensitive bed (SCSB) (1). Kripke et al (1978), used another approach for body movement recording when they introduced the wrist actigraph (11). They recorded signals from the wrist sensor by an analog cassette (tape) recorder which they later replaced by a portable solid-state system. Kayed et al 1979 (10), introduced a more comprehensive system (the acti-oculograph) which records eye and body movements in addition to the submental EMG (fig.1). The eye sensor is a miniature piezoceramic transducer (type 236 movement sensor Siemens). The analog signals were collected by a 4 channel Oxford Medilog tape recorder and played back at low speed of 2.5 mm/minute for visual scoring. The condensed printout permitted rapid scanning of the whole night to evaluate the characteristic periods of single or combined body and eye movements accompanied by high or low EMG amplitude (fig.2). A program for automatic analysis of the actioculograph was also developed using a Minc DEC/lab 23 computer. Mamelek and Hobson (12) recently introduced a portable movement-based sleep monitor (the "Nightcap") which collects digital data from an eye sensor and a head movement sensor attached to head-harness. The data is collected and stored by a portable computer via a digital interface board. The simplicity and cost effectiveness of all these systems make them very attractive candidates for large scale epidemiological sleep studies.

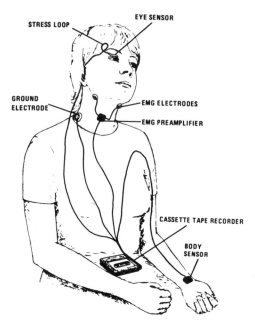

FIG. 1. The acti-oculographic monitor of sleep recording eye and body movements by microsensors and the submental EMG using 4 channel Oxford Medilog tape recorder.

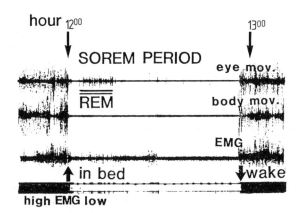

FIG. 2. A strip chart recording of Compressed acti-oculographic signals showing sleep onset rapid eye movements (SOREM) in a narcoleptic patient. Note the difference in amplitude of the eye sensor signal for eyeblinks (wake) and REM sleep.

SLEEP RECORDING BY TELEMETRIC DEVICES AND PORTABLE TAPE RECORDERS

Ambulatory sleep recording can be carried out either by telemetric systems or by analog recorders.

The "Telediagnostic" system first introduced by Coates et al 1978 (5) is a portable 8-channel telephone transmission system including a FM multiplexer and demodulation units. Some of the disadvantages of the telemetric systems are the introduction of artifacts during telephone transmission mainly due to the quality of the telephone line. As currently implemented, telemetry still requires continuous attention of a technician at the receiving station, and it also requires a polygraphic write-out.

The use of a portable four channel Oxford Medilog system for sleep monitoring was introduced by Wilkinson and Mullany in 1976 (15). Automatic scoring systems have been designed for this recorder, including the high speed hybrid automatic sleep stager by Broughton et al. 1983 (4). The main disadvantage of this 4 channel system is the availability of only 3 channels for recording biodata as the fourth channel is dedicated to time-encoding and an event marker. When all four channels are used to record biodata, the timing is not accurate.

The development of the Oxford Medilog 9000 system increased the number of the recording channels to 8 while dedicating the a ninth channel to time and event recording. The system consists of a small battery operated recorder using an ordinary C-120 cassette tape and a replay monitor for data display and scanning. There is a continuous time display on the monitor. This system has been used in our laboratory to carry out ambulatory PSG and Multiple Sleep Latency Tests (MSLT) for the diagnosis of hypersomnia. Because the MSLT is carried out at home, a standard cut-off time limit of 20 minutes is used. The application of this system to record MSLT also provided for the detection of all periods of sleepiness and microsleep episodes that can occur during the whole day. Simultaneous anterior tibial EMG monitoring can also provide information on the disorder of periodic leg movements (PMS) (Figs.3,4). When reviewing the data, the presence of anterior tibial EMG bursts typical of PMS can also be detected acoustically by playing the cassette at high speed and hearing the crackling or popping noise at regular intervals. In addition, the relation to different sleep stages and micro-arousals can be established.

The recent introduction of the Multi Parameter Analysis system (MPA) adds flexibility to the Oxford 9000 system. The tape recorder has been redesigned to include 4 channels dedicated to recording EEG, EOG and EMG according to the standard criteria, while the other 4 channels can be used to record other physiological parameters such as respiration by strain gauges, inductive plethysmography or thermistors, oximetry, EKG, nocturnal penile tumescence (NPT), temperature and anterior tibial EMG. The parameters are selected using a switch that allows ten different combinations (Figs.5,6). Data from the MPA can be transferred to the Oxford 9000 replay and display system, and subsequently to the SSMRKII Oxford Sleep Stager for automatic analysis of sleep-wake stages and other recorded physiological parameters plus the production of written results and sleep hypnograms.

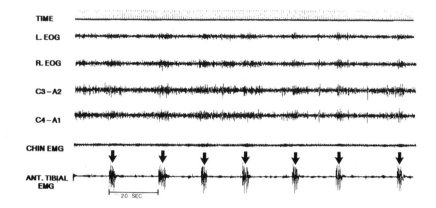

FIG. 3. Compressed display of periodic movements in sleep (PMS) recorded by the Oxford 9000 Medilog system with the typical regularly-occurring anterior tibial muscle bursts.

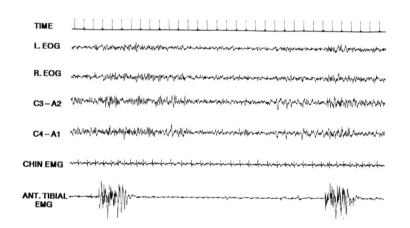

FIG. 4. Expanded display of PMS showing the EEG changes associated with the EMG bursts.

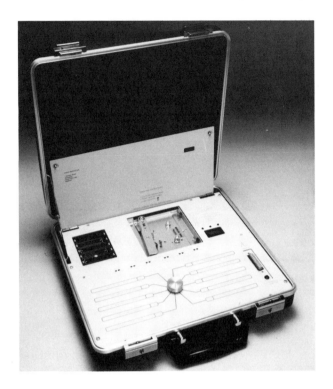

FIG. 5. The Oxford Multi-Parameter Analysis system (MPA) has 4 fixed channels for standard sleep recording, while 4 channels allow a selection of various physiological parameters including EKG, respiration, NPT and oximetry.

Some laboratories which heavily depend on ambulatory monitoring have several different devices that can be used such parameters as EKG, apnea, O2 saturation, continuous blood pressure, body position monitoring or NPT. Some devices can be programmed to record many parameters. The Vitalog "Lunch-box" (PMS-3000) monitor is a home cardio-respiratory monitor which can record O2 saturation, body and eye movements and body position, in addition to EKG and respiration. While this system does not record EEG, and therefore no sleep stages can be measured, the eye and body movement sensors can provide data on sleep states i.e. wake, NREM and REM.

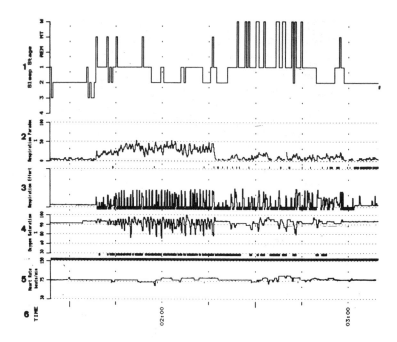

FIG. 6. Oxford MPA system. Display of data recorded from a sleep apnea patient: 1. sleep hypnogram. 2. paradoxical breathing. 3. respiration effort. 4. oxygen saturation. 5. heart rate. 6. time.

A PROTOCOL FOR EVALUATION OF SLEEP DISORDERS USING HOME MONITORS

For several years, our sleep disorders clinic has utilized the Medilog 9000 system and the Vitalog HMS-3000 monitor, to evaluate patients with sleep disorders. When the patient was suspected of having sleep apnea, the patient was recorded at home using the Vitalog monitor. When the clinical picture of the patient suggested narcolepsy, PMS or other insomnias-hypersomnias, 24 hour continuous ambulatory recording of PSG and MSLT have been carried out by the Medilog 9000 system. In the last two years, we have carried out 300 recordings for apnea detection by the Vitalog system, with a failure rate of about 2%; and 155 recording by the Medilog 9000 monitor (10 with the MPA system) with a failure rate of approximately 1%.

AMBULATORY VERSUS SUPERVISED POLYSOMNOGRAPHY

While most our patients with sleep disorders can be examined on an ambulatory basis using the above guidelines, there are still a group of patients who will require supervised PSG. The indications for supervised PSG can be summarized as follows:

1. Patients that are uncooperative, mentally disturbed or suffer from medical conditions which necessitate continuous observation during the entire night.

2. Situations requiring accurate confirmation of the relationships between certain pathological events and specific sleep stages.
3. Need for documenting simultaneous occurrence of several pathological conditions like the association of narcolepsy with sleep apnea and or PMS.
4. CPAP valve calibration before the start of obstructive apnea treatment.
5. History suggesting nocturnal epilepsy or obscure nocturnal attacks.

CONCLUDING REMARKS

Transferring EEG polysomnography to the home environment will raise important issues having to deal with the indications for supervised PSG that requires the obligatory recording of the subject in the sleep laboratory. It is evident that not all patients referred to the sleep laboratory require supervised PSG. The diagnosis of sleep related disorders can occur at several levels:

1. Central sleep laboratories with the capability of carrying-out standard PSG in addition to receiving, collecting and analyzing data.
2. Outlying hospitals using satellite data acquisition systems that can communicate with central sleep labs.
3. Dedicated systems that have been validated for recording specific parameters such as sleep apnea, oximetry or NPT.

While traditionally trained clinical polysomno-graphers tend to consider sleep disorder centers as the proper place for the diagnosis and treatment of sleep disorders, some new-comers and experts from other specialities believe that it is preferrable to have services and devices which focus on the pathological events rather than on sleep per se. Some of these dedicated systems are still in their early development phases and have not yet been fully validated. Hence, functional standards for both software and hardware, as well as guidelines for the use of ambulatory recordings in the diagnosis of sleep disorders, are required; but so far, no organization has offered to sponsor this task.

REFERENCES

1. Alihanka, J., Vaahtoranta, K. (1977): A Static Charge Sensitive Bed. A New Method for Recording Body Movement During Sleep. *Electroencephalogr. Clin. Neurophysiol*, 46:731-734.

2. Ajmone-Marasan, C. editor (1985): American Electroencephalographic Society Guidelines for Long-Term Neurodiagnostic Monitoring in Epilepsy. *Clin. Neurophysiol*, 2(4):419-452.

3. Azumi, K., Sirakawa, S., Takahashi, S. (1977): A Proposal of New Classification for Body Movement During Sleep. *Sleep Res.*, 6:49.

4. Broughton, R., Roberts, J., Suwalski, W., da Costa, B., Liddiard, S. (1983): A High Speed Hybrid System for Automatic Sleep Analyser. Accuracy Measures. *Sleep Res.*, 12:344.

5. Coates, T.J., Rosekind, M.R., Thoresen, C.E. (1978): All Night Sleep Recording in Clients Homes by Telephone. *J. Behav. Ther. & Exp. Psychiat.*, 9:157-162.

6. Coates, T.J., George, J.M., Killen, J.D., Marchini, E., Hamilton, S., Thoresen, C.E. (1981): First Night Effects in Good Sleepers and Sleep-Maintenance Insomniacs when Recorded at Home. *Sleep*, 4:293-298.

7. Erwin, C.W. (1987): Cassette Recording in Insomniac Patients (abs.). *II International Conference of Ambulatory Monitoring in Epilepsy and Sleep Disorders*. Telfs, Austria.

8. Graeber, R.L., Lauber, J.K., Cornell, L.J., Gander, P.H. (1986): International Aircrew Sleep and Wakefulness After Multiple Time Zone Flights: A Cooperative Study. *Aviation Space & Environment Med.*, 57 (12 suppl): B3-9.

9. Hoelschar, T.J., Erwin, C.W., Marsh, G.H., Webb, M.D., Radtke, R.A., Lininger, A. (1987): Ambulatory Monitoring with Oxford Medilog 9000: Technical Acceptability, Patient Acceptance and Clinical Indications. *Sleep*, 10:606-607.

10. Kayed, K., Hesla, P.E. (1979): The Actigraphic Monitor of Sleep. *Sleep*, 2:253-260.

11. Kripke, D.F., Mullaney, D.J., Messin, S., Wybocaney, G.V. (1978): Wrist Actigraphic Measurements of Sleep and Rhythm. *Electroencephol Clin Neurophysiol*, 44:674-676.

12. Mamelak, A., Hobson, J.A. (1987): Nightcap - a Portable Movement Based Sleep Monitoring System. *Sleep Res*, 16:567.

13. Sewitch, D.E., Kupfer, D.J. (1985): Polysomnographic Telemetry Using Telediagnostic and Oxford Medilog 9000 Systems. *Sleep*, 8:288-293.

14. Sharply, A.L., Solomon, R.A., Cowen, P.J. (1988): Evaluation of First Night Effect Using Ambulatory Monitoring and Automatic Sleep Stage Analysis (in press).

15. Wilkinson, R.T., Mullaney, D.J. (1976): Electroencephalogram Recording of Sleep at Home. *Post. Grad. Med. J.*, 12:344.

Medical Monitoring in the Home and Work Environment,
edited by Laughton E. Miles and Roger J. Broughton.
Raven Press, New York © 1990.

STATIC CHARGE SENSITIVE BED (SCSB) IN MONITORING OF SLEEP AND APNEAS

Tapani Salmi and *Lea Leinonen

Laboratory of Clinical Neurophysiology
Department of Neurology
Helsinki University Central Hospital
SF-00290 Helsinki, and *Department of Physiology
Helsinki University, SF-00170 Helsinki

INTRODUCTION

The static charge sensitive bed, SCSB, (Biomatt[R], Biorec Inc.) is a movement sensor designed by Dr. J. Alihanka (Department of Physiology, University of Turku, Finland) for the study of sleep (1,3). Three separate signals are obtained from SCSB which relate to movements of the heart (BCG), respiratory movements, and body movements. By analyzing the movements it is possible to distinguish between wakefulness, quiet sleep, and active sleep. Monitoring does not disturb sleep as no cables are connected to the subject. Ambulatory SCSB recording allows the study of normal and pathological sleep in a large number of subjects at low cost. When the SCSB recording is combined with monitoring of ventilatory airflow and arterial oximetry the diagnosis and quantification of sleep-related apneas becomes possible. We describe here the SCSB method and its application in computerized analysis of sleep-related movements and apneas.

THE MOVEMENT SENSOR, SCSB

SCSB is a light (2 kg) flexible plate (usually 1.5 cm x 0.9 m x 1.9 m) placed in the bed under an ordinary foam plastic mattress. SCSB consists of electrically active layers that generate static charge when deformed. The active layers induce measurable charge differences (voltage) between two isolated metal plates. The active layers and the metal plates are shielded and grounded by a metal folio to avoid electric environmental noise. According to the manufacturer the signal to noise ratio of the recording is usually better than 20:1.

SCSB is very sensitive. It detects a pea dropping on the foam plastic mattress and could be used even as a microphone detecting speech sounds as well as air pressure changes below audible frequencies. The movement forces cannot be quantified because in practice the amplitude of the signal cannot be calibrated. The amplitude and shape of the signal depend on the

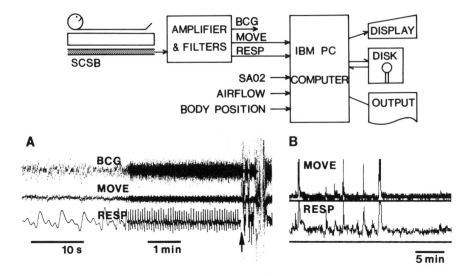

FIG. 1. Flow chart of the recording and analysis system of SCSB. In A the three signals are shown at two paper speeds. At the beginning of the recording there are no body movements (MOVE) and the BCG and respiration (RESP) have an even rhythm. Towards the end of the recording there is a period of body movements (onset indicated by the arrow). B shows a computer output graph of a 30 min recording of sleep. The high peaks on both channels (MOVE and RESP) correspond to body movements and fluctuation of the baseline in RESP corresponds to irregular breathing. This movement pattern is characteristic for REM stage. The end of the recording shows a period of quiet sleep with even breathing and no body movements.

properties of the foam plastic mattress (density, thickness, compliance), and weight and posture of the subject.

The foam plastic mattress placed on SCSB is usually 5 - 7 cm thick. Thinner mattresses may give better signals in light persons. The manufacturer has a special SCSB for children weighting less than 8 kg. SCSB has been successfully used for newborn infants weighting less than 3 kg (4,5).

AMPLIFICATION AND FILTERING OF SCSB SIGNAL

The primary SCSB signal is divided into three signals by selective filtering and amplification (3) (Fig. 1). A slow-frequency (0.05 Hz - 3 Hz) signal originates mainly from respiratory movements (RESP). A fast-frequency (3 Hz - 60 Hz) signal originates from heart beats and provides a ballistocardiogram (BCG). The third signal, with considerably lower amplification than the two others, is filtered through 0.05 Hz - 60 Hz and used for the detection of gross body and limb movements (MOVE). Although the three channels are rather selective, it is self-evident that many movements (e.g. body movements) are reproduced on all three channels. Isolated movements of a finger, toe or head may result in similar waveforms. Therefore, the origin of such movements cannot be identified with SCSB.

STORING AND DOCUMENTATION OF SCSB RECORDINGS

The first SCSB sleep recordings were done with an EEG device. The graphs were visually evaluated and compared with the movements visually observed (1). We developed computerized methods for storing and analyzing the SCSB signals and for the documentation of the results in the form of simple graphs and statistics (13). In ambulatory monitoring we previously used small cassette recorders (e.g. Oxford Medilog, Teac) and the data were later analyzed. At present most recordings are completely automated.

ANALYSIS OF SLEEP BY CATEGORIZING BODY MOVEMENTS

Alihanka was the first one to correlate the duration of body movements detected by SCSB to the type of sleep (1). He classified the movements as shorter than 5 s, 5-10 s, 10-15 s, and longer than 15 s, and found a close association between fast body movements (duration less than 15 s) and REM stage (1,8).

We have developed an automated analysis of body movements which yields criteria for the classification of any stage as "wakefulness", "quiet sleep" and "active sleep" (13). The device consists of a portable microcomputer (IBM PC) with two disc drives, an analog-digital converter (Tecmar Labmaster) and a graphic printer (Fig. 1). At present the recording and analysis can be performed on 5 channels simultaneously. RESP and MOVE are recorded from SCSB. Optional choices for the other two channels include airflow, SaO2, body position, sound, EEG, EMG and EOG.

For the analysis of MOVE, sampling rate is 30/s and the digitized values are rectified and integrated in epochs of 1 s (compressed graphic representation of MOVE in Fig. 1B and 2A). An epoch with an amplitude greater than 3 times the mean during the recording is a "movement in bed". The movements are classified according to their duration (graphic representation of MOVE durations in Fig. 2). The movements shorter than 15 s are used for scoring sleep in epochs of 3 min. A movement hypnogram signifying "wakefulness", "quiet sleep" and "active sleep" is printed together with a graph showing the distribution of movements of different durations (Fig. 2A). We compared the method with traditional polygraphic evaluation of sleep (EEG, EOG, EMG) in nine ambulatory recordings and found an agreement of 81 % (71-90 %) (13). This agreement is apparently sufficient in screening for sleep disturbances.

The amount of "quiet" and "active" sleep and the alternation of stages in the movement hypnogram are indices of sleep quality (Fig. 2). In a normal hypnogram there is a regular alternation of quiet and active sleep (Fig. 2A).

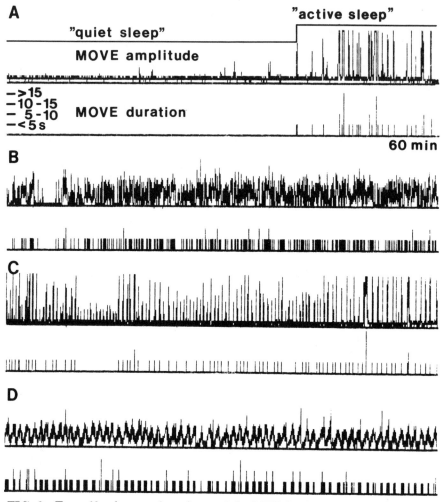

FIG. 2. Four 60 min samples of overnight SCSB body movement (MOVE) recordings. The upper graph shows the integrated amplitude of MOVE in a compressed form. The lower graph shows the distribution of movements of different durations. A: Recording classified as "quiet sleep" and "active sleep" in a healthy subject with normal sleep pattern. B: Restless sleep (waking) in a patient suffering from post-herpetic pain. C: Periodic long-lasting myoclonus of feet prevents a patient from falling into deep sleep. D: Periodic breathing (with periodic movement arousals) due to obstructive sleep apnea may completely disrupt the normal sleep pattern. The number and duration of movements during the 9 h recordings were: A: 166, 780 s, B: 1479, 6048 s, C: 731, 2062 s, D: 2848, 11832 s.

In patients with restless sleep (e.g. patients suffering from pain, or patients with primary insomnia) the pattern of sleep is disorganized and the time of sleep is reduced. In a waking subject the quiet periods characteristic for deep sleep are missing (Fig. 2B). Patients with obstructive apnea or myoclonic movements of the legs display a periodic pattern of movements (Fig. 2C,D). Analysis of the breathing pattern (next chapter) in these patients is usually sufficient to decide whether the periodicity is caused by the leg movements or by apnea. The periodicity of obstructive apneas is usually of the order of 1 min. As the computerized sleep scoring is performed in epochs of 3 min it cannot be done in these patients.

Several patient groups have been screened for sleep disturbances with SCSB. In old patients with Down's syndrome sleep was disturbed by periodic breathing due to obstructive apnea (verified with polygraphic recordings, (20)). In patients with juvenile neuronal ceroid lipofuscinosis no normal patterning of sleep was observed (18). Pathological features of sleep were also observed in SCSB-recordings of patients with dementia (either of Alzheimer or multi-infarction type; (6)), or Parkinson's disease (9), and in infants with brain damage (5).

SCSB IN DETECTION AND QUANTIFICATION OF SLEEP APNEAS

Day-time polysomnography is routinely used in our Laboratory of Clinical Neurophysiology in the diagnosis of sleep apneas. We added SCSB to these measurements during 1981 and soon found it reliable in monitoring even the smallest breathing movements (Fig. 3) (11,13,14). Sometimes the heart beats induce a slow fluctuating artefact on the RESP signal but the artefact does not disturb the analysis. The RESP signal varies with the weight of the subject. The amplification is therefore adjusted for each patient. The amplitude of the signal also varies with the position of the subject but this does not disturb the recording or its analysis.

The number of patients suffering from breathing disturbances during the night is high (10,19). For economical reasons it is not possible to study all patients suspected for these diseases with conventional all-night polygraphic recordings. To solve the problem we developed a computerized analysis system (Fig. 1) (16) for long-term monitoring of RESP and MOVE with SCSB, of airflow with a thermistor attached near the nostrils and the mouth, of SaO_2 with a pulse oximeter attached on a finger (Biox II) and of sleep position (Vitalog sensor). The recordings can be carried out in a ward, in a patient hotel, or at home, either digitized on-line or stored on tape.

Fig. 3A and B show airflow, RESP, and SaO_2 during apneic episodes with both central and obstructive features. Airflow, RESP and SaO_2 are sampled at 30/s. Digitized values of airflow and RESP are integrated in epochs of 1 s, SaO_2 in epochs of 3 s. After the recording the data are represented in a compressed form as shown in Fig. 3C and D. The whole recording is always documented in this form because various pathological states can be diagnosed from it at a glance. The data are analyzed in various ways. A significant "oxygen desaturation event" is defined as a decrease of SaO_2 by at least 4 % for 6 - 120 s followed by a return to the preceding level. Desaturation events are collected and classified into ranks at 5 % intervals. At the end of the recording various statistics from these data are calculated and plotted (eg.cumulative distribution of desaturations). The airflow signal is analyzed for local maxima and minima to detect hypoventilation or apnea and "giant breaths" following apnea.

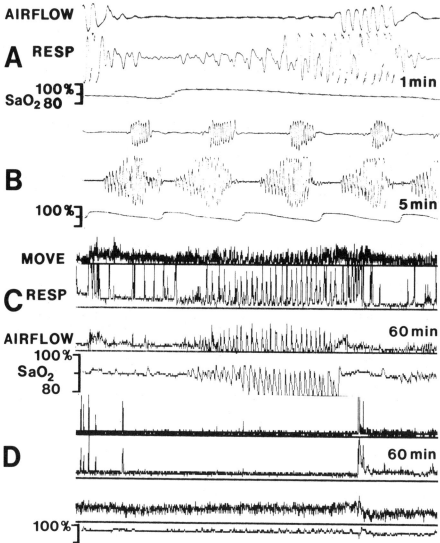

FIG. 3.   **A** and **B**: Record of airflow, SCSB respiration (RESP) and SaO2 in a patient with periodic breathing during sleep at two paper speeds. **A** illustrates an apneic episode in which RESP and airflow stop simultaneously (central apnea onset), followed by RESP activity without airflow (obstructive apnea). **B** shows the periodicity of apnea. **C**: A compressed (60 min) recording of a patient with periodic breathing and oxygen desaturation. The middle part of the record shows the same periodic breathing pattern as **B**. For comparison, a compressed output graph of 60 min of quiet sleep in a healthy subject is shown in **D**.

When the airflow signal during a minimum is less than 35 % of the mean value during the preceding 120 s, an apnea is detected, a hypopnea is defined similarly as less than 65 % of the mean. Statistics from these data are calculated and plotted (e.g. apnea index, apnea percentage).

Breathing movements are analyzed to distinguish obstructive and central apneas. If the amplitude of the SCSB signal during an apnea (detected by the thermistor) is less than 30 % of the amplitude during the preceding 120 s, the apnea is considered to be of central origin. Otherwise it is regarded as obstructive. A mixed-type apnea has usually a central onset and an obstructive end. The duration and distribution of obstructions are calculated. Statistics are calculated and plotted.

The SCSB body movement signal is analyzed as described in the previous chapter and the movement hypnogram is plotted.

The method has been compared with the conventional day-time polysomnography in 55 patients suspected for sleep apneas (16). The apneas were detected as reliably by the SCSB method as by other polygraphic means (including airflow, abdominal movements by strain gauge, submental EMG and EEG).

The computerized method is in routine use both in Department of Neurology and Department of Pulmonary Diseases, Helsinki University Central Hospital. It is used in the diagnosis of sleep apneas and hypoventilations. It is also applied in the evaluation of various treatments and in the adjustment of pressure when treating patients with nasal CPAP.

SCSB can be used alone in screening for apneas during sleep. The sensitivity of the method to detect significant periodic apneas seems to be practically 100 % (2,11,12,16,17). For differential diagnosis and evaluation of the severity of the syndrome, knowledge of the airflow and arterial oxygenation are, however, needed. Svanborg et al. (17) has used SCSB together with oximetry in screening for apneas and analyzed the records visually. They also reported high sensitivity of the method.

SPECIAL APPLICATIONS

We have developed an automatic analysis for long-term monitoring and quantifying of cough which is based on simultaneous detection of MOVE and coughing sound (15). The method is suitable for the evaluation of treatment.

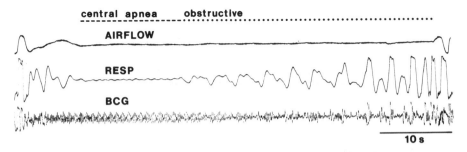

FIG. 4. Recording of airflow, SCSB respiration and BCG during an apneic episode. During the central phase of the apnea BCG has even rhythm and movement amplitude. During the obstructive phase BCG becomes irregular.

People who snore during the night have been screened for apneas by combining MOVE, RESP, oximetry and sound (19,21) The subjects with a history of habitual snoring also snored during the recordings. About 8 per cent of the subjects had periodic apneas with oxygen desaturation (19).

During an obstructive apnea BCG from SCSB shows changes related to strong fluctuation in the intrathoracic pressure and consequent disturbances in the rhythm and venous filling of the heart (Fig. 4) (2,12) similarly to changes in ECG (7). Although the signal gives additional information on apnea, we have not yet tried its automatic analysis. As also observed by users of other BCG methods, the variation of the signal with the position and weight of the patient makes the analysis difficult. The analysis could help in the detection of cardiac failure during sleep as suggested by Alihanka (2).

SUMMARY

SCSB is a cheap, easy and sensitive method for long-term monitoring of sleep and breathing. SCSB allows quantification of sleep with reliable scoring of sleep stages on the basis of movements detected by SCSB. For differential diagnosis of sleep disturbances, combination with other physiological measurements is usually necessary. Differential diagnosis of sleep-related apneas can be based on the monitoring of SCSB, airflow and arterial oxygenation.

In SCSB monitoring no cables are connected to the subject. Therefore SCSB is suitable for the monitoring of children, mentally retarded and patients with various disorders of brain function.

SCSB recording can easily be performed in surroundings where other polygraphic measurements would be difficult to carry out (home, hotel, emergency care unit, recovery room, train etc.).

SCSB signals are suitable for quantitative, computerizedanalysis because the signal to noise ratio is very good.

By combining SCSB recording with other measurements a large number of new applications can be discovered. For instance, we have used SCSB together with sound analysis in quantification of coughing during the night.

REFERENCES

1. Alihanka, J. (1982): *Acta. Physiol. Scand.,* Suppl. 511:1-85.

2. Alihanka, J. (1987): Basic principles for Analyzing and Scoring Bio-Matt (SCSB) Recordings. Annales Universitatis Turkuensis, Turku.

3. Alihanka, J., Vaahtoranta, K. and Saarikivi, I., (1981): *Am. J. Physiol.,* 240:R384-R392.

4. Erkinjuntti, M., Vaahtoranta, K., Alihanka, J. and Kero, P. (1984): *Early Hum. Dev.,* 9:119-126.

5. Erkinjuntti, M. and Kero, P. (1985): *Early Hum. Dev.,* 12:31-37.

6. Erkinjuntti, T., Partinen, M., Sulkava, R., Telakivi, T., Salmi, T. and Tilvis, R., (1987): *Sleep,* 10:419-425.

7. Guilleminault, C., Connolly, S., Winkle, R., Melvin, K. and Tilkian, A., (1984): *Lancet,* I:126-131.

8. Hasan, J. and Alihanka, J., (1981): In: *Sleep 1980,* edited by W.P. Koella, pp. 344-347. Basel, Karger.

9. Laihinen, A., Alihanka, J.,, Raitasuo, S. and Rinne UK. (1987): *Acta. Neurol. Scand.,* 76:64-68.

10. Lugaresi, E., Cirignotta, F., Coccagna, G. and Piana, C. (1980): *Sleep,* 3:221-224.

11. Partinen, M. and Alihanka, J., Hasan, J. (1983): In: *Sleep 1982,* edited by W.P. Koella, pp. 312-314. Basel, Karger.

12. Polo, O., Brissaud, L., Sales, B., Besset, A. and Billiard, M. (1988): *Eur. Respir. J.,* 1:330-336.

13. Salmi, T. and Leinonen, L. (1986): *Electroenceph. Clin. Neurophysiol.,* 64;84-87.

14. Salmi, T., Partinen, M., Hyyppä, M. and Kronholm, E. (1986): *Acta. Neurol. Scand.,* 74:360-364.

15. Salmi, T., Sovijärvi, ARA, Brander, P. and Piirilä, P. (1988): *Chest,* in press.

16. Salmi, T., Telakivi, T. and Partinen, M. (1988): submitted.

17. Svanborg, E., Carlsson-Nordlander, B., Larsson, H., Pirskanen, R. and Sterner, J. (1986): *Electroenceph. Clin. Neurophysiol.,* 64:86.

18. Telakivi, T., Partinen, M. and Salmi, T. (1985): *J. Ment. Defic. Res.,* 29:29-35.

19. Telakivi, T., Partinen, M., Koskenvuo, M., Salmi, T. and Kaprio, J. (1987): *Acta. Neurol. Scand.,* 76:69-75.

20. Telakivi, T., Partinen, M., Salmi, T., Leinonen, L. and Härkönen, T., (1987): *J. Ment. Defic. Res.,* 31;31-39.

21. Telakivi, T., Kajaste, S., Partinen, M., Salmi, T., Koskenvuo, M. and Kaprio, J. (1988): In: *Sleep 86,* edited by W.P. Koella, F. Obal, H. Schulz, P. Visser. pp. 430-431. Stuttgart, G. Fischer.

Medical Monitoring in the Home and Work Environment,
edited by Laughton E. Miles and Roger J. Broughton.
Raven Press, New York © 1990.

CYCLICAL VARIATION OF HEART RATE AND SNORING:

AN AMBULATORY DEVICE

Christian Guilleminault, *Thomas Penzel, *Riccardo Stoohs, Mary Beth
Masterson, and *J. Herman Peter

Stanford University, California 94305
*Marburg University, F.R.G.

INTRODUCTION

We have reported the presence of bradycardia during obstructive sleep apnea (OSA) followed by tachycardia at the end of each apneic event. This heart rate pattern was called "cyclical variation of heart rate" (CVHR). Several studies were initially performed, using Holter ECG in association with polygraphic recording during sleep. These studies were aimed at a better understanding of the mechanisms underlying the CVHR and the possible causes of elimination of this heart rate pattern in certain OSAS patients.

CVHR IN OBSTRUCTIVE SLEEP APNEA

Four hundred OSAS patients were investigated in succession (3). In association with them, 14 patients with a combination of OSA and autonomic nervous system lesion (heart transplant recipients, type 1 diabetic, chronic uremic-Shy-Drager syndrome), and 50 subjects with no OSA were polygraphically monitored. In each case at least one nocturnal polygraphic monitoring recorded the following variables: electroencephalogram (EEG) (C3/A2-C4/A1 of the 10-20 international placement system), electro-oculogram (EOG), diametric electromyogram (EMG), ECG (lead II). Respiration was monitored by measurement of air flow through oral and nasal thermistors and abdominal and thoracic mercury strain gauges. In the recent past, respiratory inductive plethysmography (Respitrace TM) was used. Arterial oxygen saturation was measured using a Hewlett Packard ear oximeter (model 47201A). Some cases had several recordings up to 24 hours in duration with other techniques, including the use of endoesophageal pressure transducers or balloons, hemodynamic studies with femoral arterial and pulmonary arterial pressure measurements and sampling of arterial blood gases with, at times, several successive nights of monitoring. During the hemodynamic night study, 16 OSAS patients received drugs acting on the autonomic nervous system.

The 24 hours of continuous electrocardiographic recording was originally performed with a single-channel Avionics ECG tape recording. In 1978 we switched to a two-channel ECG tape recorder. All electrocardiographic tapes were processed by computer methods previously described (2,6). Sleep monitoring was scored by 30-second epochs following the guidelines presented in Rechtschaffen and Kales' manual for the scoring of sleep states and stages (10). Apneic and hypopneic episodes were identified and scored following the criteria of Guilleminault et al. (4). Hypopnea was defined as a decrease of air exchange at nose and mouth secondary to incomplete airway obstruction or decrease of diaphragmatic output and accompanied by a simultaneous decrease in oxygen saturation (4). A correlation was made between the Holter ECG tracing and the various sleep and respiratory variables using the ECG lead on the sleep recording. To determine the statistical significance of the recordings, t test and Spearman rank order correlation were performed when appropriate.

Population

Sleep apnea syndrome population
All 400 subjects in the sleep apnea syndrome patient population had a specific pattern of sinus arrhythmia (CVHR) during sleep but not during wakefulness. This CVHR appeared during polygraphically monitored evening naps and nocturnal sleep but completely disappeared during awake periods, either during the day or the night, indicating a sleep-linked phenomenon independent of the day/night cycle. This variation was intermittent when sleep apnea or hypopnea were intermittent. On the computer print-out obtained for each patient, the swings in heart rate were easily identified.

In Figure 1, nine successive 10-minute segments are presented on a computer-generated graph. For each panel, the top line presents results of breathing sounds frequency analysis, and the bottom half presents R-R intervals. Heart rate is indicated on the left margin, and time (in minutes), on the lower line of each panel. The brady-tachycardia associated with apnea is easily seen on this figure. The mean heart rate during sleep is 70 beats per minute during non-obstructed breathing, as seen in the upper panel. Snoring is intermittent: it is indicated by black boxes above heart rate tracing for each 10-minute panel. The pattern of snoring noise-pause snoring noise is characteristic of obstructive sleep apnea. The temporal relationship between the snore and tachycardia is easily noted. Bradycardia occurs during the respiratory pause (absence of snoring). Near-continuous snoring without significant heart rate change occurs on the bottom panel, extreme right segment.

The changes in heart rate result from a progressive bradycardia associated with apnea during sleep, followed by abrupt tachycardia associated with resumption of air exchange and the arousal response. The cyclical variation in heart rate seen in sleep apneic patients differed from the sinus arrhythmia normally associated with respiration. The amplitude of each heart rate swing was greater than that seen with normal respiration, and the duration of each brady-tachycardia followed the abnormal and protracted breathing pattern (1,5). This is the heart rate pattern called cyclical variation of heart rate (CVHR).

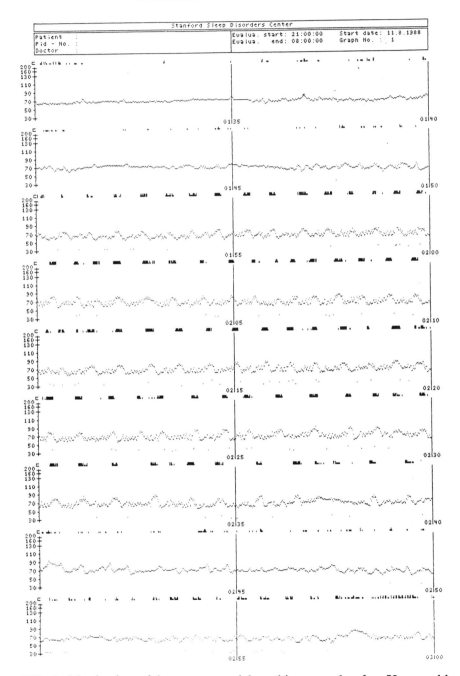

FIG. 1. Monitoring of heart rate and breathing sounds of a 52-year-old patient with obstructive sleep apnea without any autonomic nervous system lesion.

Control group

None of the fifty control patients who had been referred for sleep studies but did not have sleep apnea presented any repetitive variation of cyclical heart rate, as defined, during the 24-hour Holter ECG or sleep apnea syndrome on the polygraphic recording.

ANALYSIS OF SOME OF THE MECHANISMS INVOLVED IN CVHR

CVHR is the result of a bradycardia which occurs during sleep in association with apnea and a tachycardia seen in association with termination of apnea and an arousal response. Twenty-five sleep apneic patients with autonomic nervous system impairment or who received drugs interacting with autonomic nervous system activity during sleep-related hemodynamic studies were investigated. The effect of specific manipulations during sleep on CVHR were analyzed.

Anatomical isolation of the heart.

The three patients with heart transplant presented an Apnea-Hypopnea Index which varied between 28 and 40. Lowest oxygen saturation, between 71 and 59%, was noted during REM sleep. All monitored apnea were mixed and obstructive. No bradycardia was ever noted; no CVHR was observed. Heart rate presented a circadian rhythm-related variation with heart rate at 120 b/m near 24:00 and 80 b/m near 03:00 and progressive increase in the early morning hours.

Disease-related impairment of the autonomic nervous system (ANS).

Two insulin-dependent juvenile diabetics and one chronic uremic patient were diagnosed as having severe autonomic neuropathy and a denervated heart. Their heart rate, like heart transplant patients, was tachycardic but regular during sleep. Despite a significant Apnea Index, which oscillated between 31 and 62, with lowest oxygen saturation between 74 and 12% (12% is well below 35%, considered to be the reliability level of the ear oximeter), no bradycardia nor CVHR was noted, The three other diabetic patients, with autonomic neuropathy but without a denervated heart, presented a mild cyclical heart rate in association with obstructive apnea (Apnea Index between 15 and 40 and lowest oxygen saturation oscillating between 72 and 66%).

A similar blunting of cyclical heart rate was noted in three Shy-Drager patients. Their Apnea-Hypopnea Indices varied between 41 and 63, and lowest oxygen saturation oscillated between 51 and 39%. All apneic events were mixed and obstructive, and the cyclical heart rate was always in the mild category.

Regardless of the number and severity of obstructive sleep apneic events and amount of oxygen desaturation noted, patients with denervated heart (secondary to surgery or pathological process) never presented the cyclical heart rate pattern noted otherwise. Patients with incomplete autonomic nervous system lesions had a blunted pattern with only mild bradycardia even when oxygen desaturation was marked.

Pharmacological manipulations.

Pharmacological manipulations were performed only on sleep apneic patients without autonomic neuropathy.

Propanolol hydrochloride

A small to moderate decrease in the mean time delta between peak and trough of the cyclic swing was noted. Time delta is defined as the difference between fastest and slowest heart rate during an abnormal cyclical swing as measured in milliseconds by the computer. The reduction of this mean time delta was related to a minimum decrease in the tachycardia associated with the end of the apnea and the arousal response and also a mild decrease in the bradycardia associated with the obstructive apnea and oxygen desaturation. This change was consistent in the four patients who received propanolol hydrochloride.

Atropine sulfate and edrophonium

The most dramatic drug effect observed in all patients was noted with atropine sulfate administered to ten patients. The IV administration had an immediate effect on the sleep-apnea-related bradycardia. The dosage (1, 2, or 3 mg) had an impact on the blunting of the cyclical heart rate pattern. There was a clear drug response curve, but the decrease in the bradycardia varied depending on the subject and the administered amount. However, atropine sulfate was always the drug that, when administered alone, decreased most significantly the mean time delta compared with measurement just prior to experimental manipulation (p .01). The effect of atropine sulfate was not related to an effect on respiration or sleep. An analysis of 50 apnea prior and 50 apnea post-drug administration was performed on the ten patients. No statistically significant changes in type and duration of apnea, lowest oxygen saturation, or sleep stages were found. Edrophonium alone administered to five patients did not significantly increase the bradycardia normally seen in patients with obstructive sleep apnea syndrome but did reverse the effect of atropine sulfate at the dosage given.

Effect of oxygen

Fifteen patients received 5 to 10 l/m 100% oxygen administered by nasal prongs during NREM sleep. No change in the R-R interval pattern on Holter ECG was observed in five patients with autonomic impairment. In ten patients without autonomic impairment, 100% oxygen was administered for a mean of 20 minutes during NREM sleep. When 10 l/m 100% oxygen was administered, hyperoxia with oxygen tension oscillating between 150 and 101 mm/Hg (lowest measured values for the group) from the beginning to the end of an apneic episode was obtained in all cases. With 5 and 7 l/m, hyperoxia was also obtained but the persistence of repetitive obstructive apnea led to oxygen desaturation with lowest values of 71 and 82 mm/Hg respectively. Despite hyperoxia, the cyclical heart rate was always observed to some degree. However, in seven of the ten patients, 100% oxygen at 10 l/m led to a blunting of CVHR with a decrease of the bradycardia. There was an important variation from subject to subject of the blunting, which varied between 100 and 400 ms as compared to prior administration. No significant reduction in duration of apnea was noted when apnea measured from 5 minutes prior and 10 minutes after the start of oxygen administration were compared.

COMPARISON OF CVHR IN PATIENTS AND CONTROLS

The specific cyclical variation of heart rate (CVHR) noted in our patient population was not noted in any of our control subjects. All subjects with a normal autonomic nervous system and sleep apnea syndrome, independent of its severity or its type, presented the characteristic swings in heart rate. But CVHR was not observed in patients with denervated heart and sleep apnea, independent of the amount of oxygen desaturation. Incomplete lesion of the autonomic nervous system induces a blunting of this R-R interval pattern, with a clear decrease of bradycardia, again independent of oxygen desaturation. It was also impossible to recognize a CVHR problem in patients presenting with atrial fibrillation. Despite these known drawbacks of the technique, it was felt that CVHR could be useful in screening populations for OSA, particularly when, associated with clinical complaints and symptoms, an obstructive sleep apnea syndrome (OSAS) could be suspected.

The Marburg University research group decided to build on these initial findings (7-9). The fact that sinus arrhythmia decreases with age and that autonomic nervous system lesions or heart damage may eliminate or greatly diminish the CVHR was undoubtedly a problem, as certain patients would be missed. No attempt was first made to improve the CVHR criterion.

Constant heart rate.

Interindividual CVHR differences can be eliminated when the heart rate deviation from heart rate obtained during stable heart rate is considered. These different values can be calculated easily, and intraindividual periods of extreme heart rate variation can be determined. To do so, heart rate was determined over a 5-minute moving window. This gave a moving average value, and points of time where heart rate shows a deviation 20% from the moving average were indicated. The time period between two points with deviation <20% was called "period of constant heart rate" (7-9). Systematic investigations of OSAS patients indicated that periods of constant heart rate of short duration (i.e., (s) were significantly greater in OSAS patients than in normals. This criterion, tested on a large OSAS population, was noted as a statistically significant indicator of OSA. However, the problems related to autonomic nervous system lesions were still not resolved.

Snoring and CVHR.

It was thus decided to add another parameter that would enhance the screening potential of heart rate analysis. Considering the frequency with which patients with OSA snore, this parameter was selected and monitored simultaneously with heart rate. To extract a useful parameter from snoring, an electro-acoustic analysis was performed. Fast Fournier transforms were used, and power spectrum of sounds associated with snoring was analyzed. The power spectra of breathing sounds was calculated once every 125 s. It was shown that snoring was characterized by high power in the low-frequency range, whereas normal inspiratory and expiratory breath sounds presented with greater intensities of higher frequencies (7-9). A miniaturized filter bank allowing a continuous analysis of breathing and cross-checking with preselected specific frequencies was built up. A portable recording unit was then built, which allowed simultaneous recording of heart rate using classical ECG electrodes, and breathing sounds using a small (10 mm diameter) microphone. This device--commercially available in Europe--works on batteries and can be used to monitor a subject continuously for 14 hours. The heart rate and breath sound data can be analyzed with an IBM-compatible PC. A simple program gives a "yes" or "no" answer to the question of presence or absence of OSA, but the computer printout gives access to the data. This printout allows a visual determination of the frequency at which snoring and CVHR occur during the recording period.

Validation Study

One hundred OSAS patients were investigated at Marburg University and 20 OSAS patients and 10 patients with non- breathing related sleep disorders were monitored at Stanford University. Each subject was simultaneously monitored polygraphically during sleep and with the portable CVHR breath sound monitor. Polygraphic scoring was performed by a team of trained sleep technicians. The portable monitor printouts were scored blindly by two different individuals in Marburg and at Stanford. In this validation study, all sleep apneic patients independent of their apnea-hypopnea index were appropriately identified by the two blind scorers. In the population studied, there were also no false positives or negatives when using the automatic scoring system based on the ratio of heart rate indicator to breath sound indicator. However, the printout graph was much more informative than this ratio. A mean time of 5 minutes per blind scorer was needed to detect presence/absence of sleep apnea/hypopnea and to categorize the OSA group as "mild," "moderate," or "severe." No error was made in the subject categorization.

A more sophisticated study was performed to determine (a) periods of snoring without apnea and (b) periods of snoring with apnea and hypopnea. This study has currently been performed on 30 subjects, including OSAS and non-OSAS patients. A coefficient correlation $r = 0.92$ was noted between the Apnea/Hypopnea Index (A+HI) obtained by technicians scoring the polysomnogram and the blind ambulatory recorder printout score of "abnormal breathing event." The study is ongoing at this time.

FURTHER DEVELOPMENT

To further improve the reliability of the findings and the usefulness of the device, a light, portable ear-oximeter has been incorporated into the device. Collection of CVHR and breath sounds is associated with simultaneous collection of oximetry data. A new computer program that allows simultaneous retrieval of all collected data is now available. However, the validation study of this new system is incomplete.

COMMENTS

The ambulatory system based on analysis of heart rate and breath sound is light, easy to attach and to carry. It consists of a metallic box 12 x 6 x 2 cm contained in a case. Data are retrieved using a software based on a DOS system. Undoubtedly, the recent adjunction of ear oximetry data has increased its interest. This device is obviously very useful in performing epidemiologic studies, population surveys, and follow-up of subjects in the home environment. It has been used on a nightly basis for two years in the Marburg University Hospital and several hundreds of subjects have been studied. The device cannot replace a diagnostic polygraphic recording, but this equipment has allowed selection of subjects in need of further evaluation. It has also made possible the evaluation of home- based problems in patients equipped with nasal CPAP, the following of patients in the weight-loss program, and the surveillance of patients just released from hospital following surgery. The cost of the test has been estimated at $50.00 in the U.S.A., i.e., a low-cost informative device on heart rate and snoring.

ACKNOWLEDGMENTS

This work was supported by grants from the National Institute of Aging AG 07772 and the German Research Council.

REFERENCES

1. Anrep, G.V., Pascual, W. and Rossler, R. (1936): Respiratory Variation of the Heart. *Proc. R. Soc. London Ser. B,* 119:191-230.

2. Fitzgerald, J.W., Clappier, R.R. and Harrison, D.C. (1974): Small Computer Processing of Ambulatory Electrocardiogram Computers in Cardiology. *IEEE Biomedical Proceedings,* 3. Institute of Electrical and Electronic Engineers, Inc., Bethesda, Maryland.

3. Guilleminault, C., Connolly, S., Winkle, R., Melvin, K. and Tilkian, A. (1984): Cyclical Variation of the Heart Rate in the Sleep Apnea Syndrome. *Lancet,* i:126-131.

4. Guilleminault, C., Van den Hoed, J. and Mitler, M.M. (1978): Clinical Overview of Sleep Apnea Syndromes. In: *Sleep Apnea Syndromes,* edited by C. Guilleminault and W.C. Dement, pp.1-12. AR Liss, New York.

5. Hirsch, J.A. and Bishop, B. (1981): Respiratory Sinus Arrhythmia in Humans: How Breathing Pattern Modulates Heart Rate. *Am. J. Physiol.,* 241:H620-629.

6. Lopes, M.G., Fitzgerald, J.W., Harrison D.C. and Schroeder, J.S. (1975): Diagnosis and Quantification of Arrhythmias Using an Improved R-R Plotting System. *Am. J. Cardiol.,* 35:816-823.

7. Penzel, T., Meinzer, K. and Peter, J.H. (1987): Acquisition and Storage of Sleep-Related Biosignals. In: *Sleep-Related Disorders and Internal Diseases,* edited by J.H. Peter, T. Podszus and P. von Wichert, pp. 166-170. Springer-Verlag, Berlin, New York.

8. Penzel, T. and Peter, J.H. (1987): The Application of Time Series Analysis to the Diagnosis of Complex Internal Disorders: Sleep Apnea. In: *Sleep-related disorders and internal diseases,* edited by J.H. Peter, T. Podszus and P. von Wichert pp. 100-109. Springer-Verlag, Berlin, New York.

9. Peter, J.H,, Fuchs, E., Hugens, M., Koehler, U., Meinzer, K.,Muller, U., von Wichert, P. and Zahorka, M. (1987): An Apnea Monitoring Device Based on Variation of Heart Rate and Snoring. In: *Sleep-Related Disorders and Internal Diseases,* edited by J.H. Peter, T. Podszus and P. von Wichert, pp.140-146. Springer-Verlag, Berlin, New York.

10. Rechtschaffen, A. and Kales, A. (1968): *A Manual of Standardized Terminology, Techniques and Scoring System for Sleep Stages of Human Subjects.* Brain Information Service/Brain Research Institute, Los Angeles.

Medical Monitoring in the Home and Work Environment,
edited by Laughton E. Miles and Roger J. Broughton.
Raven Press, New York © 1990.

EVALUATING SLEEP APNEA WITH THE PORTABLE

MODIFIED MEDILOG/RESPITRACE SYSTEM

Sonia Ancoli-Israel

Department of Psychiatry
University of California, San Diego
Veterans Administration Medical Center
3350 La Jolla Village Drive
San Diego, California 92161

INTRODUCTION

Sleep apnea is a disorder characterized by complete or partial cessation of respiration during sleep. There are three types of sleep apnea (4,16,24). Obstructive apnea involves partial or complete blockage of air flow due to changes in the anatomy of pharynx and hypopharynx. The obstruction is caused by excessive relaxation of the throat muscles, and is related to an anatomically-small airway. Central sleep apnea is caused by the central nervous system failing to stimulate the diaphragm and intercostal muscles (the muscles of respiration). This can be caused by multiple factors, including neurological disorders, impairment of respiratory feedback regulation, or excessive sedation. Mixed sleep apnea is a combination of central and obstructive sleep apneas.

The diagnosis of sleep apnea is made when there are at least five apneas (complete cessation of respiration) and hypopneas (partial cessation of respiration) per hour of sleep, each lasting a minimum of 10 seconds. This is called the respiratory disturbance index (RDI). Apneic and hypopneic events are usually followed by a brief awakening. Although an RDI$\geq$5 is used as the cut-off for diagnosis, many clinical patients present with more than 70 events per hour of sleep (more than one per minute), each lasting from 10 seconds to over two minutes. Thus since some apnea patients cannot breath and sleep at the same time, it may be life-threatening.

Sleep apnea has many side effects. Blood oxygen saturation levels drop, ventricular irritability develops, and at times asystoles are seen (3,5,6,20). Hypertension (8,18) and loud snoring (9,10,13) are both very common in apnea patients, as are excessive daytime sleepiness (caused by multiple arousals during the night [17,21] and by multiple episodes of hypoxia [15]), nighttime confusion and neuro-psychological impairment (12,25).

Traditionally, patients are brought into a sleep disorders clinic to be recorded for one or more nights with a nocturnal polysomnogram.

Electroencephalography (EEG), electrooculography (EOG), and chin electromyography (EMG) are recorded to determine the different stages of sleep (19). Respiration is recorded by one of many techniques, including strain gauges, or plethysmography. Tibialis EMG is recorded (to distinguish leg jerks) as are the electrocardiogram (ECG) and blood oxygen saturation levels. A technician must watch the patient and the polygraph all night. The result of eight hours of sleep monitoring is approximately a quarter of a mile of paper, which then needs to be scored by the technician. Although the nocturnal polysomnogram is the "gold standard," it is obviously a very expensive and very cumbersome technique.

In the last 15 years, ambulatory monitors have been developed for evaluating sleep disorders, particularly sleep apnea and periodic leg movements in sleep. The first cassette recorders were able to record four channels of information. Recently, these recorders have been expanded to eight channels, allowing recording of many of the same variables recorded in the traditional polysomnogram.

Our laboratory has used the four-channel cassette recorder for over 10 years. We have recorded and evaluated over 1,000 people, both clinically and for research purposes, with a system called the modified Medilog/Respitrace recording system.

MODIFIED MEDILOG/RESPITRACE SYSTEM

The modified Medilog/Respitrace system is shown in Figure 1. Two channels of respiratory plethysmography (Respitrace), one channel of tibialis EMG and one channel of wrist activity are recorded onto a four-channel Medilog cassette recorder. Standard 120-minute cassettes are used, however the extremely slow speed of the tape drive (2 mm/sec) allows over 24 hours of recording time. Once the recording is complete, the tape is played onto a polygraph (at 60x real time) via a special playback unit, and a hard paper copy is obtained and hand-scored.

The techniques for recording respiration and leg jerks are similar to those used for polysomnography. Respiration is recorded with Respitrace(TM) bands (Ambulatory Monitoring, Inc.), which are placed around the thorax and abdomen. These transducer bands respond to inductance changes caused by chest and abdominal expansion (2). Leg jerks are measured by recording tibialis EMG with standard electrodes.

Rather than recording EEG, EOG, and chin EMG to distinguish wake from sleep, however, we record wrist activity. Wrist activity scoring has been shown to correlate highly with EEG scoring for determining wake from sleep (7,14). The wrist actigraph transducer consists of a small weight soldered off-center onto a spring-like wire, the other end of which is clamped against a piezoceramic element. The element is excited whenever the transducer is moved in any direction (7). The transducer is inside a small acrylic box (4.5 x 3.5 x 1.5 cm) which is worn on the wrist with a watchband (see Figure 1). Scoring criteria have been established (11,22,23) for distinguishing wake from sleep with the wrist actigraph. Wake is scored when activity is seen, often accompanied by movement artifact in the other three channels. Sleep is scored when there is no signal in the wrist actigraph and no movement artifact in the respiration or EMG channels. The amount of time scored asleep depends on the previous amount of wake time. For example, after four minutes of wake, the first minute that looks like sleep is still scored as wake; after 10 minutes of wake, the first three minutes that look like sleep are still scored as wake, etc. The wrist actigraph has been compared to traditional EEG (14). On a minute-by-minute basis, there was agreement for 94.5% of the minutes. The correlation between wrist activity and EEG was .98 (p.0001) for total sleep time and .97 (p.0001) for wake time.

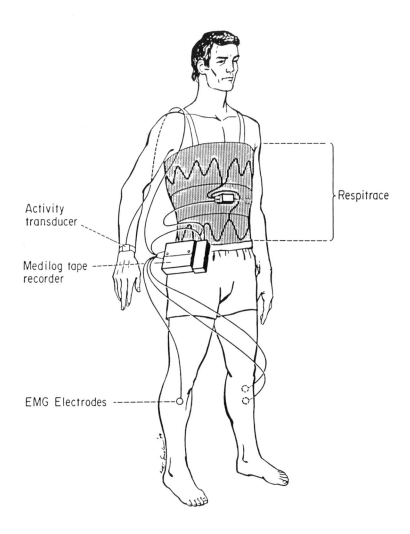

FIG. 1. The modified Medilog/Respitrace system. Reprinted with permission from Mason, et al (1986).

Figures 2-6 show samples of sleep apneas recorded with the modified Medilog/Respitrace system.

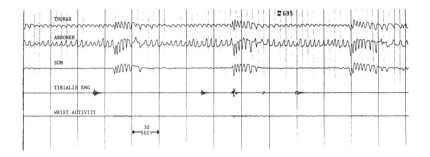

FIG. 2. Obstructive sleep apnea. The thoracic and abdominal channels are 180 degrees out-of-phase and the sum channel is < 10% of baseline.

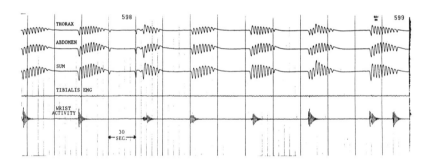

FIG. 3. Central sleep apnea. The thoracic and abdominal channels are flat and the sum channel is < 10% of baseline.

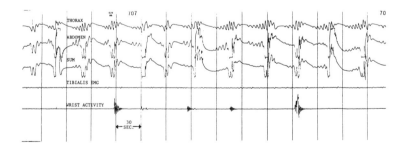

FIG. 4. Mixed sleep apnea. This apnea begins with a central component and is followed by an obstructive component.

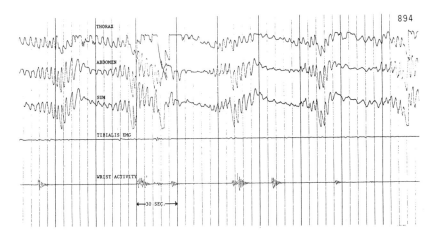

FIG. 5. Obstructive hypopnea. The thoracic and abdominal channels are 180 degrees out-of-phase and the sum channel is <50% but >10% of baseline.

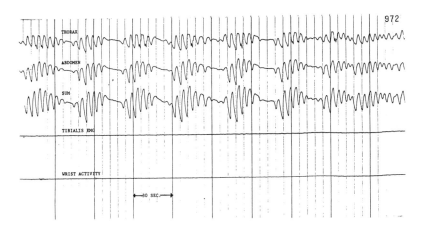

FIG. 6. Central hypopnea. The thoracic, abdominal and sum channels are all in phase and are <50% but >10% of baseline.

Note that in each figure a third channel of respiration, labeled "sum," appears. This is the sum of the thoracic and abdominal channels and is representative of tidal volume. The data of the sum channel are determined electronically by a Respitrace Calibration unit. In obstructive apnea (Figure 2), the thoracic and abdominal channels are 180° out-of-phase, and the sum channel is flat or less than 10% of the baseline respiration. Central apnea (Figure 3) is represented by flat thoracic and abdominal channels and a flat sum channel (or less than 10% of baseline). Mixed apneas (Figure 4) begin with a central component followed by an obstructive component.

Hypopneas can also be identified with the modified Medilog/Respitrace recording system. During an obstructive hypopnea (Figure 5) the thoracic and abdominal channels are 180° out-of-phase, and the sum is between 50-90% of resting. During a central hypopnea (Figure 6), the thoracic, abdominal, and sum channels are in-phase and are between 50-90% of resting.

The reliability of the modified Medilog/Respitrace recording system has been compared to the traditional polysomnogram (1). Subjects with and without sleep apnea were recorded with both techniques on the same night. The resulting reliabilities were: number of apneas, $rs = .80$ $(p < .01)$; number of leg jerks, $rs = .64$ $(p < .005)$; total sleep period, $rs = .82$ $(p < .01)$; total sleep time, $rs = .69$ $(p < .01)$; and wake time, $rs = .61$ $(p < .01)$. The sensitivity of the portable system (i.e., the ability to detect sleep apnea) was 100%, with one false positive. The inter-method agreements were therefore highly significant for the diagnoses of sleep apnea and for sleep parameters. If a portable recording is negative, we feel confident that there is no sleep apnea. A positive result is also likely to be correct but, depending on the severity, a second recording may be indicated.

Advantages of the Portable System

The main advantage includes the capacity to record for 24 hours, allowing the monitoring of patients' nighttime and daytime behavior. For example, with sleep apnea patients who complain of excessive daytime sleepiness, both napping behavior and the presence of apneas during naps can be documented. A second advantage is the possibility of studying patients in their natural environments. Since patients' sleep can be further disrupted by sleeping in a strange laboratory, allowing them to sleep in their own beds provides for a more accurate picture of their characteristic sleep. Using the actigraph instead of additional wires (EEG, EOG, EMG) also makes it comfortable for the patient. The system allows for recording patients in their hospital ward bed, intensive care unit bed, or nursing home bed when it might be difficult to move patients or bring them into the sleep laboratory. Allowing patients this flexibility also increases the compliance rate.

Another advantage is the cost-effectiveness of the portable system. While the price of a clinical polysomnogram can run over $1000, the portable recording is analogous to that of Holter monitoring, i.e., about one-third the cost of the polysomnogram. The reduced cost and increased comfort makes it easier to perform multiple recordings and to do follow-up recordings to evaluate treatment effects.

Disadvantages of the Portable System

The main disadvantage of the system is the restriction of the number of available channels. Now that an eight-channel recorder is available, other measures can be recorded. Since EEG is not recorded with our system, it is not possible to distinguish REM (rapid eye movement) sleep from NREM (non-REM) sleep. Although it is useful to show when apneas occur during REM, the clinical reality is that a diagnosis of sleep apnea and a determination of severity of apnea can be accomplished without sleep stage information.

Another disadvantage of the cassette recorder is that equipment failures are not detected until the record is played back. In our experience, the likelihood of a good recording is increased by using new batteries for each recording, using tape surgerflex material and velcro to hold the equipment in place, and checking all wires with an ohm-meter before sending the patient home (24). If there is still an equipment malfunction, the procedure is easy to repeat. The advantages of the portable system -- convenience and low cost -- still outweigh the disadvantage that a recording may be lost.

CONCLUSION

In summary, the advantages of the convenience and low cost of the Medilog/Respitrace system outweigh the few disadvantages. This portable system has been shown to be reliable as a screening device for sleep apnea.

ACKNOWLEDGEMENTS

Supported by: NIA AGO2711, NIA TNH AGO3990, and the Veterans Administration.

REFERENCES

1. Ancoli-Israel, S., Kripke, D.F., Mason, W. and Messin, S. (1981): Comparisons of Home Sleep Recordings and Polysomnograms in Older Adults with Sleep Disorders. *Sleep*, 4:283-91.

2. Cohn, M., Weisshaut, R., Scott, F. and Slacker, M.A. (1978): A Transducer for Non-Invasive Monitoring of Respiration. In: *International Symposium on Ambulatory Monitoring*, edited by F.D. Scott, E.B. Raftery, P. Sleight and L. Goulding pp. 119-128. Academic Press, London.

3. Guilleminault, C., Eldridge, F.L., Simmons, F.B. and Dement, W.C. (1975): Sleep Apnea Syndrome. Can It Induce Hemodynamic Changes?. *West. J. Med.*, 123:7-16.

4. Guilleminault, C. and Dement, W.C. (1978): *Sleep Apnea Syndromes*, pp. 1-372. Alan R. Liss, Inc., New York.

5. Guilleminault, C., Connolly, S.J. and Winkle, R.A. (1983): Cardiac Arrhythmia and Conduction Disturbances During Sleep in 400 Patients with Sleep Apnea Syndrome. *Am. J. Cardiol.*, 52:490-494.

6. Guilleminault, C., Motta, J., Mihm, F. and Melvin, K. (1986): Obstructive Sleep Apnea and Cardiac Index. *Chest*, 89:331-334.

7. Kripke, D.F., Mullaney, D.J., Messin, S. and Wyborney, V.G. (1978): Wrist Actigraphic Measures of Sleep and Rhythms. *Electroencephalogr. Clin. Neurophysiol.*, 44:674-76.

8. Lavie, P., Ben-Yosef, R. and Rubin, A.E. (1984): Prevalence of Sleep Apnea Syndrome Among Patients with Essential Hypertension. *Am. Heart J.*, 108:373.

9. Lugaresi, E., Coccagna, G. and Cirignotta, F. Snoring and Its Clinical Implications. (1978): In: *Sleep Apnea Syndromes*, edited by C. Guilleminault and W.C. Dement pp. 13-22. Alan R. Liss, Inc., New York.

10. Lugaresi, E. and Coccagna, G. (1980): Hypersomnia with Periodic Apneas. *Z EEG EMG*, 11:167-72.

11. Mason, W.J., Kripke, D.F., Messin, S. and Ancoli-Israel, S. (1986): The Application and Utilization of an Ambulatory Recording System for the Screening of Sleep Disorders. *Am. J. EEG. Technol.*, 26:145-6.

12. Moldofsky, H., Goldstein, R., McNicholas, W.T., Lue, F., Zamel, N. and Phillipson, E. (1983): Disordered Breathing During Sleep and Overnight Intellectual Deterioration in Patients with Pathological Aging. In: *Sleep/Wake Disorders: Natural History, Epidemiology, and Long-Term Evolution*, edited by C. Guilleminault, and E. Lugaresi, pp. 143-150. Raven Press, New York.

13. Mondini, S., Zucconi, M., Cirignotta, F., et al. (1983): Snoring as a Risk Factor for Cardiac and Circulatory Problems: an Epidemiological Study. In: *Sleep/Wake Disorders; Natural History, Epidemiology and Long Term Evolution*, edited by C. Guilleminault and E. Lugaresi pp. 99-106. Raven Press, New York.

14. Mullaney, D.J., Kripke, D.F. and Messin, S. (1980): Wrist-Actigraphic Estimation of Sleep Time. *Sleep*, 3:83-92.

15. Orr, W.C., Martin, R.J., Imes, N.K., Rogers, R.M. and Stahl, M.L. (1979): Hypersomnolent and NonHypersomnolent Patients with Upper Airway Obstruction During Sleep. *Chest*, 75:418-422.

16. Phillipson, E.A. (1978): Control of Breathing During Sleep. *Am. Rev. Respir. Dis.*, 118:909-939

17. Phillipson, E.A., Bowes, G., Sullivan, C.E. and Woolf, G.M. (1980): The Influence of Sleep Fragmentation on Arousal and Ventilatory Responses to Respiratory Stimuli. *Sleep*, 3:281-8.

18. Pollak, C.P., Bradlow, H, G., Spielman, A.J. and Weitzman, E.D. (1979): A Pilot Survey of the Symptoms of Hypersomnia-Sleep Apnea Syndrome as Possible Prediction Factors for Hypertension. *Sleep Res.*, 8:210.

19. Rechtschaffen, A. and Kales, A. (1973): *A Manual of Standardized Terminology, Techniques and Scoring System for Sleep Stages of Human Subjects.* Los Angeles, Brain Information Service. (Third Edition)

20. Romaker, A.M. and Ancoli-Israel, S. (1987): The Diagnosis of Sleep-Related Breathing Disorders. *Clin. Chest Med.*, 8:105-17.

21. Stepanski, E., Lamphere, J., Badia, P., Zorick, F. and Roth, T. (1984): Sleep Fragmentation and Daytime Sleepiness. *Sleep*, 7:18-26.

22. Webster, J.B., Kripke, D.F., Messin, S., Mullaney, D.J. and Wyborney, G. (1982): An Activity-Based Sleep Monitor System for Ambulatory Use. *Sleep*, 5:389-99.

23. Webster, J.B., Messin, S., Mullaney, D.J. and Kripke, D.F. (1982): Transducer Design and Placement for Activity Recording. *Med. Biol. Eng. Comput.*, 20:741-744.

24. Weitzman, E.D., Pollak, C., Borowiecki, B., Burack, B., Shprintzen, R. and Rakoff, S. (1977): The Hypersomnia Sleep-Apnea Syndrome: Site and Mechanism of Upper Airway Obstruction. *Trans. Am. Neurol. Assoc.*, 102:1-3.

25. Yesavage, J., Bliwise, D., Guilleminault, C., Carskadon, M. and Dement, W. (1985): Preliminary Communication: Intellectual Deficit and Sleep-Related Respiratory Disturbance in the Elderly. *Sleep*, 8:30-33.

Medical Monitoring in the Home and Work Environment,
edited by Laughton E. Miles and Roger J. Broughton.
Raven Press, New York © 1990.

THE SOMNOLOG SYSTEM: HOME MONITORING OF SLEEP-EEG, OTHER PHYSIOLOGIC DATA, AND SOUND PRESSURE LEVEL

Gordon Wildschiødtz, Jesper Clausen,
and *Michael Langemark

Sleep Laboratory
Department of Clinical Neurophysiology
Copenhagen County Hospital, 2600 Glostrup
*Department of Neurology and Department of Clinical Neurophysiology,
Copenhagen County University Hospital, 2900 Hellerup, Denmark.

INTRODUCTION

In recent years increasing interest in sleep medicine and the discoveries of well defined sleep disorders have raised an enormous need for sleep recording facilities. Until now sleep recording have mainly been performed in hospital settings, using sleep laboratories and by the classical polygraphic technique with manual visual scoring according to the criteria described by Rechtschaffen and Kales (9) in 1968. Several well known disadvantages of the classical sleep recording clearly restrict their usefulness.

Paper polysomnography is very expensive and time consuming. The recording takes place in a special designed laboratory, where the technical staff has to take care of both the equipment and the patients. The disturbing effect of the first night is more pronounced in the laboratory than in the familiar surroundings in the patients home or stationary ward. If the environment plays a role in the sleep disturbance the recording has to take place "on location" to get a true picture of the disturbed sleep. Home recordings can be applied nearly without limitations, if the recording equipment are cheap and easy to handle for the patients (11).

Data reduction through online pre-analysis makes homesleep recordings even more convenient. Scoring of standard sleep recordings are laborious and neither the interrater nor the intrarater reliability are satisfactory (7). With computerized sleep analyses the results will be identical when repeated; and the resolution of such analysis gives a much better dynamic description of both the EEG, EMG and eye movement data. In the Rechtschaffen and Kales analyses micro events (micro arousals, K-complexes, sleep spindles) are very poorly described.

AMBULATORY MONITORING

Radiotelemetry was the first step towards extrication from the leads of the polygraph. The range of the radiotransmitter is usually around 100 meter and restricts the use to the closest environment of the laboratory (6). Transfer of analog data through the telephone is another possibility; but it is quite expensive and not reliable.

Taperecorders made home monitoring of sleep possible and small tape recorders using standard cartridges has been used. Unfortunately, the low signal to noise ratio of this equipment reduces the signal information, especially a problem in further computerized analyses. The analog replay units have until now not been satisfactory.

Digital storage of the full signal demands a very large memory, but for pre-analyzed data CMOS storage of reasonable size has been used in our first delta analysis system. The filtered delta waves turned a counter on or off and delta time per minute could be calculated (13,14). Eye movements and hand movements were digitized using a voltage controlled oscillator (VCO) controlled by the output voltage from a piezo-electric sensor. Output pulses were counted per minute and stored. EMG was recorded the same way using the rectified EMG as controlvoltage (12,14).

COMPUTERIZED SLEEP ANALYSES

To overcome the shortcomings of the standard sleep recording technique a lot of computerized methods have been applied in sleep research in the last 15 years. Unfortunately, no system has until now gained widespread recognition and no system has eliminated visual analyses completely. The first attempts to perform automatic sleep analysis used analog techniques such as filtering and measurement of the peak to peak amplitude (2).

Digital analysis has in common the first step of analog to digital conversion of the EEG signal and after that either a signal analysis in the frequency domain (Fourier analysis) or the time domain (period amplitude analysis) (3). Finally, several systems have used a combination of analog and digital technique.

GENERAL OVERVIEW OF THE SOMNOLOG[1]

The Somnolog recording unit contains the hardware necessary for user interface with the patient, analysis of sleep EEG and various physiological data, recording of sound pressure level and finally a set up for several types of reaction time measurements (15). The unit is powered by nickel cadmium rechargeable batteries and the operating time in sleep recording mode is more than 20 hours on fully charged batteries. The recording unit is constructed mainly on two printed circuit boards. Signal input comes from various sensors and electrodes connected to an input unit with a 120 cm shielded cable.

---

[1]   SOMNOLOG is a trademark of VENTEC aps, Brønlunds Alle 47, DK 2900 Hellerup, Denmark.

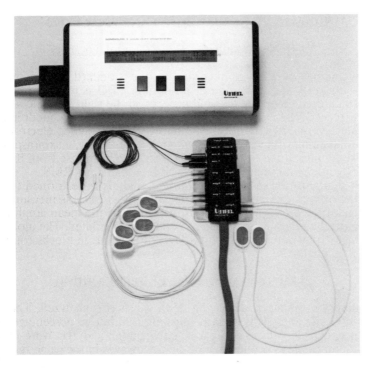

FIG. 1. The Somnolog recording unit with LCD display and 3 buttons for user interface and connecting cable with 7 disposable electrodes and 2 piezo-electric sensors for standard recording.

The signals are led into the amplifier board, a printed circuit board (PCB) with amplifiers for EEG, EMG, ECG and movement sensors. The signals are conducted through amplifiers, the EMG through envelope generators and ECG through an R-wave detector placed on the same PCB. The analog signals are then conducted to a computer print circuit board, where the analog to digital converter is placed together with the Intel 8085 CPU (central processing unit) memory, clock calender, and I/O (input output) unit. A third small board contains the buttons to control the unit and the supertwisted LCD display with 2 lines of 40 characters.

All the boards and connections are arranged in an optimal way so the final size is minimized. It is packed into an aluminum case measuring 270 x 125 x 45 millimeters. The weight is 1300 grams. The investigators' communication with the recording unit takes place through an RS 232 interface. Before the recording starts, the patient's identification has to be loaded into the recording unit; and after the recording the analyzed sleep data has to be transferred to a diskette either directly to the computer or through a modem.

SIGNALS TO BE RECORDED AND ANALYZED

Electroencephalography (EEG), alpha activity

One channel of EEG is recorded in the standard set up, but two channels are available in the unit as an option. EEG is recorded bipolarly between an electrode on the mastoid process on the right side and a frontal electrode placed close to the hairline on the left side (a modified F3). Disposable silver-silver-chloride, self-adhesive and pre-gelled electrodes are used after cleaning with water and soap and, if necessary, a skinrasp. EEG-signals are amplified and filtered with a frequency response from 0.5 to 30 Hz (-3 dB) and the noise of the amplifier is less than 1 uV RMS.

After digitalization a period-amplitude analysis is performed (10). To enable the analysis of wakefulness alpha waves (8-12 Hz) is measured as a percentage of the 6 seconds epoch (alpha-time) and the mean amplitude of the recognized alpha waves in the same epoch is calculated. The alpha-time and average alpha amplitude is stored every 6 seconds in blocks containing data from all channels.

Electroencephalography (EEG), delta activity

To describe the sleep depth the delta waves are analyzed. The same period-amplitude analysis is used to calculate the time in percentage of the 6 seconds epochs in which EEG waves between 0,5 and 2Hz were present. The delta amplitude is the average of the deltawaves in the same time. The signal is recorded, amplified and filtered as described above under alpha activity.

Eye movements (EM)

Detection of eye movements are necessary to determine the stages REM and Wake. In the traditional sleep recording set up, variation in the eye movement generated potentials are measured from electrodes placed at the outer canthi (OEG). Unfortunately these signals can not clearly be separated from EEG activity. In this system a mechanical sensor designed for detection of eye movement artifacts is used (Siemens, Zak), first employed in sleep research to detect REM's by Kayed et al. (4).

The sensor consists of a small (15 x 4 x 2mm) piezo-electric ceramic transducer connected through a thin coaxial cable. The sensor is placed on the upper eyelid on the top of the bulging of the cornea; and eye movements generate a voltage proportional to the bending of the sensor. Both horizontal and vertical eye movements are easily detected and eye blinks give very high signals. The method is more sensitive than the standard EOG recording and, because it is undisturbed from the EEG, it is much more specific and easier to quantify. The activity can be compared to that activity measured using the well-defined calibration procedure. (Fig. 2).

The signal is amplified with a noise level less than 1 microvolt, bandpass filtered within 0,5 and 3 Hz (-3dB) and the activity is again integrated in 6 seconds epochs. The results are stored logarithmically in the memory.

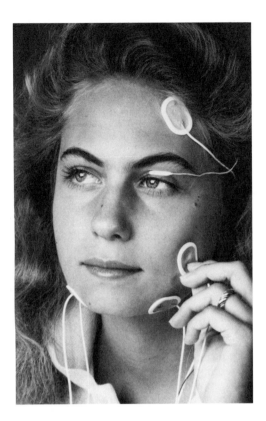

FIG. 2. A normal control subject demonstrates the electrode set up with disposable, pre-gelled, self-adhesive electrodes and piezo-electric eye movement transducer. All the sensors and electrodes can be mounted by normal controls and younger patients.

Hand movements (HM)

The promising results from Kripke et al.(5) and Mullaney et al. (8) that demonstrated a 95% correlation between hand movements and wakefulness were the reason to include this parameter in the sleep analysis system. The very sensitive piezo-electric sensor (identical to the eye movement sensor) is placed dorsally to the proximal joint of the left index finger. The great number of normal arousals are detected and especially pathological movements in sleep, as nocturnal myoclonus or obstructive sleep apnea, are well described and quantified (Fig. 5).

Electromyography (EMG)

Although EMG until now has been poorly quantified in sleep recordings, the relative EMG level is of importance to differentiate between the stages Wake and REM. In addition EMG is valuable in the diagnosis of movement and arousal disorders of sleep as for example obtructive sleep apnea, nocturnal myoclonus and bruxism (Fig. 5)

EMG is measured bipolarly with silver-silver chloride, disposable, self-adhesive, pre-gelled electrodes placed under the base of the mandible (Fig. 2). The signal is amplified and filtered through a band pass filter between 100 Hz and 10KHz with a noise level lower than 5 microvolt. The signal is rectified, enveloped and integrated in 6 seconds epochs and stored logarithmically.

Electrocardiography (ECG)

Two standard disposable electrodes (the same as used for EEG and EMG) are placed at least 15 cm vertically apart over the sternum. The ECG is amplified and bandpass filtered between 10 and 20 Hz and conducted to an analog QRS detector with adaptive threshold and peak detector. The heart rate per minute is calculated and stored every 30 second, which is enough to demonstrate the difference between the stable low level in delta sleep and the faster and fluctuating level in REM sleep. The brady-tachycardia seen in many patients with obstructive sleep apnea is also clearly detected.

Sound pressure level (SPL)

Noise is very important for all sleep recordings. Even in the sleep laboratories the sound insulation is not perfect and the patients can be aroused from exterior noise. When sleep recordings take place in the natural daily settings, recording of the sound is very important to describe the environmental disturbances. Sound emitted from the patient is also measured and is valuable especially in the diagnosis of snoring and obstructive sleep apnea.

The sound is recorded from a standard unidirectional electret microphone. The microphone is usually placed 1 meter above the patient directed against the head. The sound is amplified and filtered with a filter characteristic close to that of the human ear (A-curve). The peak level is detected every 6 second and stored. The sound measurement is very helpful in detection of obstructive sleep apneas (Fig. 5).

DISPLAY AND ANALYSIS OF DATA

When the sleep recording is terminated the somnolog recording unit is connected to a standard PC and data are transferred using the somnolog operating program. Handling of data is menu driven. The transfer of data from the somnolog to a diskette takes a few minutes. To protect data against identification error they can only be stored in the patients own "file area", normally a diskette.

Any files in the patients directory can be selected for further display and analysis. First step is an overview of the total sleep data for the whole night (maximum 10 hours) and histograms of the various data are

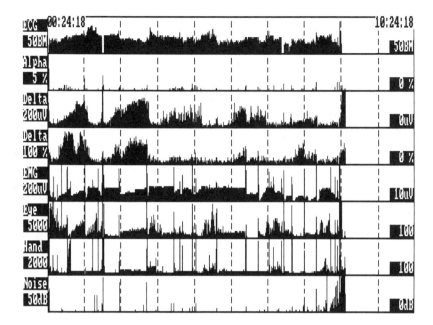

FIG. 3. Compressed overview of 8 hours sleep recording. The signal description is in the left edge of the print together with the window span. At the right edge the baseline level is indicated. In the delta channel 200 microvolts is the span and the display of this channel clearly shows the two first slow-wave sleep periods within the first 3 hours.

automatically calculated and can be shown on the screen for further evaluation. In this way, it is possible to accomplish the best visualization of all data channels by scaling in windows (base line and span) (Fig. 3).

The operating program can show any part of the night in an extended version (zooming in) and one hour is shown on the screen. This mode shows the data in maximal resolution with 600 6 second epochs. The whole night can be reviewed on the screen or printed out on a matrix printer with the same resolution with different colors for different signals.

In the standard version the data displayed are from the bottom noise, hand movement, eye movement, EMG, EEG delta activity time, EEG delta amplitude, EEG alpha time, ECG (Fig. 4). In a special version it is possible to perform sleep staging using a moving cursor. A full sleep scoring approximated to the rules of Rechtschaffen and Kales can be performed, shown on the screen printed out or stored in a special data file. Finally, a report of all the relevant sleep data can be printed out from the data file, and the data files can be placed in any data base program or statistical packages for further analyses of group data or comparison to a normative data base.

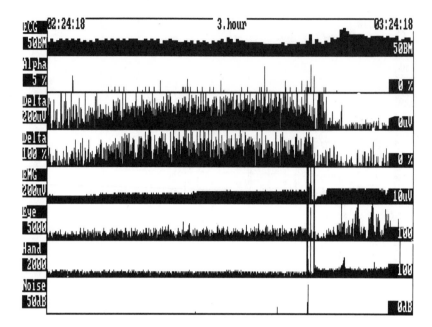

FIG. 4. Extended print of 1 hours sleep recording, in this case the third hour from figure 3. In the first 45 minutes both delta percentage and delta amplitude clearly show the second delta sleep period. In the last 10 minutes high activity in the eye movement channel indicate REM period.

Algorithms for automatic analysis are under development to be used as the first step in the scoring procedure or as the final objective scoring results.

REACTION TIME TEST

Most severe sleep disturbances result in fatigue, sleepiness, and in many cases, impaired daytime performance. Use of hypnotic medication may improve the sleep but worsen the daytime performance.

Performance tests are built into the somnolog unit to enable a day to day control of psychomotor performance. Three different tests are available. The Wilkinson reaction time test provides a simple reaction time to light (LED) or a sound. The signal occurs in random intervals from 1 to 4 seconds. The LCD displays the test number and the reaction time): and both waiting times and reaction times are stored. Up to 100 test signals can be performed per recording session and 24 reaction time sessions can be stored before read out. After transfer of the data to a diskette the somnolog program can calculate means, medians, standard deviations and variation in reaction time according to the number of tests or according to the waiting time.

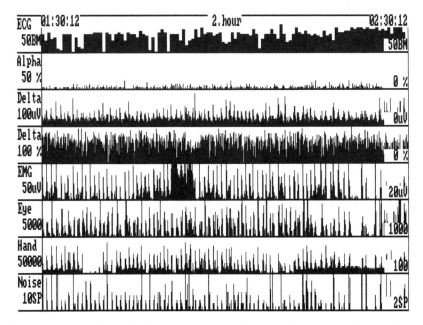

FIG. 5. An overview of 1 hour recording from a patient with obstructive sleep apnea. The arousals terminating the apneic events result in hand movements, eye movements, EMG and delta artifacts, and increasing (snoring) noise measured by the microphone. The heart rate fluctuates widely as a result of the brady-tachycardia.

CONCLUSION

The Somnolog sleep recording system is a totally integrated system for full sleep recording in the home environment or in facilities outside sleep recording centers. The system is portable and the patient can operate the system and apply the electrodes by himself after a brief instruction. The data is easily recovered through a modem or by connecting the Somnolog device directly a computer. The displayed data provides a sleep recording with scoring possibilities close to Rechtschaffen and Kales criteria. The system gives a quantitative and dynamic resolution of alpha and delta activity, and eye movement density. Other physiological data can be monitored simultaneously and sound pressure level appears to be a valuable parameter.

REFERENCES

1. Borbély, A.A. (1986): *Brain Dev.,* 8: 482-488.

2. Hasan, J. (1983): *Acta Physiol. Scand.,* Suppl. 526

3. Hasan, J. (1985): *Ann. Clin. Res.*, 17: 280-287.

4. Kayed, K., Hesla, P.E. and Rosjo, O.(1979): *Sleep*, 2:253-60

5. Kripke, D.F., Mullaney, D.J., Messin, S. and Wyborney, V.G.(1978): *Electroencephalogr. Clin. Neurophysiol.*, 44:674-76

6. Kupfer, D.J. et al. (1972): *Behav. Biol.*, 7:525-590.

7. Monroe, L.J. (1972): *Psychophysiology*, 5:376-384.

8. Mullaney, D.J. et al. (1980): *Sleep*, 3:83-92.

9. Rechtschaffen, A. and Kales, A., editors (1968): *A Manual of Standardized Terminology, Techniques and Scoring System for Sleep Stages of human Subjects.* BIS/UCLA, Los Angeles.

10. Stigsby, B. (1981): *Thesis*, University of Lund

11. Webster, J.B., Kripke, D.F., Messin, S., Mullaney, D.J. and Wyborney, G. (1982): *Sleep*, 5: 389-399.

12. Wildschiødtz, G. (1983): *Sleep Research*, 12:357.

13. Wildschiødtz, G. (1984): *Sleep Research*, 13:216.

14. Wildschiødtz, G. (1984): *Proc.2nd European Symposium on Life Sciences Research in Space.* pp.275-278.

15. Wildschiødtz, G., Vendelbo, L., Langemark, M., Clausen, J. and Taagholdt, S. (1987): *Abstr. 5th International Congress of Sleep research*, Copenhagen: p 770

Medical Monitoring in the Home and Work Environment,
edited by Laughton E. Miles and Roger J. Broughton.
Raven Press, New York © 1990.

PORTABLE MONITORING OF SLEEP-RELATED PENILE TUMESCENCE AND THE EVALUATION OF PENILE ERECTILE IMPAIRMENT

Sabri Derman

Sleep Disorders Center
University of Texas Health Science Center
San Antonio, Texas 78212

INTRODUCTION

During the last 20 years since Karacan (10) and Fisher (5) independently described REM-sleep related cyclic penile erections, much research has been devoted to understanding this phenomenon. Earlier studies, some of them including large patient series (8), suffered from imperfections of recording techniques and incomplete definitions of patient/subject populations. Karacan's ontogeny study (11) published in 1976 has since been widely used as a guideline and normative data in evaluation of Sleep-Related Penile Tumescence (SRPT). After more than twenty-five thousand recording nights in normals of all ages and patients with various disorders, the working assumption now is that penile tumescence monitoring represents an objective, reliable, non-invasive means of differential diagnosis of male erectile impairment. If a person is complaining of erectile dysfunction, but has normal sleep-related erections, his impotence has a high likelihood of being psychogenic. On the other hand, if sleep-related erections are absent or grossly impaired, the problem has an organic or mixed genesis. Some recent studies however, question the specificity and accuracy of sleep-related penile tumescence in the differential diagnosis of erectile impairment since in some patients abnormal circumference changes and rigidity may be associated with depression and might be reversible (15,16). Discussion on the theoretical and practical aspects of SRPT is beyond the scope of this chapter, which will instead briefly review the portable monitoring of it.

A comprehensive way of assessing sleep-related erections is a multi-night polysomnographic study in a sleep laboratory (12). Penile circumference changes at the base and behind the glands of the penis are continuously recorded using mercury-strain gauge transducers, together with EEG, EOG, EMG, ECG, respiration and other physiological parameters. Assessments of the erection episode are made when the penis is at maximal circumference increase. Photographic and/or video recordings are obtained, and both patient and investigator rate the erection on a range of 0 to 100% compared to the subjects best previous erection.

Rigidity measurement is also performed, usually measuring buckling pressure in grams per square centimeter or mmHg. At the end of the recording, both sleep and tumescence data are scored and reduced for clinical interpretation.

Recently, on-line analysis of penile tumescence data with appropriate hardware and computer programs has become available. For example the CASS system from CNS, Inc. (Minneapolis, Minnesota) and CAPS system from Areca Corporation (Palo Alto, California) both allow the investigator to set certain parameters, then automatically score, analyze and print-out data in easily useable clinical reports. Although time saving and comprehensive, these techniques still require technologists or doctors to carefully review the data and reject various artifacts. They do help generate several parameters, provide graphic displays of the data, and correlations with other polysomnographic variables that are otherwise time consuming and often difficult to produce.

Circumference monitoring alone has the short-coming of not accurately predicting penile rigidity. Although rather rare, Pelvic Steal Syndrome and severe sensory deficits of the genitalia can also lead to false positive tumescence interpretations. To enhance the reliability of the tumescence monitoring, rigidity measurements are necessary. This can be done by manually applying a pressure gauge to measure the resistance of the penis to longitudinal buckling, or by using a series of snap-bands to measure different levels of circumferential rigidity (4). Another technique uses a loop placed about the penis. This loop is automatically constricted at intervals in order to measure the radial loading (2); and the device is commercially available under the name of Rigiscan from Dacomed Corporation (Minneapolis, MN). Another system using volummetric pleythysmography as the basis for continuous rigidity assessment has become commercially available from Texas Medical Instruments (Houston, Texas). When combined with a data recorder, it can be used as a portable monitor.

Currently-available portable (or home) penile tumescence assessment equipment can be classified as follows:

1. Devices that detect only the presence or absence of penile rigidity, such as nocturnal penile tumescence stamps (1) and snap-gauges (4).
2. Devices that continuously record only circumference changes, such as Vitalog and MMS LFT 212 monitors.
3. Devices that continuously record both circumference changes and axial rigidity, such as Rigiscan by Dacomed Corporation and SPP-1 Monitor by Texas Medical Instruments.

MMS-LFT-212, from Medical Monitoring Systems Inc. (Teaneck, New Jersey), is a small, ruggedly housed NPT monitor with a microcomputer processor and mini-cassette data recorder, that can record 2 channels of NPT data from mercury strain gauges for about 72 hours. It has an easy to use, excellent calibration feature. Data can be displayed, reproduced on any paper recorder, or dumped to a computer for further analysis. This device has been on the market for several years and has received favorable comments from users.

At the time this review was prepared, the Rigiscan monitor has been used more than any other system. Since its introduction in 1985 (2), there have been several studies investigating Rigiscan's application in the field of erectile dysfunction (3,13,17,9,7), including a methodological review of external computer-based monitoring of penile circumference and rigidity (6). Rigiscan has good computer software, is compact and is easy to use.

Although not on the market at this time, Oxford Medilog Company is reportedly in the process of integrating penile tumescence recordings into their 9000 series portable recorder and data processor, which will enable the user to perform simultaneous polysomnography and sleep related penile tumescence assessment.

More complicated devices provide the user with more detailed information, but it is often more difficult to descriminate artifact and interpret the record.

ADVANTAGES OF PORTABLE (HOME) PENILE TUMESCENCE MONITORING EQUIPMENT.

1. The cost of the study per night is less than hospital based full polysomnographic evaluation. Long-term monitoring is less expensive compared to sleep laboratory studies.
2. The patients' sleep in their home environment may be more typical of their usual sleep, i.e. with less REM fragmentation, fewer awakenings, and longer REM episodes.
3. Since home monitoring for sleep-related penile tumescence uses a limited number of transducers, it is more comfortable for the patient.
4. Results can be obtained more rapidly, speeding up the assessment by the physician.
5. Longer duration recordings (multiple nights) are more feasible.
6. Initial evaluation or screening of erectile impairment can be performed in private settings and smaller hospitals where extensive polysomnographic study facilities are not available.

DISADVANTAGES OF PORTABLE (HOME) PENILE TUMESCENCE MONITORING EQUIPMENT.

1. It fails to assess sleep in general, and REM sleep in particular. The working hypothesis of sleep-related penile tumescence has the prerequisite of fairly normal sleep structure, with particular emphasis of normal REM on percentage and continuity in each REM episodes. Without objective documentation of sleep, reliability of the data is questionable.
2. Portable tumescence monitoring fails to uncover concomittant pathology, e.g. sleep apnea or nocturnal myoclonus (14), which can interfere with the results.
3. The patient can bias the results by tampering with the equipment, thereby jeopardizing the objectivity of the technique (an important feature of sleep-related penile tumescence assessment).

4. Preliminary results indicate that technical reliability of home monitoring is questionable (18). Artifact recognition in borderline cases is difficult, sometimes impossible.
5. Recorders with microprocessors are relatively expensive and fairly fragile, prone to costly repairs and prolonged down time. A problem with the Rigiscan device is that it has no external calibration capabilities and does not have on-line outputs to correlate tumescence and rigidity with other physiological measures.

Portable penile tumescence monitoring equipment is becoming popular for recording erections induced by audio-visual stimulation for research and diagnostic purposes; and for the intracavernous injection of various pharmacologic agents, such as papaverine, phentolamine or prostaglandin E1, for diagnostic and treatment purposes. Although few studies have been done, the current literature suggests that such on-line monitoring may provide for better dose assessment of pharmacological agents (3,17,7), since there is considerable variability in sensitivity to intracavernous injection of these agents from one patient to another.

At present, portable monitors appear to be useful in providing basic information for screening purposes in which accuracy and reliability are not crucial. For research, assessment before various penile surgeries, and cases with medico/legal implications, however, polysomnographic studies under controlled conditions seem to be essential. Portable monitoring can be used for long-term monitoring and follow-up purposes which might be otherwise cost-inefficient and/or undesirable from the patients point of view, if performed in sleep laboratories.

There is the need for well controlled large scale studies involving normals and patients with various types of erectile impairment at laboratory and home monitoring settings. Other improvements would be further miniaturization of monitors, improvement of transducers and cross-correlation with other relevent polysomnographic parameters.

Home monitoring for penile tumescence is promising to become a significant part of the differential diagnostic work-up for erectile dysfunction. Furthermore, sleep-related penile tumescence, like comparable changes in vaginal blood flow, represent the integrated function of the common final pathways of autonomic nervous system. In this context, SRPT can become a valuable test in assessing autonomic nervous system functions both under natural states, such as in sleep, or with audio-visual and/or pharmacological manipulation. Better erectile monitoring devices will certainly contribute to further understanding of this complex phenomenon.

There is no single test procedure which sufficiently differentiates organic from psychogenic erectile dysfunction. Sleep-related tumescence and rigidity measurement provide the most reliable non-invasive measurement technique for initial evaluation as well as for monitoring of treatment in both clinical and research contexts. There is very little discomfort for the patient, and if coordinated with further psychological and physical examinations, SRPT evaluation is a fast, cost-effective and comprehensive way of evaluating erectile impairment. Furthermore, developments in portable monitoring of polysomnographic variables are expected to make sleep- related penile tumescence evaluation easily accessible in areas where fully equipped sleep disorder centers or sexual disfunction clinics are not yet established. As with any new technology and methodology, it is crucial that the physician using SRPT be completely familiar with its capabilities and limitations, and recognize it as part of a comprehensive evaluation.

REFERENCES

1. Barry, J.M., Blank, B., and Boileau, M. (1980): Nocturnal Penile Tumescence Monitoring With Stamps. *Urology*, 15:171-172.

2. Bradley, W.E., Timm, G.W., Gallagher, J.M., Johnson B.K. (1985): New Method for Continuous Measurement of Nocturnal Penile Tumescence and Rigidity. *Urology.*, 26:4-9.

3. Derman, S. and Nadig, P. (1986): Continuous Rigidity and Size Assessment During Sleep-Related and Pharmacologically Induced Tumescence (Abstr). *Proceedings of the Second World Meeting on Impotence*, (3;3), June 17-20, Praha, Czechoslovakia.

4. Ellis, D.J., Dogramji, K., Bagley, D.H. (1988): Snap-Gauge Band Versus Penile Rigidity in Impotence Assessment. *J. Urol.*, 140:60-63.

5. Fisher, C., Gross, J., and Zuch, J. (1965): Cycle of Penile Erections Synchronous with Dreaming (REM) Sleep. *Arch. Gen. Psychiat.*, 12:29-45.

6. Frohrib, D.A., Goldstein, I., Payton, T.R., Padma-Nathan, H., and Krane, J.R. (1987): Characterization of Penile Erectile States Using External Computer-Based Monitoring. *J. Biomechanical Eng.*, 109:110-114.

7. Giesbers, A.A., Bruins, J.L., Kramer, J.L., Jonas, U. (1987): New Methods in the Diagnosis of Impotence: Rigiscan Penile Tumescence and Rigidity Monitoring and Diagnostic Papaverine Hydrochloride Injection. *World J. Urol.*, 5:173-176.

8. Jovanovic, U.J. (1972): *Sexuelle Reaktionen and Schlafperiodik bei Menschen: Ergebnisse Experimenteller Untersuchungen*. Ferdinand Enke Verlag, Stuttgart.

9. Kaneko, S. and Bradley, W.E. (1986): Evaluation of Erectile Dysfunction With Continuous Monitoring of Penile Rigidity, *J. Urol.*, 136:1026-1029.

10. Karacan, I. (1965): The effect of Exciting Presleep Events on Dream Reporting and Penile Erections During Sleep. *Doctoral Dissertation*, New York: State University of New York, Downstate Medical Center.

11. Karacan, I., Salis, P.J., Thornby, J.I. and Williams, R.L. (1976): The Ontogeny of Nocturnal Penile Tumescence. *Waking and Sleeping,* 1:27-44.

12. Karacan, I (1982): Evaluation of Nocturnal Penile Tumescence and Impotence. In: *Sleeping and Waking Disorders-Indications and Techniques,* edited by C. Guilleminault. Addison-Wesley, Menlo Park

13. Kessler, W.O. (1988): Nocturnal Penile Tumescence, *Urol. Clin. North Am.,* 15(1):81-85.

14. Pressman, M.R., DiPhillipo, M.A., Kendrick, J.I., Genrey, K., and Fry, J.M. (1986): Problems in the Interpretation of Nocturnal Penile Tumescence Studies: Disruption of Sleep by Occult Sleep Disorders. *J. Urol.* 136:595-598.

15. Thase, M.E., Reynolds, C.F., Glanz, L.M., Jennings, J.R., Sewitch, D.E., Kupfer, D.J., and Frank, E. (1987): Nocturnal Penile Tumescence in Depressed Men. *Am. J. Psychiat.,* 144(1):89-92.

16. Thase, M.E., Reynolds, C.F., Jennings, J.R., Frank, E., Howell J., Houck, P.R., and Kupfer, D.J. (1987): Diminished Nocturnal Penile Tumescence in Depression. *Sleep Res.,* 16:57.

17. Weinberg, J.J. and Badlani, G.H. (1988): Utility of Rigiscan and Papaverine in Diagnosis of Erectile Impotence. *Urology,* 31:526-529.

18. Wooten, V., and Fields, T.J. (1987): Evaluation of the Dacomed Rigiscan Device. (Abstracted) *Presented to the Southern Sleep Society Meeting,* Feb. 5-7, New Orleans, LA.

Medical Monitoring in the Home and Work Environment,
edited by Laughton E. Miles and Roger J. Broughton.
Raven Press, New York © 1990.

AMBULATORY MONITORING FROM THE
GASTROINTESTINAL TRACT

William C. Orr

Baptist Medical Center of Oklahoma Foundation
3300 Northwest Expressway
Oklahoma City, Oklahoma 73112-4481

INTRODUCTION

The gastrointestinal tract presents formidable problems with regard to physiological monitoring in general, more specifically ambulatory monitoring. In contrast to a number of physiological signals such as respiration and EKG, the smooth muscle of the GI tract is relatively inaccessible and requires a nasal intubation for monitoring. Thus, our knowledge of in vivo studies of gastrointestinal functioning have been somewhat limited. Certainly, ambulatory studies of the GI tract have lagged far behind advances in ambulatory monitoring of the cardiovascular system. The success and subsequent popularity of Holter monitoring has, perhaps more than any other single stimulus, promoted the growth and development of ambulatory monitoring. The increment in knowledge obtained by evaluating the cardiac patient in a natural setting has proven to be of considerable clinical utility. It has seemed apparent from these studies that the standard laboratory evaluation of such patients did not satisfactorily predict cardiac functioning in the patient's natural environment.

Interest in ambulatory monitoring, therefore, has spread particularly to areas of medicine and physiology felt to be especially susceptible to the emotional and physical stress of daily living. Certainly, among the most notable physiological systems felt to be quite sensitive to environmental and physical stress is the gastrointestinal system. For reasons noted above, ambulatory monitoring of important gastrointestinal physiological parameters has been difficult, and therefore our understanding of gastrointestinal physiology and its alteration by the physical and emotional environment remains on a less than solid footing.

Perhaps the most assessible and easily measured gastrointestinal phenomenon would be gastroesophageal reflux via esophageal pH monitoring. A pH probe in the distal esophagus (pH=approximately 6) can detect the reflux of acidic gastric contents (pH approx. 2). By standard convention, any drop in distal esophageal pH to below 4 on pH monitoring is considered an episode of gastroesophageal reflux in the absence of any other obvious stimulus such as acidic food.

Distal esophageal pH monitoring has long been established as a technique for assessing esophageal function. The primary methods were to load the stomach with 300 cc's of acid, and have the patient engage in a variety of provocative maneuvers (i.e. leg elevation, Valsalva maneuver, etc.) in order to provoke the reflux of acid into the distal esophagus. This was felt to be a test of lower esophageal sphincter (LES) competence. The Standard Acid Clearance Test (SACT) was designed to assess the ability of the esophagus to adequately neutralize refluxed acid. This test is also done by placing a pH probe in the distal esophagus and subsequently instilling 15 cc's of 0.1 N.HCl. This would produce a pH drop to below 4, and the patient was instructed to swallow every 30 seconds until the pH was reestablished to 4.0. Esophageal function was considered normal if the pH was reestablished within seven swallows. Both of these tests are provocative tests which assess the functioning of the LES and the body of the esophagus under somewhat contrived and unphysiologic circumstances. Neither actually measures the occurrence and clearance of spontaneous episodes of gastroesophageal reflux (GER).

Prolonged monitoring of the pH of the distal esophagus in order to directly assess the occurrence of episodes of GER has been developed only recently and pioneered by Drs. Lawrence Johnson and Thomas DeMeester (7). Their studies were done in a hospital setting with the patient actually tethered to a recording device. In the last half of the 1970's devices were devised to acquire pH data from the distal esophagus while the patient was ambulant in his/her natural environment. These data were subsequently computer analyzed. The computer analysis revealed the number of reflux episodes, whether the events occurred in the upright or supine position, the actual percent of acid exposure time (that is the percent of time the esophageal pH was below 4), and the number of episodes exceeding 5 minutes in duration. A number of units are now commercially available which provide essentially similar information.

RECORDING AND ANALYSIS TECHNIQUES

All of the commercially available units for recording ambulatory esophageal pH signals use essentially similar techniques of data acquisition and analysis. The pH probe itself is placed trans-nasally into the distal esophagus. This placement is generally 5 centimeters above the manometrically determined LES; or alternatively it can be withdrawn from the stomach (with an acidic pH of less than 3) to the level of the esophagus at which the pH becomes 4 or above. In general, when this occurs the probe is withdrawn another 3 to 5 centimeters. Either technique ensures a distal esophageal placement 3 to 5 centimeters above the LES. There are a variety of pH probes available ranging from glass-tipped to antimony and antimony crystal. Technical advantages and disadvantages of each of these probes is beyond the scope of this paper. The esophageal pH is generally sampled several times per second and the result stored in a small unit which is generally worn around the waist or carried with a shoulder strap.

Patients are given instructions concerning diet (if the patient is to follow a specified diet to avoid foods with an acidic pH), and the specific technique for indicating the presence of heart-burn, chest pain, regurgitation, or dysphagia. In addition, the patient indicates on a log all meal times, sleep times, and any other unusual events. The 24 hours after the initiation of the study, the patient returns to the laboratory and is extubated. Subsequently, the data are downloaded onto a computer for data analysis. Data analysis periods are divided into three segments, i.e. total 24 hour interval, upright interval (primarily awake time), and supine interval (predominately sleeping). The number of reflux episodes occurring during each interval, and the percent acid exposure time (time the pH is less than 4) are computed for each interval. In addition, the number of episodes exceeding 5 minutes in duration, and the episodes with the longest duration are also noted for each analysis segment. The actual data printout can be accomplished for the entire 24 hour segment, or nearly any desirable subsegment such as every hour, every three hours, etc. Symptoms, mealtimes, and sleeping intervals are all identified in the computer output.

PATTERNS OF GASTROESOPHAGEAL REFLUX

Ambulatory pH studies of the esophagus has allowed an understanding of the phenomenon of gastroesophageal reflux (GER) and gastroesophageal reflux disease (GERD) which would have otherwise been quite unobtainable. For example, the phenomenon of GER is now known to be quite common particularly post-prandially. That is most individuals have a tendency to belch after meals and experience short episodes of GER. These are usually asymptomatic, but the average individual will experience occasional heartburn in association with these reflux events. Ambulatory studies in normal individuals has also revealed the general absence of GER during sleep (2). Thus, it would appear that normality and abnormality are defined not so much on the occurrence of GER, but when it occurs (i.e. sleeping vs. waking).

That is not to say, however, that abnormal waking reflux does not exist. Studies by Johnson and colleagues have shown a close relationship between the pattern of GER, and the severity of endoscopic distal esophageal changes (8). These investigators found that individuals identified with predominately waking reflux had minimal changes in the distal esophagus. Those who were identified as predominately sleep refluxers (with minimal reflux during the day) had somewhat more severe changes in the distal esophageal mucosa, and those with both upright and supine reflux (termed combined refluxers), had the greatest incidence of mild, moderate, and severe alterations in the distal esophagus. This is a landmark study in conceptualizing the importance of identifying the specific pattern and time of GER events, and specifically relating these to the severity of esophageal mucosal damage.

Ambulatory studies, as well as studies from our sleep laboratory, have documented that acid clearance during sleep is markedly prolonged when compared with the waking state (7,9,10). Although, as alluded to above, sleep related episodes of GER are relatively uncommon in normals, their presence and the associated prolongation of acid clearance is felt to play a major role in the development of the more severe complications of GERD (8,11).

Unmasking these fundamental differences in the incidence and clearance of episodes of gastroesophageal reflux during different states of consciousness has lead to a more global understanding of GERD and its associated clinical complaints and complications.

CLINICAL APPLICATIONS

The clinical utilization of 24 hour ambulatory esophageal pH recording is increasing rapidly, and indications for its use appear to be expanding (4). As the clinical use of this test is in a state of evolution, precise indications have not been developed. However, most gastroenterologists and sophisticated users of this technique would prbably agree to the following indications for 24 hour esophageal pH monitoring: refractory heartburn; atypical chest pain; recurrent nocturnal cough/wheezing; and suspected pulmonary aspiration (recurrent pneumonia). In a recent study by DeMeester and colleagues (3), 27% of 179 patients with typical symptoms of heartburn had a normal pH study. On the other hand, 54% of 146 patients with normal endoscopy exhibited an abnormal ambulatory pH study. Of 18 patients with respiratory symptoms, 61% had an abnormal ambulatory pH evaluation. This study eloquently addresses the extreme complexity of esophageal disease in terms of the relative inability to predict esophageal disease on the basis of the presence or absence of symptoms. Again, this argues very strongly in favor of acquiring these ambulatory data since a knowledge of the presence or absence of clinically significant GER would certainly weigh more heavily in a treatment decision irrespective of the presence or absence of symptoms. Similarly, in a study of a group of 53 patients with normal endoscopy and symptoms of either reflux, atypical chest pain or respiratory problems, 47% were shown by ambulatory 24 hour pH monitoring to have abnormal GER (4). Thus, although certainly not indicated in patients with routine heartburn, the utilization of ambulatory 24 hour pH monitoring would seem to have applications in a wide variety of symptoms related to the many manifestations of GER.

The extra-esophageal complications of GER are becoming increasingly well documented. For example, it is now well established that GER can exacerbate bronchial asthma, and contribute to the development of laryngopharyngitis and symptoms of chronic nocturnal cough; and it is felt to be a major pathogenetic agent in recurrent pulmonary aspiration and/or chronic pulmonary fibrosis (1,5,11,15). The identification of nocturnal GER and the concomitant association of asthma attacks can lead to a more focused treatment approach (5).

Ambulatory 24 hour esophageal monitoring studies have played a major role in delineating the role of GER in these seemingly unrelated medical conditions. For example, in asthmatic patients it has been documented that distal esophageal acid contact will produce a reflex bronchoconstriction which would be capable of triggering an asthmatic attack (14). Other studies have documented the presence of nocturnal GER particularly in patients with asthmatic patients who demonstrate nocturnal wheezing (12). Thus, the identification of daytime, but particularly nocturnal GER in asthmatic patients can, in many instances, significantly enhance the understanding of the etiology of the asthmatic attacks and thereby develop a more focused treatment regimen.

This technique allows not only the assessment of the degree of distal acid exposure, but also the relationship between symptom production and

GER. Clearly, there are situations in which a normal degree of reflux can cause symptoms; or, conversely, an abnormal degree of acid exposure time may not be associated with particularly impressive symptoms. Ambulatory data which provides information concerning the actual physiological event (in this case reflux) and its specific relationship to symptoms (i.e. heartburn, regurgitation, or chest pain), allows the clinician to focus more precisely within the treatment regimen. For example, if daytime reflux and heartburn are the predominant problem, and the patient is without nocturnal GER, the treatment can be focused exclusively in the daytime. On the other hand, if nocturnal reflux can be identified, with or without symptoms, it would be prudent for the clinician to treat the patient throughout the 24 hour day. This type of assessment can only be accomplished via the simultaneous assessment of symptoms plus GER by ambulatory recording.

The pulmonary aspiration of gastric contents is a well known, but relatively rare, phenomenon. Clinically, it is suspected in a setting of recurrent pneumonia, unexplained pulmonary fibrosis, or chronic nocturnal cough. Obviously, for this to occur gastric contents must migrate from the distal esophagus to the proximal esophagus and spill over into the tracheo-bronchial tree. If pH monitoring were occurring under such circumstances, it would obviously be associated with a markedly prolonged episode of GER. The relatively rare incidence of actual aspiration dictates that the assessment of the role of GER in the particular symptoms under investigation would be presumptive.

Ambulatory pH monitoring can be particularly helpful in that it can identify fairly frequent episodes of prolonged GER during sleep, or perhaps even associate this with symptoms of chronic cough and choking. The index of suspicion then would be increased in terms of associating GER with the particular pathologic entity of interest. Here again, the clinician must make a judgment as to the likelihood that the events noted on ambulatory pH monitoring are specifically related to the symptom complex under investigation. Thus, as with any other diagnostic tool, it is ultimately the judgment of the clinician which is paramount. However, the availability of ambulatory pH monitoring certainly gives the thoughtful clinician much additional information which would otherwise be unavailable.

AMBULATORY ESOPHAGEAL MOTILITY RECORDING

Disorders of esophageal motility, to include esophageal spasm, and extremely high amplitude peristaltic contractions (commonly referred to as the "nutcracker" esophagus), are thought to produce symptoms of chest pain mimicking those of classical angina or disecting aortic aneurysm. Since these episodes of non-cardiac chest pain are episodic, the documentation of an esophageal motor disorder via a laboratory study, or the documentation of the motor disorder in the presence of the production of a typical symptom is rare in laboratory evaluations with such patients. In order to determine that the patient's chest pain is indeed attributable to some esophageal motor disorder, an ambulatory study which allows continuous monitoring of motor function and symptoms is mandatory.

Esophageal probes allowing continuous ambulatory monitoring of esophageal motor function are commercially available. Although these studies have been utilized in various research studies on patients with non-cardiac chest pain, their routine clinical utility has yet to be effectively demonstrated. In fact, in virtually every study, the majority of patients with non-cardiac chest pain in whom an esophageal disorder is documented have GER as the primary pathologic entity (6,13).

SUMMARY

In summary, then, it would appear that in terms of ambulatory monitoring from the gastrointestinal system, certainly ambulatory esophageal pH monitoring has the greatest promise in terms of its application to the evaluation of patients with the common symptoms of heartburn and chest pain.

REFERENCES

1. Allen, C.J. and Newhouse, M.T. (1984): Gastroesophageal Reflux and Chronic Respiratory Disease. *Am. Rev. Respir. Dis.*, 129:645-647.

2. DeMeester, T.R., Johnson, L.F. and Guy, J.J., et al. (1976): Patterns of Gastroesophageal Reflux in Health and Disease. *Annals of Surgery*, 184:459-470.

3. DeMeester, T.R., Wang, C.T. and Werny, J.A., et al. (1980): Techniques, Indications, and Clinical Use of 24 Hour Esophageal pH Monitoring. *J. Thorac. Cardiovasc. Surg.*, 79(5):656-670.

4. Donald, I.P., Ford, G.A. and Wilkinson, SP: Is 24hr Ambulatory Oesophageal pH Monitoring Useful in a District General Hospital? *Lancet*, Vol. 1:89-91.

5. Harper, P.C., Bergner, A. and Kaye, M.D. (1987): Antireflux Treatment for Asthma: Improvement in Patients with Associated Gastroesophageal Reflux. *Arch. Intern. Med.*, 147:56-60.

6. Janssens, J., Vantrappen, G. and Ghillebert, A. (1986): 24 Hour Recording of Esophageal Pressure and pH in Patients with Non-Cardiac Chest Pain. *Gastroenterology*, 90:1978-1984.

7. Johnson, L.F. and DeMeester, T.R. (1974): Twenty-Four Hour pH Monitoring of the Distal Esophagus. *Am. J. Gastroenterol*, 62:325-332.

8. Johnson, L.F., DeMeester, T.R. and Haggitt, R.C. (1978): Esophageal Epithelial Response to Gastroesophageal Reflux, a Quantitative Study. *Am. J. Dig. Dis.*, 23:498-509.

9. Orr, W.C., Robinson, M.G. and Johnson, L.F. (1981): Acid Clearing During Sleep in the Pathogenesis of Reflux Esophagitis. *Dig. Dis. Sci.*, 26(5):423.

10. Orr, W.C., Johnson, L.F. and Robinson, M.G. (1984): The Effect of Sleep on Swallowing, Esophageal Peristalsis, and Acid Clearance. *Gastroenterology*, 86:110-119.

11. Pelligrini, C.A., DeMeester, T.R., Johnson, L.F. and Skinner, D.B. (1979): Gastroesophageal Reflux and Pulmonary Aspiration: Incidence, Functional Abnormality, and Results of Surgical Therapy. *Surgery*, 86:110-119.

12. Perrin-Foyalle, M., Bell, A. and Kofman, J., et al. (1980): Asthma and Gastroesophageal Reflux. Results of a Survey of Over 250 Cases. *Poumon Couer*, 36:225-230.

13. Peters, L.J., Maas, L.C. and Dalton, D.B. et al. (1988): Spontaneous Non-Cardiac Chest Pain: Evaluation by 24 Hour Ambulatory Esophageal Motility and pH Monitoring. *Gastroenterology*, 94:878-886.

14. Spaulding, H.S., Mansfield, L.E. and Stein, M.R., et al. (1982) Further Investigation of the Association Between Gastroesophageal Reflux and Bronchoconstriction. *J. Allergy Clin. Immunol.*, 69:516-521.

15. Wiener, G.J., Koufman, J.A. and Wu, W.C., et al. (1987): The Pharyngo-Esophageal Dual Ambulatory pH Probe for Evaluation of Atypical Manifestations of Gastroesophageal Reflux (GER). *Gastroenterology*, 92(5):1694.

Medical Monitoring in the Home and Work Environment,
edited by Laughton E. Miles and Roger J. Broughton.
Raven Press, New York © 1990.

CARDIORESPIRATORY MONITORING OF INFANTS IN THE HOME ENVIRONMENT

Dorothy H. Kelly

Pediatric Pulmonary Laboratory
Massachusetts General Hospital
Boston, Massachusetts 02114

INTRODUCTION

For more than a decade, infants have been treated at home with cardiorespiratory monitors which alert the parents to apnea or bradycardia that their baby may be experiencing. In this chapter, I will discuss the types of equipment currently used and review the criteria for determining which infants should be monitored at home. I will also review the outcome of this treatment modality.

EQUIPMENT

Monitors

During the last decade various home monitors have been made available to physicians. There are three basic types: a)impedance, b)mattress, and c)acoustic.

The *impedance monitor* has been used most extensively for infant monitoring. There are many different impedance monitors, but all follow the same principle of measuring the change of impedance across the thorax to determine when a breath has occurred. The monitor is programmed so that, if a breath does not occur within a certain number of seconds, it will alarm. The settings for this alarm range from 10, 15, 20 to 25 sec. delays. In addition to monitoring changes in thoracic air volume by impedance, they generally monitor the heart rate by routine electrocardiography. The *mattress monitor* has been used infrequently in this country. These devices monitor movement of the infant. When the infant is asleep, the major movement that is sensed by these monitors is that of respiration. These monitors have no contact with the infants skin and they generally do not monitor the heart rate. *Acoustic monitors* use a microphone to detect air entry. These are currently being developed.

Recording Devices

There are several means of recording physiologic data in infants who are being monitored. The recording can be done in the home or hospital for short or long period. One long-term method appropriate for the hospital or home is the 12 hour pneumogram (8). Respiration and heart rate are recorded onto a magnetic tape cassette with a small, slow speed recorder. If desired, oxygen saturation can also be recorded. The magnetic tape is played through a replay unit to generate a hard copy and through a computer for analysis of the physiologic signals. The hard copy can be analyzed and interpreted by physicians. Short-term recordings can be done at home and in the hospital. Polygraphic recordings may last 4-12 hours. Since a polygraph has multiple channels, many physiologic signals can be recorded simultaneously to determine if there are any abnormalities, and if they are influencing physiologic events in other channels could result in an abnormality in the respiratory channel such as central or obstructive apnea. The respiratory abnormalities could lead to an abnormality in the O2 saturation channel reflecting desaturation (Fig. 1).

A second type of short-term recording is the event recording. This is done by attaching the event recorder to the monitor. The recorder is activated

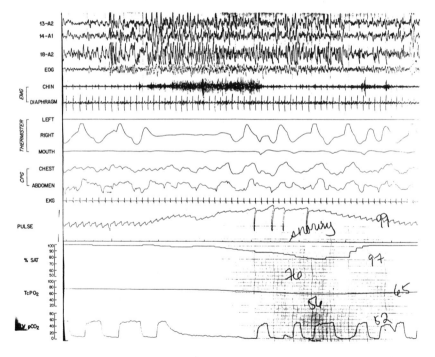

FIG. 1. Polygraph tracing demonstrating initial seizure discharge in EEG leads followed by obstructive apnea (chest and abdominal movement with no air flow) which is then followed by oxygen desaturation to 76 mmHg.

by the monitor alarm to record the current physiologic signals onto paper, magnetic tape or diskette. The record then remains available for analysis and interpretation of the physiologic changes occurring at the time of the monitor alarm. This type of recording is helpful to determine if the monitor alarms are due to physiologic or mechanical problems, that is, "true" or "false" alarms respectively. A pneumogram can provide similar information.

Thus, at present there is a moderate amount of equipment available to assist the physician in monitoring infants in the home environment and for initially evaluating infants in the hospital.

Any physician who is treating infants with home monitors must be fully aware of the specifications of the equipment that s/he uses so that s/he understands its limitations and the normal functioning.

S/he should be able to prescribe the specific piece of equipment that will safely aid in the care of the patient. In addition, if physiologic recordings are used, s/he must also acquire the specific skills necessary to interpret the recording so that s/he will be able to use them in the treatment of these patients.

WHOM TO MONITOR

In 1986 the National Institutes of Health convened a panel to review the available data on infant monitoring evaluating which infants should be monitored and the outcome of those infants who were and were not monitored. The consensus panel published a statement (5) which recommended that all infants who have had an unexplained apneic event should be monitored. In addition, they recommend that infants who are subsequent siblings of a Sudden Infant Death Syndrome (SIDS) infant, should be considered for monitoring, if they have symptoms of apnea or bradycardia or if the parents and physicians together decide that they wish to monitor the infant. In addition we will monitor at home preterm infants who are ready for discharge but continue to have apnea and/or bradycardia despite treatment with theophyllin.

For sixteen years we have evaluated and managed infants who have had an event that was frightening to the parents and of concern to their physician. These infants are evaluated by a thorough history of the event from all observers such as the caretaker, neighbors, relatives, emergency medical technicians and emergency room personnel. This includes information of the event, the intervention that is used to terminate the event, and the abnormalities in the infant which continue following resumption of breathing (Fig. 2).

The remaining evaluation consists of a thorough history, physical examination and laboratory tests appropriate for the event. In general, laboratory tests that will be performed are a complete blood count, urinalysis, serum electrolytes, calcium, blood sugar, electrocardiogram, chest x-ray, electroencephalogram, barium swallow, pneumogram, and polygraph recording. In addition, a 24 hour pH probe recording the pH in the esophagus is obtained, if the history is consistent with gastroesophageal reflux.

Name _____

HISTORY OF EVENT (leading to evaluation): Please circle features and complete as needed.

Date: _____ ; Age: _____ ; # hours after feed: _____

Last Immunization (specify date / type): _____ ; Medications; _____

Recent illness: _____

OBSERVER	LOCATION	INFANT POSITION	STATE	COLOR	COLOR CHANGE
Parent	Holding infant	Prone	Asleep	Cyanotic	Entire body
MD	Same room	Supine	Awake	Grey	Extremities
RN	Audible distance	Upright	Drowsy	Pale	Face
Other _____	In car	Infant seat	Feeding	Red	Perioral
	Other _____	Other _____	Other _____	Purple	Lips
				Normal	Other _____

BREATHING	TONE	EYES	NOISE	FLUID	HEART RATE
No effort	Limp	Closed	Cough	Milk	Bradycardia @ ___bpm
Shallow	Stiff	Dazed	Choke	Vomitus	Tachycardia @ ___bpm
Struggling	Tonic/clonic	Scared	Stridor	Mucus	Normal
Rapid	Normal	Rolled	Gasp	Blood	Unknown
Normal	Other _____	Staring	Cry	None	
Other _____		Normal	None	Other _____	
		Other _____	Other _____		

STIMULATION	DURATION OF EVENT:	ABNORMALITIES FOLLOWING EVENT
None	_____ sec / min	Abnormal breathing x _____ min / hrs
Gentle		Color change x _____ min / hrs
Vigorous		Behavior _____
MTM: # breaths _____		None
CPR: # cycles _____		

EMT/ER Observations:

FIG. 2. History form used to obtain details of the apneic event from all observers.

If the history or physical examination were consistent with upper airway obstruction, a sleep airway fluroscopy and possibly a bronschoscopy would be done. Other studies such as septic workup are obtained if indicated (3).

Based on this assessment, we would recommend monitoring all infants who had an unexplained episode of apnea while awake or asleep that was terminated by resuscitation or vigorous stimulation. Monitoring is recommended in infants who had apnea which resolved with gentle stimulation, if there are physiologic abnormalities on the pneumogram or polygraph. Also, any infant who has a family history of apnea and/or SIDS and an unexplained episode of apnea is monitored. Based on the above evaluation, in our program we have monitored 11% of 13,401 infants referred to us. An additional 24% were treated with theophylline and 34% were treated for identified abnormalities. In the remainder, monitoring was not recommended since no abnormality was found and the history was not consistent with significant event (4).

HOW TO INSTITUTE MONITORING

When one decides to monitor an infant at home, the home care dealer usually supplies the equipment. The parents must be thoroughly instructed in the use of the equipment. The teaching can be done by nurses who work with the physician in their home monitoring program or with the dealer. The physician must be assured that the parents understand the use of all equipment so that they will be able to: a)interpret if the alarms are real or due to equipment problems such as lead misplacement and b)troubleshoot in case of equipment alarms. Parents must also be taught: a)the observations that should be made of both the infant and the equipment at the time of each alarm, and b)how to intervene appropriately for the alarm. If the alarm is an equipment alarm, they must make the small adjustments necessary to terminate the alarm and allow the equipment to function correctly. If the alarm is a true patient alarm, they must determine the type of intervention necessary. If there is a color change, they should stimulate immediately: but, if the infant has no color change, they may wait ten seconds from the onset of the alarm before beginning intervention. If the alarm persists, they should first place a hand on the infant's back and gently shake the infant. If this is not adequate to restore normal heart rate and/or normal breathing, they should pick the infant up, supporting his head carefully, and vigorously stimulate him in an attempt to establish respirations or normalize the heart rate. Finally, if these interventions fail, they should institute mouth-to-mouth resuscitation and proceed to full cardiopulmonary resuscitation (CPR), if necessary. These types of intervention including infant CPR should be taught to the parents. The parents must be able to demonstrate the proper use of these techniques prior to discharge. This material should be reviewed again during the first few weeks after discharge for better retention.

The teaching program is extremely important. No equipment should be placed into the home unless the caretakers have been instructed in its use. If proper teaching is not done, there is a large amount of anxiety at the time of discharge and during the weeks at home. The stress that the parents experience is significant and may impact on their family life as well as on their ability to care for their infant and use the equipment. Teaching and support can minimize this anxiety (1,2).

OUTCOME OF MONITORING

Infants monitored through the program at Massachusetts General Hospital have been categorized based on the characteristics of their presenting episode (awake or asleep) and the intervention used (mouth-to mouth resuscitation, vigorous stimulation, gentle or no stimulation). Using these characteristics, all infants who presented with a sleep onset apnea that resolved with only mouth-to-mouth resuscitation were reviewed. During the course of monitoring, 13.2% died and 33% of these infants had subsequent severe events at home, defined as a sleep onset apnea which resolved with either vigorous stimulation or resuscitation and (6). Those infants that presented with sleep onset apnea which was terminated with vigorous stimulation had a low mortality rate (0.8%), but 33% did have at least one subsequent severe event. None of the infants that presented sleep onset apnea with gentle or no stimulation died, but 19% did have significant severe events. Awake onset apnea was divided similarly into three groups depending on the intervention used to terminate the episode: a)resuscitation; b)vigorous stimulation; c)gentle or no stimulation. Thirty-three percent of Groups 1 and 2 babies did have subsequent severe apnea during sleep, whereas only 2.5% of Group 3 had a subsequent severe event. In our program no deaths have occurred among those infants who were monitored because they presented with an awake onset episode of apnea.

Reviewing the circumstances of death in all infants that died during monitoring in our program, we found that 72% of the deaths occurred when there was a breakdown in the system of monitoring, usually parental delay in responding to the alarm. The remainder (28%) died when all reportedly was performed correctly. Thus the majority of deaths during monitoring may be preventable. Based on this, in our teaching program we strongly emphasize the necessity of responding to alarms quickly and adequately. Hopefully, this will decrease the mortality rate especially in the high risk group of babies.

Finally, we also monitor some infants with a family history of SIDS. Any sibling of a SIDS infant who is having unexplained apnea or bradycardia is monitored. Any sibling of a SIDS infant who has unexplained prolonged apnea. bradycardia, increased periodic breathing or hypercarbia on recording, or who has two or more siblings who have died of SIDS (mortality 18% in our program (7)) will also be monitored. We monitor siblings of SIDS infants whose parents request monitoring because of anxiety. Complete teaching of all caretakers about equipment and methods of observation and intervention including infant CPR is essential so that the anxiety present in these parents, who have already suffered the death of one child, will be somewhat diminished.

SUMMARY

Home monitoring is available in our country for: a)infants who have had an inexplicable life threatening event, and b)infants whose sibling has died of SIDS. One may use one of several types of monitors, but the home monitor in general usage in this country is the cardiorespiratory impedance monitor. If monitoring is to be undertaken, it must be done with the knowledge that the physician and the parents are a team. All team members must understand the normal functioning of the devices that will be used and the methods of observation and intervention. With proper teaching and support during monitoring, several studies have shown a decrease in anxiety during the course of monitoring (1,2). Without proper teaching or support it is our experience that monitoring has been extremely stressful.

The outcome of infants who are monitored generally is excellent except for three groups of high risk babies: a)infants who have had a sleep onset episode of apnea requiring resuscitation and during the course of monitoring had a repeat severe apneic event, b)siblings of SIDS who have a sleep onset apnea requiring resuscitation, and c)infants who have had two or more previous siblings die of SIDS. The mortality rates of these groups of infants in our program are 28%, 25% and 18%, respectively. In reviewing the circumstances surrounding these deaths, we have found that deaths (72%) occurred when there was not complete compliance with the method of monitoring, usually involving a delay in initiating intervention for the infant. In the remaining infants (28%) the caretaker response to the alarm and method of intervention reportedly was correct.

We recommend that parents be told that their infants are at high risk and that it is extremely important that they monitor them correctly. For those parents who feel that they are unable to assume this responsibility, long-term hospitalization should be offered for infants in the high risk groups. More research is needed to identify the causes of these unexplained deaths and to decrease the mortality rates.

REFERENCES

1. Black, L., Hersher, L. and Steinschneider, A.L. (1978): Impact of the Apnea Monitor on Family Life. *Pediatrics,* 62:681-685.

2. Deykin, E., et al. (1984): Apnea of Infancy and Subsequent Neurologic, Cognitive, and Behavioral Status. *Pediatrics,* 73:638-645.

3. Kelly, D.H. (1988): In: *Ambulatory Pediatric Care: Apnea of Infancy,* edited by R. Dershewitz. pp. 843-847. J.B. Lippincott Company, Philadelphia, PA.

4. Kelly, D.H. (1988): In: *Sudden Infant Death Syndrome Cardiac and Respiratory Mechanisms and Intervention: Home Monitoring For The Sudden Infant Death Syndrome: The Case For,* edited by P.J. Schwartz, D.P. Southall, and M. Valdes-Dapena pp. 158-163. New York Academy of Sciences, New York.

5. National Institutes of Health Consensus Development Conference on Infantile Apnea and Home Monitoring, Sept. 29 to Oct. 1, 1986: Consensus statement. *Pediatrics,* 1987; 79:292-299.

6. Oren, J., Kelly, D.H. and Shannon, D.C. (1986): Identification of a High Risk Group for SIDS Among Infants Who Were Resuscitated for Sleep Apnea. *Pediatrics,* 77:495-499.

7. Oren, J., Kelly, D.H. and Shannon, D.C. (1987): Familial Occurrence of Sudden Infant Death Syndrome and Apnea of Infancy. *Pediatrics,* 80:355-358.

8. Stein, I.M. and Shannon, D.C. (1975): The Pediatric Pneumogram: A New Method for Detecting and Quantitating Apnea in Infants. *Pediatrics,* 55:599.

Medical Monitoring in the Home and Work Environment,
edited by Laughton E. Miles and Roger J. Broughton.
Raven Press, New York © 1990.

LIFELINE AND OTHER PERSONAL EMERGENCY RESPONSE SYSTEMS

Cynthia Pearson, Marymae Seward, and Margaret Gatz

Psychology Department
University of Southern California
Los Angeles, California   90089-1061

INTRODUCTION

The number of older adults in the population is rapidly expanding. In 1986, 12.1% of the U.S. population were 65 and older. The fastest growing segment of all are those aged 85 and older (2). Chronic illnesses and debilitating conditions are frequent among elders (heart disease, hypertension, arthritis, respiratory problems, impaired mobility).

While many older adults require institutional long term care--5% of those aged 65 to 74, 10% of those aged 75 to 84, and 20% of those aged 85 and older (3)--others remain living in the community. Of those aged 65 and older living in the community, about 30% live alone. This group is at especially high risk of needing long term care or institutionalization in case of physical health difficulties.

Thus, a big concern for older adults and for their relatives is availability of immediate medical assistance, even at times when the older person is not able to place a telephone call. It is this need that constitutes the primary rationale for personal emergency response systems (PERS).

Personal emergency response systems are designed to signal when help is needed. The elements of a PERS include a transmitter (portable help button or emergency "trigger") and a unit connected to the user's telephone. The unit contains an automatic dialing machine that sends an electronic message whenever the button is pressed. The largest manufacturer, and the prototype for the service concept, is Lifeline Systems of Watertown, Massachusetts.

DESCRIPTION OF EQUIPMENT

Lifeline uses an electronic monitoring unit that is hooked by means of modular jacks to the telephone of the user, who is called a subscriber. An emergency may be signalled by pressing a button on the unit itself or by using a remote control "trigger". When an emergency is signalled, the phone line is seized and the unit automatically dials a central response station, frequently located at a hospital. Upon receiving an alarm, the emergency operator first phones the user. If there is an emergency or if the user cannot be reached, the operator calls a list of emergency responders, typically beginning with a next- door neighbor who has a key. As needed, paramedics or other emergency personnel are called. Another feature of the equipment is a passive monitoring timer, which can be set to 12 or 24 hours. If the subscriber does not use the telephone or press a reset button in that time interval, an emergency is signalled.

Lifeline emphasizes that it is not just equipment; it is a program that involves electronic equipment, central emergency coordinators, and neighborhood responders. It is important to the Lifeline concept that the central response stations are located in community agencies and that volunteer assistance is used to help staff the programs. Hospital personnel typically are very involved with the subscribers, beginning with in-home instruction when the system is installed, and continuing through monthly phone calls to subscribers at which time the equipment is checked. Moreover, the use of neighbors as responders is a crucial way in which Lifeline uses existing informal social networks to promote the ability to live in the community.

As Lifeline has developed, it has been used not only for the aged, but also for chronically disabled individuals of all ages. The rationale is similar; that in order to live in the community rather than in an institution, the availability of emergency assistance is a necessary service element.

There have also been advances in the Lifeline equipment. Initially the call button was a rather cumbersome item. It can now be made much smaller and worn on a watchband or as a pendant without being intrusive, and is now being made fully waterproof. Voice-operated units are also available that permit two-way voice communication with the operator even if the subscriber is on the floor in another room. Great attention goes into making the units reliable. An evaluation by Cominos and Sekler (5) found very few examples of equipment malfunctioning. Underwriters Laboratories (UL) is developing standards to insure safety and reliability, and PERS manufacturers seeking UL approval must meet rigorous functional and environmental tests.

Lifeline is not the only manufacturer. AARP (American Association of Retired Persons) issued a brochure in 1987 that describes 12 different PERS that are available nationally (1). Within various locales, there may be other major competitors. In Washington, D.C., for example, there is a service called Life Safety Systems, Inc.; and in Los Angeles, Emergency Response Systems, Inc.

The two major variations of PERS are systems that signal an emergency response center (like Lifeline) and systems that send prerecorded emergency messages directly to prearranged emergency responders (1,19). Some systems are installed by the provider and others by the user. For systems with a central response station, there are also two major variations, those located at health or social service agencies and those where the manufacturer has a national or regional center (1,19). Lifeline now offers both variations of the central response station: To accommodate persons who cannot be served by a community program, their national emergency response center can accept calls by means of 800 telephone lines.

There are differences in the design of the portable triggers and electronic consoles for various PERS manufacturers (1,19). For example, some consoles have different buttons for medical emergency, fire, and police. Not all systems have the inactivity timer as an option. More complex monitoring is also possible, such as an automatic signal if the subscriber falls down.

COSTS

Lifeline home units originally cost $495; however, typically the hospital purchases the units and leases them to the subscribers. Stafford and Dibner (24) found that the typical charge to the subscriber was $10 or $15 per month. In many programs, however, units are offered free through the sponsoring agency. The central response station costs $7000. Costs are similar for other companies, although most have an option for the consumer to purchase or to rent and/or lease.

RESEARCH ON LIFELINE AND OTHER PERS

The Lifeline concept was invented by Dibner in 1973. Sherwood and Morris (23) published the results of a demonstration project conducted in 1976-1979. By 1982 there were 438 Lifeline programs in 46 states. By 1988 there were over 2000. There have been a number of evaluation studies. The main questions asked include: (a) characteristics of users, (b) whether the system provides the advertised service of getting help to subscribers in case of emergency, (c) psychosocial effects, i.e., sense of security, (d) delay of nursing home entry, (e) savings in health care dollars. General effectiveness will be treated in this section, while a section below will focus specifically on cost-benefit.

The Original Demonstration Project

Sherwood and Morris (23) conducted the initial evaluation. They established 3 target groups: target group 1 is severely functionally impaired and socially isolated; target group 2 is severely functionally impaired but not socially isolated; target group 3 is moderately functionally impaired or medically vulnerable and socially isolated. These target groups have been used in much subsequent Lifeline research, while the screening instrument that assigns individuals to target groups is often used by hospitals in interviewing prospective Lifeline clients.

Sherwood and Morris (23) found that benefits were most pronounced for target group 2. All groups felt an increased likelihood that they would get help, if it was needed. Target group 2 showed reduced anxiety about living alone and a more positive feeling about independent living, while the other two groups showed some paradoxical elevation of anxiety. The investigators wondered whether the Lifeline intervention inadvertently had served to heighten the socially isolated individuals' awareness of their frailty and vulnerability, rather than to reassure them that having help in the form of Lifeline could make them more independent.

Gabovitch and Batra (13) analyzed the types of emergencies for which subscribers used Lifeline, using the data from the Sherwood and Morris evaluation. They found that 69% of the emergencies were medical; 20.7% were environmental (e.g., someone breaking and entering, apartment flooding); 2.7% were psychiatric (e.g., making bizarre claims about being persecuted); and 5.4% were precautionary medical (e.g., feeling weak and worried that it may worsen). They also found examples of medical and environmental emergencies of individuals other than the subscribers (e.g., someone getting stuck in an elevator). Of all subscribers, 29.7% had at least one emergency. A few had multiple emergencies, leading to a figure of .44 emergencies per subscriber per year.

The single most frequent type of emergency was falling. The most frequent illnesses were chest pains or heart attacks or just not feeling well. There were also other mobility-related problems, such as not being able to get out of the wheelchair.

Subsequent Field Studies

Gatz et al. (14) and Gatz and Pearson (15) presented an evaluation of Lifeline in Los Angeles. One of the concerns of these investigators was that demonstration projects often study programs that are organized around the evaluation, whereas programs that subsequently spring up may operate under very different conditions. For example, the system in the Sherwood and Morris (23) evaluation used an alarm company for a central response station, whereas hospital emergency rooms were the location for central response stations in Los Angeles. Sherwood and Morris (23) identified impaired elders and tried to enroll everyone. In Los Angeles the programs advertised and accepted those who responded. As a consequence of this different recruitment strategy, Gatz and Pearson (15) found many subscribers who were moderately functionally impaired or medically vulnerable but not socially isolated. They were called "target group 4."

Across all subscribers, 32% had an emergency within a one-year period. Some had multiple incidents, leading to an annual rate of .48. The most common emergency was falls and other mobility problems (48%) followed by cardiovascular complaints (16%). Between pretest and post test, there was a significant decline in anxiety about medical emergencies. However, changes on measures of the psychological attributes supposedly functioning to allay anxiety were not statistically significant.

Gatz and Pearson (15) focused in particular on the families of the subscribers, noting their importance in the decision of whether or not to institutionalize a frail elder. They found some evidence of lessened sense of burden on the part of family members as a consequence of having Lifeline.

Dibner (7) presents a national survey of 72 Lifeline programs, and Stafford and Dibner (24) and Dibner (9) present the results of a national survey of 335 Lifeline programs. Both surveys found that hospitals were the most common central response station for a Lifeline system (93% in 1982; 91% in 1984). The funds for program coordinator, personnel to perform monthly phone calls to check on equipment, and so forth typically came from a combination of the hospital itself, government funding, and volunteer agencies. In 1984, the 335 programs monitored a total of 11,598 subscribers.

The average number of emergencies in the 1984 survey was .60 per subscriber per year. This figure compares to .44 (24), .84 (7), .288 (12), .48 (15). The distribution of emergencies is not equal; most subscribers have none, a few subscribers have several. For instance, Dibner (7) found only

30% of subscribers had emergencies, but multiple emergencies were common, leading to the higher annual rate per person.

Consistent with other studies, the 1984 survey identified the most common type of emergency as falling, followed by cardiovascular-related problems (heart attack or chest pain). Compared to Sherwood and Morris (23), the national surveys revealed that the proportion of medical emergencies was higher while the proportion of environmental emergencies was correspondingly lower.

Stafford and Dibner (24) reported that subscribers who were more likely to have emergencies were those who had the greatest number of disabilities. There were no differences in the number of emergencies for subscribers who lived alone as compared to subscribers who lived with their spouses. Those subscribers who had more emergencies were also reported to be more satisfied with the system, although level of satisfaction with Lifeline was quite high overall.

According to the Stafford and Dibner survey, Lifeline subscribers tend to be old, with 78% aged 70 and older, and 46% aged 80 and older (24). Medical condition and social isolation are the most common screening criteria (in 72% and 52% of the programs, respectively), which is not surprising given that these two characteristics were emphasized in the screening instrument used in the Sherwood and Morris evaluation. History of falling was mentioned only 8% of the time as a criterion. Eighty percent of subscribers lived alone, mainly in their own homes. A quarter lived in apartments. Forty-three percent were referred by their families.

Cominos and Sekler (5) studied a Lifeline program based in one Los Angeles County hospital. It was typical of other local programs in its level of support. One part-time hospital employee was the program coordinator, and the only paid staff working on the Lifeline program. She was assisted by three part-time volunteers, who installed the units in subscribers' homes and who performed the monthly equipment test calls. The evaluators concluded that this was not a sufficient level of staffing. Of interest was that 39% of subscribers had not received a test call in over one month, while 7% had not received a test call in over two months. Twenty-two test calls were observed; personnel had difficulty completing 14 of these calls on the first attempt. None of these 22 subscribers were wearing their emergency triggers at the time of their check (5).

Gettings (16) focused on the control-enhancing potential of the Lifeline service. In another Southern California community, she compared 30 Lifeline subscribers to 30 users of other aging services at two times of measurement. She found Lifeline subscribers to have increased significantly in their sense of control concerning emergency situations. She did not find change in scales designed to assess sense of well-being.

While studies indicate that the most common use of the system is for quite prosaic emergencies, a few dramatic emergencies have made for impressive human interest stories. Newspapers (the Jamestown, ND, <u>Sun</u>; The Norman, OK, <u>Transcript</u>; the Rancho Bernardo, CA, <u>News Chieftain</u>) have carried testimonials to the effect that without Lifeline the subscriber might have died or could not have continued to live independently. Numerous quotations assert that Lifeline has replaced a sense of vulnerability with peace of mind. Most of the stories concern someone who fell, fainted, had a heart attack, or had a stroke, and, without Lifeline, might have lain for hours without being discovered.

Taken together, these various surveys and evaluation studies indicate that PERS do meet the goal of insuring availability of emergency medical services and reducing anxiety about living alone. Satisfaction is consistently high. Psychometric analyses of social gerontologic measures usually failed to find significant change, probably because the instruments were too broad for assessing the phenomenon. One of the constructs that has proved most appealing is the idea that PERS can lead to a reduced sense of vulnerability or an increased sense of personal control. Again, while scales purported to assess mastery or control have not yielded significant findings, other evidence has accumulated that does support the notion that the "peace of mind" insured by PERS involves a reduction in feeling vulnerable and an expanded sense of being the master of one's own life.

Cost-Benefit and Delay of Institutionalization

Ruchlin and Morris (21), using the Sherwood and Morris (23) data, compared matched groups of 139 subjects who were Lifeline subscribers and 139 controls. They determined use of institutional care and use of community support services in both groups over a 13-month period in order to arrive at an estimate of benefits of the program. Institutional care included acute hospitals, chronic and rehabilitation hospitals, skilled nursing facilities, and intermediate care facilities. Controls were found to use 10 times as much nursing home care as experimental subjects. The effect was strongest for target group 2, for whom Sherwood and Morris (23) reported 1 day of long term institutional care compared to 13 days for their matched controls.

Formal community support services included physician care, mental health care, social counseling, at-home nursing care, physical therapy, nutritional counseling, home health aide care, homemaking service, meal provision, friendly visitor service, daily checking, and transportation. There was no overall significant difference between system users and controls in use of formal community services. Informal community support services included help provided by family and friends, including supervision of home physical therapy programs, provision of meals, homemaking, daily checking, and transportation. Not surprisingly, controls had someone checking in daily more often than did system users.

Costs of all services were estimated. The total resource consumption of controls exceeded that of experimentals by over $62,000. The cost of Lifeline was extrapolated from an estimate of $24.97 per month per subscriber. The total costs were just over $33,000, leading to a benefit-cost ratio of 1.87. When the results were examined within target groups, the benefit-cost ratio for target group 2 was very large (according to Sherwood and Morris, each $1 spent on Lifeline saved $7.19 in long term care costs), while the ratios for the socially isolated subscribers (groups 1 and 3) were small to negligible.

Lifeline program coordinators responding to the Dibner (7) and Stafford and Dibner (24) surveys were asked to estimate reduction in institutional care. Both surveys indicated that 9% had hospital stays shortened while 16% had entrance into a nursing home delayed due to Lifeline.

Koch (18) and Ross (20) described a Canadian program where the focus was on discharging inpatients who no longer needed acute care but who were waiting for long term care beds. Lifeline was used in the patients' homes as an intermediate step during this waiting period. A second purpose was to offer Lifeline as an alternative to hospital admission to selected patients who presented themselves to the emergency room. Towards these goals, physicians estimated that 29% of Lifeline patients could not have been discharged as soon from the hospital without the program, while 38% were able to delay institutional placement (20). Three-quarters of the patients had a heart condition and two-thirds had impaired mobility.

Koch (18) presented data to support reduced use of acute care hospital facilities. Given that these patients obviously were becoming increasingly frail, it was not surprising that they showed increasing use of hospital facilities in the 3 years preceding installation of Lifeline. Nonetheless, hospital use actually decreased following installation of Lifeline, compared to the year before its installation (18).

Dibner (8) did an in-depth retrospective study of hospital utilization by Lifeline subscribers at 4 hospitals. The data were the subscribers' actual hospital records. Subscribers' hospital use was compared before and after installation of Lifeline. The general pattern was for use to increase annually for the 3 years preceding installation of Lifeline, undoubtedly reflecting an increased level of impairment. During the year after Lifeline was installed, hospital use was greatly reduced, returning to approximately the level that characterized these respondents 2 years before receiving Lifeline. Given that projections based on health status alone would have predicted a continued upward trend in hospital use, the reversal was impressive.

Dixon (12) described a program that supplemented home attendant services with a PERS. A survey found that once personal care tasks had been performed, many individuals preferred PERS to the constant presence of a home attendant because of the privacy afforded. By having a PERS, monthly personal attendant hours were reduced an average of 91.2 hours per client, with estimated savings of $533.35 after subtracting the cost of the PERS (12). Another report found monthly savings of $956 when a PERS was used in conjunction with personal care attendants (6). Among moderately to highly dependent clients, an average of 4.8 hours of attendant care was saved per client per day. The authors report that not all clients had reduced attendant care following installation of the PERS; instead, the PERS served to increase the monitoring of especially physically frail clients and to maintain them outside of the hospital without further increase in number of attendant care hours (6).

Cost-benefit is a concern for all who are interested in the expanded use of PERS and in the improvement of the long term care system for older adults. The import of the various studies, taken together, is that PERS do have the potential of saving health care dollars.

PROBLEMS AND NON-PROBLEMS

The main categories of problems envisioned by those first considering PERS include: (a) whether an older person would want such a device, (b) whether there would be many false alarms, (c) whether hospital staff at the central response station would be burdened or annoyed by having to respond to the alarm, and (d) whether neighbors would be willing to serve as responders. The studies to date have addressed each of these areas, documenting some difficulties and laying other worries to rest.

Acceptance of Electronic Equipment

Jarvis (17) and Dibner et al. (10) described user acceptance of the Lifeline system by examining the Sherwood and Morris (23) data from the point of view of characterizing those who accepted the system and those who declined it. A needs assessment identified potential users. When Lifeline was offered at no cost, 65% accepted it. Target group 3 contained the most refusers; target group 2, the fewest. Within target groups 1 and 2, acceptors were more limited in activities of daily living and received more assistance than refusers; in other words, acceptors were more personally dependent and more accepting of services. Dibner et al. found that reasons for rejection included concern about the device, about the agency, and about hidden costs or obligations. Jarvis concluded that it is important to discuss with new clients what it means to need and use the service.

These findings are consistent with other observations about older adults and service use. Perhaps counter-intuitively, older people have been found to deny quite pressing needs, ignore serious symptoms (or report less serious, although undoubtedly annoying, symptoms), and use fewer health, psychological, and social services than their health status would suggest appropriate (4,22).

Cominos (5) wrote: "I personally feel that one of the most interesting questions would be to look at subscribers who have not themselves requested the system but have it because a friend or relative procured it for them or badgered them into asking for it. Do these subscribers feel that the machine symbolizes abdication of family and friends--that having Lifeline will mean fewer visits and social contacts since the family no longer has to `worry' about Aunt Lydia and stop in once a day to see how she is doing. Do these kinds of Lifeline enrollees have more problems mastering the system? What could be done to make them see the positive aspects of having Lifeline?"

Gatz and Pearson (15) compared subscribers whose family played a role in convincing them to get Lifeline with subscribers whose family were not primarily involved. They found some evidence of increased anxiety on the part of the "family choice" as compared to the "own choice" group. They suggested that a sense of choice over having the system could also have played a role in explaining the heightened anxiety in the socially isolated subscribers of Sherwood and Morris (23).

Another form of nonacceptance may be to have the equipment in the house but not to use it. For instance, a phenomenon frequently occurring in the Gatz and Pearson study was that someone other than the subscriber would actually press the emergency button. Gatz et al. (14) also inquired about emergencies for which Lifeline was not used, but which were handled in some other fashion, such as waiting to see if things got better or phoning a relative directly or phoning the hospital rather than using Lifeline to contact the hospital. Gabovitch and Batra (13) counted as emergencies those times that the subscriber or a friend or relative telephoned the central emergency station. These instances accounted for over 20% of all emergencies. Gatz et al. (14) would have considered these events as examples of emergencies in which Lifeline was not used.

Similar findings were reported by Wolf-Klein and Silverstone (25), who studied a 24-hour hot-line for patients discharged from hospitals to day health care. The operator could always reach an on-call physician if necessary. The annual use rate was 7% of the patients; 85% of calls were placed by relatives, 15% by the patients. Over one-third of the calls resulted in hospitalization. If anything, the authors concluded, patients did not use the service enough.

False Alarms

Many people hearing about Lifeline for the first time suspect that there would be many false alarms, primarily older people pressing the button to relieve loneliness. This has not been the experience reported in any of the evaluation studies. Dibner, Lowy, and Morris (10) found .56 false alarms per client per month. Forgetting to reset the passive timer was the most frequent cause. Ninety-six percent of all false alarms were able to be handled without involving any formal service system; the others led to unnecessarily alerting police or other personnel.

Cominos and Sekler (5) distinguished between false alarms and inactivity alarms due to failure to reset the timer. The rate of accidental alarms of both types was 3 per day for a system of 200 subscribers. They found false alarms to predominate. However, Gatz and Pearson (15), like Dibner et al. (10), found failure to reset predominated. Cominos and Sekler pointed out that inactivity alarms typically take longer than false alarms to resolve. Gatz and Pearson (15) cited two instances in which paramedics eventually were summoned to deal with situations that turned out to be accidental inactivity alarms.

Frivolous signalling was exceedingly rare. Gabovitch and Batra (13) found that in 47% of all emergencies, the subscriber did receive medical treatment. Stafford and Dibner (24) found that 55% of emergencies resulted in the subscriber's needing to be brought to the hospital, indicating the serious nature of the emergencies experienced. Typically, whenever a new subscriber seems to press the button at a time other than an emergency, hospital personnel will help establish an alternative outlet for the need for contact. Screening also eliminates potential subscribers who would not be able to respond to instruction. S.S. Dibner (11) reported that, over several years, one large hospital had to remove a unit from only one subscriber. This subscriber had become too confused to use it properly.

The observations of Gatz et al. (14) about emergencies for which Lifeline is not used, bear as well on the question of false alarms. Not only is the rate of false alarms smaller than might be expected; if anything there may be a reluctance to use the system even when it might be warranted.

Hospital Staff Burden

Another major concern has been that the hospital will be burdened by serving as the central response station. S. S. Dibner (11) reported that the experience of one hospital was that nursing staff were not overwhelmed by having the Lifeline central response station in the emergency department, although prior to the system's installation they had been concerned about the time commitment and level of responsibility.

Cominos and Sekler (5) commented on the problem of having programs based in hospitals, particularly in communities in which the health care industry is very competitive. Discharge planners at hospitals that do not have programs may be reluctant to recommend a service that is seen as a promotional tool for another hospital. Indeed, literature from hospitals with Lifeline confirms that the marketing angle has not gone unused.

Burden on Neighbor Responders

Another concern is the role of neighbors as responders. Will they be available when there is an emergency? Will they be willing to serve in the role that is needed to make the system work? Gabovitch and Batra (13) found that central emergency operators had some difficulty reaching these informal responders and began to rely more on formal responders (such as police, paramedics, and visiting nurses), unless it was clear that there was no dire need for immediate help.

Gatz and Pearson's (15) findings about reluctance to use Lifeline in some emergencies are relevant to the neighbor's role. One major reason subscribers gave for not using Lifeline was concern about bothering the neighbor. Considerable turnover in responders was also noted. Nonetheless, responders who were interviewed after the subscriber had been on the system for a year spoke positively about the program and their role.

SUMMARY

Personal emergency response systems (such as Lifeline) offer an excellent example of the convergence of two contemporary events: the increasingly old population, and the rapid rate of technological advances. PERS demonstrate how technology can be used in a helpful way to benefit elders and their families. PERS are tremendously appealing to health care providers as well as to some elders and those who care for and about them. They don't cost a great deal, and clear instances of benefits are obvious. No harmful side effects have become apparent, even after considerable study and proliferation of use. Problems that were predicted are proving to be considerably less troublesome than anticipated. Importantly, several such problems would seem to be amenable to intensifying the education provided to the different persons involved in a PERS program--subscribers family, emergency personnel. Presenting PERS programs as enhancing frail elders' options, rather than as further complicating and constraining their lives, may enable the benefits to be appreciated more fully by current users and extended to others whose reluctance prevents their participation.

REFERENCES

1. American Association of Retired Persons, (1987): *Meeting the Need for Security and Independence With Personal Emergency Response Systems (PERS)*.

2. American Association of Retired Persons. (1987): *A Profile of Older Americans.*

3. Blazer, D. and Siegler, I.C. (1984): *A Family Approach to Health Care for the Elderly.* Addison-Wesley Publishing Co., Menlo Park, California.

4. Brody, E.M. (1985): *Mental and Physical Health Practices of Older People.* Springer Publishing Co., New York.

5. Cominos, E. and Sekler, J. (1987): An Evaluation of Lifeline. *Paper for UCLA School of Public Health.*

6. Coordinated Care Management Corporation. (1987): Emergency Response System Demonstration Project: *Preliminary Report.* Buffalo, New York.

7. Dibner, A.S. (1982): *A National Survey of Lifeline Programs.* Lifeline Systems Inc., Waltham, Massachusetts.

8. Dibner, A.S. (1985): *Effects of Personal Emergency Response Service on Hospital Use.* Lifeline Systems, Inc., Watertown, Massachusetts.

9. Dibner, A.S. (1986): Lifeline Emergencies. *Paper Presented at the Annual Meeting of the American Public Health Association*, Las Vegas, Nevada.

10. Dibner, A.S., Lowy, L. and Morris, J.N. (1982): Usage and Acceptance of an Emergency Alarm System By the Frail Elderly. *Gerontologist*, 22:538-539.

11. Dibner, S.S. (1984): Lifeline: Monitoring Home-bound Patients From the Emergency Department. *Journal of Emergency Nursing*, 10 (6):294-297.

12. Dixon, L. (1987): *Evaluation of Electronic Call Device Pilot Project.* Medical Assistance Program, City of New York Human Resources Administration.

13. Gabovitch, R.M. and Batra, G.R. (1978): An Analysis of the Emergency Events Experienced By Users of an Emergency Alarm and Response System. *Paper Presented at the Annual Meeting of Gerontological Society*, Houston, Texas.

14. Gatz, M., Eiler, J., Pearson, C., Gilewski, M., Fuentes, M., Zemansky, M., Emery, C. and Dougherty, L. (1984): Evaluation of a Personal Emergency Response System. In: *Aging and Technological Advances*, edited by P.K. Robinson, J. Livingston and J.E. Birren. Plenum Press, New York.

15. Gatz, M. and Pearson, C. (1988): Evaluation of an Emergency Alert Response System from the Point of View of Subscribers and Family Members: *Final Report.* University of Southern California, Los Angeles, California.

16. Gettings, S. (1981): An Investigation of the Effects of Perceived Environmental Control Through the Use of an Emergency Alarm System on the Psychological Well-Being of Elderly Community Residents. *Masters Thesis*, California State University, Los Angeles, California.

17. Jarvis, M.L. (1988): Factors Associated With the Acceptance of an Emergency Alarm System for the Elderly. *Masters Thesis*, Boston University School of Social Work.

18. Koch, W. J. (1984): Emergency Response System Assists in Discharge Planning. *Dimensions in Health Service*, 61 (11):30-31.

19. Lerner, J.C. and Stevens, R.B. (1986): Personal Emergency Response Systems. The Commonwealth Fund, *Commission on Elderly People Living Alone*, Baltimore.

20. Ross, I.W.A. (1985): The Preliminary Development of an "Integrated Program Monitoring System" for a Personal Emergency Response Program. *Masters Thesis*, University of Oregon, Interdisciplinary Studies Program.

21. Ruchlin, H.S. and Morris, J.N. (1981): Cost-Benefit Analysis of an Emergency Alarm and Response System: A Case Study of a Long-Term Care Program. *Health Services Research,* 16(1):65-80.

22. Shanas, E., Townsend, P., Wedderburn, D., Friis, H., Milhoj, P. and Stehouwer, J. (1968): *Old People in Three Industrial Societies.* Atherton Press, New York; Routledge and Kegan Paul, London.

23. Sherwood, S. and Morris, J.N. (1981): A Study of the Effects of an Emergency Alarm and Response System for the Aged: *Final Report.* National Center for Health Services Research.

24. Stafford, J.L. and Dibner, A.S. (1984): *Lifeline Programs in 1984: Stability and Growth.* Lifeline Systems, Inc. Watertown, Massachusetts.

25. Wolf-Klein, G.P. and Silverstone, F.A. (1987): A Hot-Line Emergency Service for the Ambulatory Frail Elderly. *Gerontologist*, 27:437-439.

Subject Index